A Mind Body Perspective

HEALTH

AND

DISEASE

SYMBOLOGY

HANDBOOK

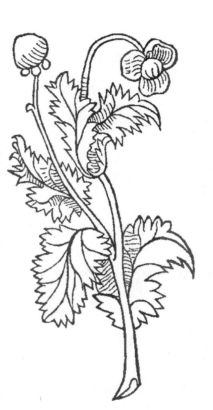

Michael Schwartz

Health and Disease Symbology Handbook

By Michael Schwartz

symbolreader@msn.com

Published by: Inner Health Books, 8400 Menaul Blvd. NE, Box 176, Albuquerque, NM 87112

DISCLAIMER:

This publication is designed to educate and provide information regarding the subject matter covered. It is not intended to replace the counsel of other professional advisors. The reader is encouraged to consult with his or her own advisors regarding specific situations. While the author has taken reasonable precautions in the preparation of this book and believes the facts presented within the book are accurate, neither the publisher nor author assumes any responsibility for errors or omissions. The publisher and author specifically disclaim any liability resulting from the use or application of the information contained in this book.

Publisher's Cataloging-in-Publication (Provided by Quality Books, Inc.)

    Schwartz, Michael, 1943-

        Health and disease symbology handbook / by Michael

    Schwartz.

        p. cm.

        Includes bibliographical references and index.

        LCCN 2007929674

        ISBN-13: 978-0-9796884-0-9

        ISBN-10: 0-9796884-0-X

        1. Nutrition--Handbooks, manuals, etc. 2. Mind and body--Handbooks, manuals, etc.   I. Title.

RA784.S39 2007   613.2

        QBI07-600168

Acknowledgements

First and foremost, I'd like to thank my wife, Phyllis, for her understandings, as well as her support through this journey that we have both experienced; Gene and Rhona Capshaw, who opened up the door to the information and the Alpha Group we have talked about in this Work; Dr. Peter Rothschild, certainly the major instructor in medical information and understandings in my life; Elizabeth Burmeister and Roxanne Llewellyn for their editorial skills and help, as well as Dr. Holly Lucille for her medical and nutritional editing.

Contents

SECTION IV: BASIC NUTRIENTS AND THEIR SYMBOLOGIES

Section V: Tomorrow—A New Future

Preface

I am an eternal optimist who believes that all things are possible. In particular, I believe that you and I can attain excellent health—physical, material, emotional, social and spiritual.

Excellent health is based on understanding all the factors in one's life. In my own life, this understanding is predicated on the Universal Teachings. These are the fundamental Laws and Teachings channeled through Gene and Rhona Capshaw imparted to me and to my wife, Phyllis, over a twelve year period through a clairvoyant channel. Through this channel, we were introduced to the Alpha Group, comprising entities from a different plane of reality, entities that are symbolically representative of a level of consciousness that can be attained through mastery of the Universal Teachings. Through incorporating and applying the Universal Teachings, mastery, including good health, is achieved on a personal level.

The Alpha Group's purpose is to help mankind gain greater awareness in order for the true Spiritual Self to prevail and master all aspects of material life, including physical health. The Alpha Group taught us how to think about and understand life from a metaphysical perspective, based on a set of principles that govern life and the human mind. These principles comprise steps for insightful growth and self-development, providing clarity about the energies involved in every human transaction.

The Alpha Group is the name that was presented to us through the clairvoyant channel. The Alpha Group is composed of enlightened souls/beings that dwell in a different dimension/plane of existence. They have the ability to "read" from the Akashic records as well as look at the skeins of time. The information provided was both personal as well as guidance for all of humanity. The Akashic records are the term applied to a matrix of impressions. They are the impressions of everything that has ever happened in the material plane and they cover all time. Everything that was ever done by anyone is recorded in these records.

In this Work I want to stimulate your thinking and encourage you to question and seek answers and guidance from within. Through application of the Universal Principles that I will explain, it will become easier to control your emotions, thus leading to growth and an ability to understand and use the power of your Spiritual Self to create what you desire.

I will offer symbolic interpretations of each part of the body, and the metaphysical causes and cures of ailments, beyond their obvious physical components. These metaphysical elements include your existing belief systems, patterns of learned behavioral responses, and the cycles in which they flow, all of which are reflected in your physical health and well-being. As your understanding and thinking expands, you will begin to exercise greater control—only then will your health improve on all levels.

I have experienced firsthand the enhanced ability to gain control of my life through understanding the subconscious concepts that form the foundation of my personal belief system. From understanding comes growth and insight on how to control detrimental emotional energy and habits, a particularly crucial part of this process. Control over emotional responses leads to mastery, which is reflected in well-being and excellent health on all levels.

It is my fervent hope that you will find this information thought provoking, and that you will use it to achieve balance and harmony, which will be reflected in your good health.

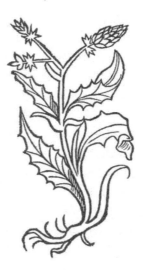

Introduction

As a nutritional counselor I had a client who wanted to lose weight. She had tried many times to reduce her weight without great success. I asked her what weight she wanted to attain, and once we established what that level was, I asked her the important questions beyond the normal diet and exercise ones. When I questioned her occupation, she said that she was a principal at the elementary school. I asked when the last time was that she was the weight she was now seeking to achieve, and she stated that it was when she was a third grade teacher. I asked her if she was willing to give up her authority (weight) and go back to the time when she was a third grade teacher. Once she understood that giving up the weight was not a reflection of a loss of power, she was able to lose the weight and achieve her goal.

Although we know that life, in both its physical and psychological manifestations, is a simple process that develops from the inside out according to specific lines of creation, few of us learn how the process unfolds. By explaining that process, this Work will help you sort out the what and the why of your life. Understanding the process of accepting concepts, values and standards (this is done on a subconscious level) and adhering to, or rejecting, them as a form of approval is the first step. Seeing the concepts in action through behavioral patterns is the second step. The last step is the fulfillment of expectations, which is reflected in your everyday life and health.

Here is some background to selected sections, chapters and headings:

- ♦ **From the Inside Out** provides a framework upon which to build your understandings, and defines key concepts and terms used throughout this Work.

♦ **The Fundamental Principles** examines the principles that are creating your current life, and the reasons for their specific applications.

♦ **How the Mind Works and Why** also explores reasons for the principles' specific applications. You will come to see a distinct similarity in that often-cited law of physics, that for every action in life, there is an equal and opposite reaction. The similarity is that not all reactions are the opposite of the initial action. Some reactions create imbalances and disharmonies; as you read and process the material here, you will recognize the causes and outcomes of these reactions, and you will achieve the clarity needed to interrupt the cycles that lead to imbalances and disharmonies, thus gaining an outcome that is more in keeping with what you truly want to create.

If you are seeking self-healing on any level—health, financial, social, or psychological—this section offers ways to help you achieve it. For example, if you are dealing with a health problem, you can examine it and discover what dietary changes and specific nutrients would be beneficial in promoting healing and recovery. You will also learn ways to increase overall well-being.

Through exploring the symbology of nutrients and diseases, this part of the material will spark insights into why you are dealing with particular health concerns.

This Work teaches that all ailments result from conflict between the two selves: the Inner/Spiritual Self and the Outer Self, or ego. As you begin to understand the symbolic significance of diseases and other ailments, you, too, will embrace this belief.

Often, we have a conscious desire to make a change—go back to college, return to an ideal weight or find the perfect love. And yet, subconsciously, we may not feel that we have the right, the authority or even the power to succeed. A conflict arises, pitting our desires against our doubts. Desire is an aspect of faith, and doubt is a part of ego. The manifestation of such a conflict can range from a nagging discomfort to a medical condition and even disease (*dis*-ease).

♦ **Concepts, Patterns of Behavior, and Cycles** examines what the events in your life reflect and symbolize. Coupled with self-examination, the insights you will gain in this section will lead to a greater personal understanding of why you think the way you do, why you act the way you do, and why your personal history repeats itself.

♦ **The Multiple Selves** presents understandings based on the Universal Teachings as laid out at the beginning of the first section. Through them, the Inner/True Self becomes harmonious with the Outer/Ego Self, in the sense that the Ego Self becomes less dominant in the intrapersonal relationship. The energy and consciousness of the True Self prevails, bringing balance and harmony into all aspects of a person's life.

♦ **Symbols: The Living Language** shows you how to work with symbols as guides to developing a clearer perception of life as it unfolds. Symbols, because they are pre-cognitive, will also provide you with guidance as to how certain situations will unfold in the near future. Learning the techniques for discerning and analyzing the symbols will allow you to gain even greater control over your life's energies.

Insights lead to understandings, and understandings ultimately lead to gaining control over patterns of behavior. When that occurs, you will be on a true path to mastery over every aspect in your life.

If your desire is to help others as a healing arts practitioner, working through this book will increase your knowledge and enhance your communication skills. From a practitioner's point of view, the information will help you construct conversations that will provide your client and you with greater harmony in the communication.

An example of this approach would be in working with an arthritic client. Fundamentally, these people are pretty set in their ways of looking at and doing things. Knowing this in advance helps the practitioner in listening for an opportunity to present what they need in a way that will be acceptable to those of inflexible thinking.

Often when we speak with one another about a physical condition or a disease—or about anything on an emotional level—defenses are raised, and the defensive individual ceases to hear clearly what is being said. For him or her, it becomes about defending the self, while at the same time, looking for an opening to attack the "accuser."

For instance, I was counseling a husband and wife about their diet and the fact that the husband had diabetes. When I said that he needed to reduce his sugar intake, his wife chimed in with, "he never listens to me when I tell him the same thing." Within a heartbeat he said to her that she never cooks anything without using sugar, and is always eating the foods that she says he should not be eating. Explaining the symbology enables you to get past these defenses.

Practitioners will gain an increased ability to guide clients through new, deeper understandings of the symbology of their condition, the affected body parts and how nutrients relate.

♦ **Symbolic Significance of the Body** presents the symbology of the human body and describes the conflicts that reside within the body on emotional levels as well as the diseases that these conflicts create. This knowledge will lead to greater communication skills and the ability to guide clients to quick resolutions, not just temporarily, but on a permanent and more consistent basis.

♦ **Physical Manifestations in the Body and Understanding Their Cure** maps out the symbolic associations for common ailments and conditions as well as the nutrients, vitamins, herbs, minerals and amino acids helpful to these conditions.

As symbology is a relatively new concept, keep in mind it is a work in progress. While a lot has been identified, there remains more to be uncovered.

This book will help you recognize the root causes at work on every level of your life. By becoming attuned to the symbolic significance of physical distress, you can begin to bring about balance and harmony between the body and the mind.

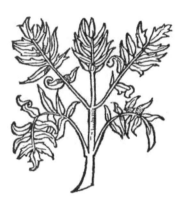

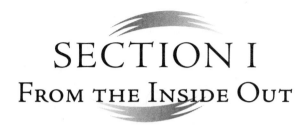

SECTION I
FROM THE INSIDE OUT

1. THE GUIDING PRINCIPLES: UNIVERSAL TEACHINGS

Throughout this Work, I refer to "Universal Teachings" as the fundamental principles upon which this information is based. Although you may not realize it, examples of these principles thread throughout your life. "What goes around, comes around" and "you get what you give," for instance, are heard in everyday life, while "ask and you shall receive," and "turn the other cheek" are part of our religious experience.

These aphorisms are termed Universal Teachings because, regardless of a person's religious convictions or spiritual bent, they can be meaningful for each of us.

The scriptural admonishment of "casting your bread upon the water" is equivalent to the secular "you get back what you give out." So, by giving out good energy, love, tolerance, and acceptance, is their return automatically guaranteed? No, but when that does not happen, it is because one has a deep-seated need to hear, see, or feel something else. This fulfilling of subconscious expectations is a theme that we will explore throughout this Work.

"Turn the other cheek" and "resist not, evil" are Universal Teachings to which almost everyone can relate. If you have ever argued with someone, you may have found that the more you responded in the argument, the worse it became. Regrettable, even unforgettable and unforgivable things may have been said. Yet, if you walk away from the argument, the energy simply dissipates—thus, the wisdom of turning the other cheek.

My wife, Phyllis, and I have another favorite Teaching with which we maintain our perspective: "Take the speck out of your eye before you look at the mote in your brother's eye." In short, we should all examine our own belief systems first. In our own minds, we are absolutely, 100 percent right, just as all other persons believe that they, too, are right.

The human propensity for seeing things from one's own perspective as filtered through a personal belief system, and created and shaded by subconscious constructs, makes right a relative term. That is why it is so important to understand the concepts at work in your own life. Otherwise, we may pursue goals as might "the blind lead the blind."

"Know what is before your eyes, and all the mysteries will be revealed" implies that if you are attuned and aware when you look at your surroundings, you are seeing and recognizing your concepts in action. Implicit in this is accepting that we are the co-creators of everything around us, based on our subconscious expectations.

The Creative Continuum was a term that the Alpha Group often used to describe an aspect of the God Force. It is a constant creative energy that dwells within as well as outside of us. It is the energy that is within everything. It is this energy that we use to co-create our personal reality.

The Creative Continuum and all actions are "imprinted" in the Akashic records, the plane wherein is recorded everything that has ever been written or spoken across the skeins of time. The Creative Continuum, within and without, seeks to manifest balance and harmony in all things.

The Akashic records are like a natural sponge complete with an infinite number of chambers and channels that contain all of the information and energy of everything that has ever transpired since the beginning of time. Those who are spiritually developed beyond this plane of existence have the ability to read from these records and through clairvoyant channels provide information that can become a source of guidance for those in the material plane.

Our partner, the Creative Continuum, has roots in the mind. The mind is the operator of a powerful electromagnetic generator—the brain—that constantly emits electromagnetic waves that attract positively charged particles called ions. These particles form molecules, the building blocks of both people and things. Thus, like a magnet, we draw people and things to us, co-creating the events in which our relationships play out based on our concepts and patterns of behavior. Conversely, by carefully focusing the mind's energy, we can repel or deflect people or situations not beneficial to our higher good.

Finally, there is "ask and ye shall receive." Keep in mind that left unexplored and unchecked, it is your subconscious mind that is doing the asking, seeking to fulfill subconscious expectations. Are you seeing, attracting, and manifesting what you truly desire?

2. Fundamental Principles

Spirit, Mind, and Emotions

Almost every philosophy and religion talks about the "spirit," yet beliefs diverge around just what spirit is and where it dwells. Some sects view it as being a thing above and beyond the reach of man…something external. For others, the spirit is very much an indwelling energy force at the center of all life and experience.

Many people believe that mankind is powerless to control this internal energy, the environment and our lives in general. Yet, the fact that we have the ability to think is proof that we always have the freedom to choose. The Inner Self knows this to be true. Any disbelief arises within the Outer Self, an ego-driven construct.

Your Inner Self follows a master plan, a kind of primary spiritual directive. That plan is to express the harmony of the Creative Continuum through the understandings and practice of the Universal Teachings.

The ego-fed Outer Self, on the other hand, is on a different tack, one guided by man-made concepts, programs, and teachings passed on by our parents and patterned in childhood. We are vulnerable in our youth because we seek acceptance from our mothers. We look first to our birth mother for this approval, for it was she who provided our doorway into the material plane. Because we are spiritual beings, we have a natural desire to return to the tranquility of the spiritual plane, and because of that deep, subconscious drive, no one wants to be rejected or shut off from the "doorway" back home. Therefore, all children naturally want and seek their mother's acceptance and strive to be what she expects them to be. We readily accepted this programming. Through their actions, reactions, deeds, and attitudes, our parents revealed what was expected of us. As we grew, the concepts and patterns were reinforced by our own actions and interactions with society: extended family, friends, peers, teachers, and even cultural norms.

But concepts, either man-made or spiritual, are designed to promote a particular belief system or structure, and some of these idealized notions and beliefs can actually be misconceptions. For example:

♦ *Males have the dominant, provider's role.*

♦ *Females are subservient, relegated to the mundane.*

♦ *Competition is necessary for growth and development.*

♦ *Material possessions make one whole and complete.*

It is an understatement to say these particular concepts have been, and continue to be, the source of miscommunications.

The Outer/Emotional Self is affected by what is seen and heard, and we see, hear, evaluate, and act according to the ego's subconscious directives, which are designed to validate what we believe to be true about our manifest selves.

Physical problems occur when misconceptions held in the subconscious belief system contradict the Inner Self's directives. Mentally, we may feel incapable of handling a given situation after evaluating it, particularly if this evaluation is based on doubt or another man-made concept programmed into us as children.

Unchecked, the mental conflict spurred by an inner-outer battle will eventually result in physical problems. When a person works with concepts that tell him or her that he or she is inadequate and cannot communicate effectively, then that person may subconsciously create any number of ailments to avoid a project requiring communication or the person may avoid communicating in general.

The ailment likely will take the form of something familiar and comfortable, often from one's family background. While it can be anything, by far the most common response is the cold, complete with sore throat, high fever, and nausea. The person in this situation perceives the project (communicating) as difficult, creating charged emotions (anger/fever) and distress (nausea). The concepts that stimulate subconscious feelings of inadequacy, a lack of authority to speak, and the inability to communicate will set conditions in motion to create an ailment that will prevent communicating. Some of these concepts/energies will direct the immune system to let down its guard and bring about the physical condition.

I remember a client who developed pneumonia because of financial pressure that was placed upon him. He had just recently bought a new home on fifteen acres of land complete with a one acre lake. His parents wanted to build a house on the property overlooking the lake, which was fine until they said that they wanted him to finance the transaction. The door had originally been opened for them to live on the land, but with the understanding that they had the money to pay for the construction. He wanted to finance the deal for his parents, but being in ill health made my client feel that he would not be able to afford the expense of this new house. He realized that he did not have the faith in himself to be able to pay for everything because he was also having trouble with his business. The self doubt combined with the financial burdens were more than he could handle and so he developed pneumonia.

When disharmony occurs within the body, the result is a specific energy blockage that sets in motion biochemical and physiological changes that affect a particular system or part of the body. This is where conditions, diseases, and accidents originate. The mind is the cause, but it is also the cure. Once the reason for the blockage is understood and resolved, the energy can flow properly, restoring the area to harmony and health.

Disharmonies within are the direct result of conflict between the subconscious and conscious minds. The mind sets in motion biochemical changes that affect the physiological status of the body. Knowing the symbolic significance of the condition and the body part affected allows the mind, the cause, to become the cure.

In order for the mind to create the physical reflections of the disharmony within, it must communicate to the brain the conflict at hand. The brain and mind work together to alert us by presenting the proper symbols that a disturbance is occurring within. Once we have the "symbolic viewing," we then gain deeper insight regarding both what is out of balance and the source of the conflict. This in turn provides us with an opportunity for change.

The True Self

The True/Spiritual Self is part of the God Force, the Creative Continuum. This self and the Creative Continuum direct the flow of energy to make us who we are. More precisely, they guide our spiritual essence toward our purpose.

The Spiritual Self directs the flow of the creative energy that defines us. The mind of the Inner Self encases the Spiritual Self in a layer of ego, which sends spiritual energy to the brain, and there, converts those energetic thoughts into electromagnetic impulses and biochemical changes experienced throughout the body. What emerges is filtered through the Outer Self's egocentric concepts: man-made values, ideas, and standards. The person then seeks to experience life from those perspectives.

Put another way, the brain takes directives from the Spiritual Self and the Outer and Inner Selves. They pass through the ego's expectations and affect the body accordingly. The body is a reflection of the concepts and directives at work. We seek to fulfill our ego's subconscious expectations of ourselves. We also see the world as we think it should be—a reflection of our inner-thoughts and expectations at work.

Look at your body, and then think back to ailments you have experienced. What situations were going on in your life at that time? Once you learn to see from a different point of view the situations that previously caused you difficulties, you will begin to understand the problem's root cause, and, thus, prevent future ailments.

Brain-Body Connection

The mind has no clear properties of physical matter. It takes up no space, nor does it have perceptible weight. The brain, on the other hand, has all the properties of matter. This fascinating organ that controls the animate body is, in fact, the prototype after which all computers are designed. The brain computes each and every situation we face, scanning the mind's memory banks for information on how we handled similar ones in the past.

The brain then converts the retrieved memories into a mental "language" for the mind to use. If a physical reaction is necessary, the mind "tells" the brain what to do, most likely directing it to a programmed response.

The brain then goes about setting up the conditions within the body that will allow it to cope, based on similar experiences from the past. "History repeats itself" is the Teaching applicable to this process. Ecclesiastes 3:15 states: "That which hath been is now; and that which is to be hath already been…"

Human behavior is based on patterned responses to stimuli. If your finger comes close to a flame, you automatically withdraw the finger because of the memory of pain learned from past experiences with intense heat.

In every situation, your mind scans back for a mental picture of the proper or acceptable course of action to take. That course might entail an ailment, an accident, or whatever the mind thinks is necessary to resolve the conflict. Some people use ailments as a means of getting attention. Others use them to avoid certain situations or to withdraw or even reject.

The subconscious mind spawns countless reasons for an individual to engage in transactions to avoid or resolve conflict. In that process, the mind uses the body as a barometer, the ultimate mirror with which to reflect a concept at work, often repeatedly.

You have the power to change the concept and stop its cyclic actions, once you see it at work. This can occur only when your man-made ideas of what "should be" are discarded and replaced with the Universal Teachings' True Concepts. True Concepts are those that people should be living by because they allow for perceptions, insights and understandings without the bias of gender, cultural or religious influence.

One caution: such change does not come passively. An individual must actively seek to understand the true goal of living, which is to bring balance and harmony to all tasks and all aspects of life, especially within the self.

When you live in harmony with the Universal Teachings, and are practicing the True Concepts, you will enjoy good health, prosperity, and peaceful living all the time.

Metaphysical Body-Mind Nutrition

Good nutrition plays a key part in enabling the body and mind to find balance and good health; even nutrients have their symbology (presented in Section IV). Knowing and understanding this information can be a powerful tool in halting the progress of a physical condition or disease.

Metaphysical body-mind nutrition offers a unified, in-depth way of examining diseases and conditions of life from two different and distinct perspectives. First there is the corporal, or body, aspect that comprises physical elements such as conditions, diseases, and nutritional states. The mind aspect, on the other hand, looks to emotional factors.

Remember that the mind influences the brain to perform certain functions or create situations. For example, under the mind's subconscious directives, the brain will alter the body's biochemistry, creating the right internal conditions to bring about a particular result. This would be a metaphysical result, an impact or outcome that occurs beyond the physical.

Likewise, your mind sets in motion all of the energies needed to create a desired result consistent with subconscious expectations. Although the result may only be one aspect of the concept at work, it will provide a symbolic perspective of where you are in any given pattern of behavior.

Your mind wants to help you understand these patterns so that you can begin to change your attitudes and thoughts, thus altering the outcome and setting the stage to create a new result.

By using the information in this Work, you should be able to identify negative patterns of behavioral responses and prevent them from returning on a consistent basis. I say "consistent basis" because of the Universal Teaching: "Life flows in cycles."

Every time you see a particular symbol, or a similar energy manifestation, it triggers a concept and stimulates a pattern of behavior. It also lets you know where in the patterned response you are. By adjusting your thoughts and attitudes you change your energy, and that changes the outcome.

Your mind reflects back on how you have dealt with that energy before and creates a "how to deal with it now" scenario. Your mind is also telling you what energies are at work. An example from my own life is the symbol of a black cocker spaniel.

When I was about ten years old I was attacked by a black cocker spaniel. Once I became involved with this Work and understood symbols I had a source of guidance I could work with. Every time I saw a black cocker spaniel, I knew that fear was at work in my life. At that point I wanted to understand what was going on. What was I engaged in? Who was I dealing with? What was upcoming that I felt I could not do and yet had to face?

Through "reading" the symbols and knowing that life flows in cycles and that "history repeats itself," I was better prepared to deal with upcoming situations. Symbols are based on the Teaching "forewarned is forearmed."

3. HOW THE MIND WORKS AND WHY

How Life Works

Living life is a complex matter of fulfilling subconscious expectations, driven by the human need for acceptance and approval. We look first to our birth mother for this approval, for it was she who provided our doorway into the material plane.

Because we are spiritual beings, we have a natural desire to return to the tranquility of the spiritual plane. And because of that deep, subconscious drive, no one wants to be rejected, or to be shut off from the "doorway" back home. Therefore, all children naturally want and seek their mother's acceptance and strive to be what she expects us to be.

Those who actively seek to emulate mother and the concepts she presents might be described as taking the "Goody Two-Shoes" approach to approval... doing all the "right" things "correctly." After all, being "just like mom" is the ultimate form of acceptance. It is one reason men seek a wife or companion with the same manifest ideals and behaviors as those of their mothers.

Conversely, dad represents mom's manifest concept of a male. Everything that mom believes and expects a man to be can be found in dad. Daughters usually choose someone possessed of the same or similar male concepts that mom held to be true.

Rejection as a Form of Approval

There are children who follow another avenue to acceptance: rejection. It can be difficult to see beyond the paradox of rejection as a form of acceptance because when we think about seeking acceptance from others, we think about doing everything that is correct in their eyes.

Rejection as a form of acceptance is something the soul chooses even before it is born, because this course offers something the soul needs to understand.

To this end, each child chooses their parents, and every set of parents provides that child's soul with opportunities for mastery. This is not often seen or appreciated by the child because in some instances children are born into horrible situations, while others find more favorable conditions. The circumstances depend upon what that particular soul needs to understand, resolve, and master.

Even being born into a positive situation could be the most difficult of all paths simply because it is so easy. Consider the lament of the poor little rich girl or boy. Just because a path has the appearance of being easy does not mean that it is the most beneficial thing for the soul in question.

Sometimes a soul/person will make bad, wrong or unhealthy choices while under the influence of a particular concept or pattern of behavior. After all, the soul would never voluntarily choose something that it inherently knew was bad for it.

Life-long patterns of behavior, both good and bad, trace their foundations to the soul's first "awareness of conception," tied to the very moment the woman becomes cognizant of her pregnancy. If the pregnancy is unwanted, it generates feelings of resentment and rejection toward the developing child. The same thing can happen with an unplanned pregnancy. This may manifest with the second or third child.

There is a very subtle energy, perhaps even a conscious energy, generated through the woman's negative thoughts, fears, or concerns about her pregnancy. Although the woman may not welcome it, her religious and moral convictions may compel her to go through with the pregnancy.

During this pregnancy, rejection will manifest in different ways and on different levels. It may become more pronounced when the soul enters the fetus, at around three months of gestation. The fetus begins to move around this time, setting the stage for even stronger feelings of rejection from the mother as she realizes the pregnancy is real and will change her life forever.

Operating through not yet understood karmic patterns and concepts, that energy may affect the developing fetus to the point that the child may be born deformed or sickly. The mother may experience severe morning sickness or other complications up to and during labor and delivery. Invariably there will be some issues surrounding the birth.

What the child understands and experiences from all of this is the energy of rejection. Since that energy is dominant at such a crucial time, the association is made that maternal rejection is a form of security, a form of approval.

Such a soul invariably will end up going through life creating scenarios that will manifest in rejection, cycle after cycle.

Such rejection takes many forms: procrastination, indecision, confrontation, avoidance, and non-completion are but a few of the behaviors that can evoke rejection, thus validating their expectations.

This brings us back to mother, our portal to spiritual serenity. We are driven to maintain access to the doorway that spurs creation of all our modes of behavior, drawn from the very concepts we learned from our parents through observing their gender-based deeds and attitudes.

These concepts become the foundations for our internalized expectations of what we believe we should be. We then live our lives seeking to fulfill them, thus validating what we think we should be.

But the truth is you are living for so much more than that. You are here to participate in the harmonizing of both mankind and nature, which begins with harmonizing within one's self.

Keep in mind that life is a continual cleansing process intended to eliminate the misconceptions that we live by: man-made ideals, values, and standards. In doing so, the Inner Self can once again learn, express, and manifest the benefits and gifts that lie deep within the Spiritual Self.

Concepts, Patterns of Behavior and Cycles: Co-creating Your Reality

How are personal belief systems built, and why do people live to sustain them at all costs? How does the mind work with regard to this process? In answering these questions, we look at three interrelated key elements:

- ◆ *Concepts—ideas, standards, values, and guides that you hold to be true and live by*

- ◆ *Patterns—repetitive acts of behavior based upon those concepts*

- ◆ *Cycles—the basic movement of life*

Concepts mold the way you think and feel about yourself, other people, and the world. Thus, your actions and reactions are stimulated and governed by your concepts.

Concepts are the foundation of patterns. Each idea or concept that you maintain about yourself represents a stone in the foundation of your belief system. Stone upon stone, each concept is joined together to form the whole. You build your belief system on what you expect and accept to be true or real. Behavioral patterns soon form around these central beliefs about how to act in every situation, eventually flowing into cycles and influencing each aspect of self accordingly.

These are the four aspects of the self:

- ◆ *The Physical/Material Self is the direct result of your thoughts; i.e., being thin, heavy, sickly, healthy, rich or poor.*

- ◆ *The Social Self is an outward manifestation of personality.*

- ◆ *The Emotional Self is capable of the full range of "human" feelings and how you feel about your self (faith in self).*

♦ *The Spiritual Self may show complete obedience to religious dogma or follow the path of the agnostic, the atheist, or the seeker of spiritual truths.*

4. The Spiritual Self and Belief Systems

The Spiritual Self may show complete obedience to religious dogma or follow the path of the agnostic, the atheist, or the seeker of spiritual truths.

Concepts are the root cause of all disharmonies, the conflict between the Inner/Spiritual Self that is perfect and in balance, and what the Outer/Emotional Self wants to be or do. This conflict manifests in various forms of self-destructive behavior including emotional outbursts, an inability to complete tasks, and violence. Often, such subconscious conflicts lead to illness.

When I first became involved with this Work I was asked to give a lecture on some of the Teachings. The weekend before I was supposed to give my presentation I developed a severe cold, ran a high fever, and had heavy congestion and a sore throat. I could not communicate. As I worked with the symbology of my own condition I came to understand that my doubt in my ability combined with my feelings of a lack of authority was the cause of my condition. Once I understood this I had a rapid recovery. I did deliver my presentation without a hitch.

Your concepts influence and determine your feelings, thoughts, attitudes, and preferences in every area of life. What you hold to be of value, what you feel to be true, and what you are willing or unwilling to accept all spring from your belief system, which shades your perception of everything in life.

For example, your belief system determines self-confidence and what you think you can or cannot accomplish. Let's say as a child you were told repeatedly that you were sloppy, that everything you did was messy. Over time, you began to accept those suggestions as truth. They became a concept that you made into an aspect of your self-image. That aspect may still manifest today, in an unkempt appearance and disorganized home and office.

Another way of looking at the personal self-image belief system is based on understanding the concepts that you maintain about yourself. These will be influenced by your gender as well as the mode of acceptance that you use, whether it is approval or rejection. To gain even greater insight, look at your parents and then to project into the future. This will give you a clearer picture of who you are evolving into if patterns are not understood and worked with. With that said here is another example of a pattern at work. We have a situation where as an individual is maturing, he is becoming more and more withdrawn and quiet. If you look at his lineage, grandfather and father you see the same exact pattern at work. The very same concept is passed on generation after generation. The concept of a man, an aging man, is that he becomes quiet and withdrawn. The son has learned this by observation.

Had you been told you would never amount to anything, then that suggestion may have borne the fruit of incompletion. By that, I mean you may have begun a hundred projects yet never finished one because the completion would equate to being "something," which would be counter to your acquired self-concept.

Finally, had you been labeled a selfish brat as a child, today you likely would be an individual who is overly concerned with self, someone who becomes testy when things don't go your way. These concepts were suggestions given to you and reinforced by the comments, actions, inferences, and innuendos of your parents. Consequently, although not true reflections of your Inner Self, you have accepted them as such.

Remember that parents are meant to be guides, not to impose but to point the way toward reunification with the Creative Continuum. It is through this parent-child relationship that concepts are passed along. You accept your parents' concepts as "the way to be" because you want approval. This is why, if your parents say or imply, for example, that you are stupid, then you will accept that image as true. After all, they love you, and you do not want to be rejected—no one does!

The Creative Continuum was the term used by the Alpha Group to express a fundamental aspect of God. That God/IT is a creative force, a creative energy, hence the Creative Continuum. IT is infinite and beyond our comprehension. IT is constantly creating, which brings us back to ourselves. In this dimension we are co-creating our reality. We are doing so through the Creative Continuum that flows within us as well as without.

Yet, recall there are those who have become conditioned, even before birth to seeking rejection as a form of approval. They seek it in every relationship, every project, and every endeavor. This is what they were taught, and it satisfies their needs.

Every soul that enters into the material plane brings with it gifts, abilities and understandings that it has acquired. Additionally, every soul has an agenda. This agenda is the framework, on a very subconscious level, of what it needs to understand in this life cycle. In that regard there is somewhat of a conditioning of what is necessary for growth in the next life cycle. So every soul comes into the material plane with something to master in order to continue their spiritual growth towards unification with the Creative Continuum, the God Force. To understand how the process works picture yourself sitting in a room with one hundred TV monitors and your agenda on your lap. As you are sitting there you are looking for the perfect opportunity to understand and master what needs to be resolved. You are looking for that perfect couple that will present you with the opportunity to achieve your goals. The objective is to understand your goals so that you can evolve out of the concepts, in as many life cycles as it takes, that your parents have presented to you, through words, attitudes and examples. It is through being an example that we teach children how they should handle every situation that confronts them. Through the mastery of each concept you will know the truth about yourself and "the truth will set you free" (another Universal Teaching).

You accept the concepts presented to you. You incorporate them into your life and build your belief system and image around them. The concepts manifest according to how you have been conditioned to seek approval. For instance, what if mom believed women to be independent, authoritative, and dominant, and men, weak, non-supportive, and non-authoritative? Daughters in this family who work under the concept of acceptance for approval would be very much like mom, viewing men and women in the same way as her mother. If, on the other hand, the daughter's form of approval was rejection, then she would be the opposite of mom with opposite perspectives.

If a son in this family is working on acceptance for approval, he will be like his father because this is the accepted image of men. Yet, if he is seeking rejection for approval, then he will be the opposite of his father.

Now, you can take this example and interchange the concepts, where the daughter is like the father and the son like the mother, and find which mode you fit into.

Patterns of behavior: everything you experience is influenced by stimuli that direct the Outer/Emotional Self to a particular path of expression, to a pattern of behavior.

How the Outer Self responds is based on past responses and reactions to similar stimuli. Reactions to stimuli are based on how you were shown to handle a situation. For example, if a person's self-concept is that of being a failure, in every situation—a relationship, work, projects, hobbies—something will take place to fulfill that concept. And of course, the Outer Self will find a logical, rational reason for the non-completion, or failure. The mind is truly wonderful in that way. It can and will rationalize and justify every action and reaction it takes.

When a person fails to complete an assignment or show up for an appointment, this will create rejection by the others, satisfying the pattern of behavior centered on rejection as a form of approval.

If you could predict the outcome of a situation based on your particular patterns, the chances are you will not become so upset, and it is possible to make such predictions, based on your past experiences and knowledge. The Universal Teaching at work here is "look back in order to see ahead." The mind stores experiences in its memory banks and when a situation arises, scans the brain cells like a computer for memories of dealing with similar situations triggered by the same root cause. Some situations will trigger love, courage, and perseverance. Others may evoke withdrawal, escape, sickness, aggression, or rejection.

In each of the ways that the mind looks back will determine the outcome of the pattern. So let us take as an example the concept of men disappointing women. If a woman has the concept that men disappoint, as each new situation and relationship is encountered, a particular kind of expectation is placed upon the relationship. Usually it will be an expectation that cannot be achieved; therefore, it sets the woman up for disappointment. This could lead to rejection because rejection is a part of the same energy of emotions, feelings and concepts. Love runs from total acceptance, no matter what, to abject rejection, hate. Let us not forget that the male would fit into this scenario because of his patterns to disappoint.

These and other types of behavioral responses are set patterns to given situations or stimuli. How can that be, given the variables of time and environment for each occurrence? These variables do change situations only outwardly, not in a substantive way. The same basic ingredients are present, the same basic stimuli triggering responses from the same basic root cause, and the very same fundamental energy is present.

By way of illustration consider the child that grows up in a very authoritative household. Here the father is the dominate person always meting out punishment for any and all infractions. As time goes on, whenever this individual begins to stray from the path of what is expected of them, as they move forward they may, depending upon the situation, have an encounter with authority. The underlying affect is to stop any forward movement. Another possibility is that the authority will derail or hinder them and slow them down. Then later in life different things would happen where authority would block them from forward movement. The mind knowing the concepts and patterns at work will constantly give guidance to the individual to understand the concept and master the pattern. Part of the guidance system the mind uses, symbols, are indications the mind is communicating with the person.

Here is another example that this is happening. One day driving to work a person notices three police cars, one after the other. Those police cars, those symbols, would tell the person that the concept of authority is at work. Now they would need to question how that would affect them based on what they were working on at the time.

Another pattern at work occurs when someone is generating resources to move upward, yet as a result of bad decisions ends by depleting the resources without achieving the anticipated growth.

A perfect example of this is the business owner that is seeking to grow his business through increased marketing and advertising. At the same time he buys a building for the company because of anticipated growth. This was determined by "looking back in order to see ahead." However, by not considering a personal pattern of depletion he also embarked upon an aggressive advertising campaign. Advertising is a long term investment and may not yield the return that one expects immediately, and it is very expensive. Therefore, it ended up creating a depletion of dollars, in addition to the new level of overhead, which in turn created massive out of stocks within the inventory, which further reduced income. Something along those lines could put a person out of business.

Every pattern is triggered by something associated with something else. For instance, if you were bitten by a black cocker spaniel, simply seeing one could trigger your fear. So, in a precognitive sense, the black cocker spaniel becomes a symbol that reflects the energy of fear. All precognitive symbols are based on the Universal Teaching: "Know what is before your eyes and all the mysteries will be revealed."

This precognitive symbolic communication gives you time to stop and think about everything that is going on. It affords opportunity to change your attitude or energy regarding a situation, especially when you know how the pattern operates. By changing an attitude and reinforcing the change with positive energy and the knowledge of understandings, it is possible to move to a new level of being.

Cycles: people sometimes feel they are stuck in a revolving door...that their lives are repeating themselves. It is true. Life does go in circles, or at least, in cycles, driven by our own patterns of behavior.

Remember that all patterns of behavior flow in cycles. As a pattern unfolds, symbols are being generated, symbols that help you see where you are in the cyclic flow. They will also help you to identify which pattern is at work. That, in turn, can help you understand which concept has been triggered. Through a perceptive understanding of the symbols combined with the understanding of cycles, it is possible to change any situation. You can begin to express your freedom of choice and stop history from repeating itself.

Consider this cycle: you argue with a friend and say something hurtful. Later, you realize you are wrong and apologize. The friend accepts your apology, only now you feel he should respond by acknowledging your apology, but he does not. You are disappointed, and that leads to resentment for having apologized, and now you feel guilty for feeling resentful. Your guilt feelings make you angry with the friend for making you feel guilty because he did not respond the way that you thought appropriate. You attack with anger again, and the cycle repeats itself.

Your subconscious concepts create your patterns of behavior; your behavioral patterns influence your flow of life: cycles. "Cycles are an immutable law of nature," a Universal Teaching. Just look around to see this Teaching in action. The Moon circles the Earth and the Earth circles the Sun, while the Sun itself circles an even greater star in the universe.

Closer to home are the seasons of the year. With spring, summer, fall, and winter always following one another in the same sequence, their cyclic flow never changes. This demonstrates the Universal Teaching that "every end is but a beginning." Cycles have no beginning and no ending—they flow into one another.

Although the seasons follow a particular sequence, their appearance, or essence, changes. Some summers are hotter than others, some springs, wetter, and some winters, harsher. Just as individual thought patterns influence our individual lives, the collective thought patterns of the general populace also influence our "weather" patterns.

There are four cycles, just as there are four aspects of the self: Emotional, Spiritual, Social/Intellectual, and Physical/Material. Every human passes through these cycles on a daily, weekly, monthly, and yearly basis. Some cycles take a decade to traverse.

The Emotional cycle deals with thoughts and feelings about self-image. The Emotional Self is the container filled with courage, doubt, insecurity, strength, and the faith in one's ability for self-expression. In the Emotional cycle, all of these energies take on an "emotional" hue.

The Spiritual cycle refers to faith in self, much different than having faith in an external source. While faith in the Creator is an example of blind faith, or believing that some external force will provide for individual needs, faith in self is a "working" faith. Based on knowledge and experience, it is a direct reflection of self-confidence. So, in this aspect of the cycle, you have the opportunity to express your ability to aspire, grow, and change.

The Social cycle deals with one's ability to relate to others and influences communication and relationships.

The Material/Physical cycle concerns worldly possessions, health, financial security, and sustenance.

There are cycles within cycles within cycles. For example, all disharmonies and diseases begin in the emotional part of any cycle but manifest in the cycle's material aspect. This happens when you have missed all of the symbols along the path of the pattern.

As an example, one of the causes for nearsightedness could be based on the fear of death. The closer you get to the unknown and finality of your life you become terrified and don't want to see it coming. Thus, the muscles adjust to create the condition.

By missing cycles—not seeing them or not reading the symbols—you do not change an attitude; therefore, the pattern continues unabated. When that happens, it manifests itself in material reality. This can take many different forms, including accidents, conditions and diseases. Losing things such as a wallet, purse, or keys are other examples. This doesn't mean it takes a year for something to manifest—remember there are cycles within cycles. Sound confusing? Then consider the following scenario.

When someone is in a highly active social situation, the Social Self is prominent, along with all of the concepts maintained about that self. Suddenly, something is said that triggers an emotional reaction. This evokes an emotional response, albeit in a social setting. The "attack" then moves on to the person's Spiritual Self, as faith in self is called to task. This could lead to a social, but highly emotional, response that, if internalized, could result in a physical response, either illness, such as an upset stomach, or a physical assault on the person who verbalized the attack.

For example, we were at my granddaughter's birthday party at her father's parent's house. One of the children invited to the party was in the kitchen and I walked in just in time to hear her mother say, "Get out. You are always in the way." I immediately looked at the child and saw that she was embarrassed and crushed. The look on her face said it all, one moment she was talking away and laughing and the next minute she was quiet and sullen. She walked out of the kitchen looking very sad because this event caused her to question her own value and actions in a social setting. If she is constantly told that she is "always in the way" then she will seek to be "out of the way" by becoming withdrawn from social situations. Of course, there could have been another response, instead of walking out of the room she could have turned to anger and taken that form of expression, either way the pattern would manifest based on those types of situations. How the child responded and handled the situation will become the way that those types of situations will be handled in all future events of that nature. Depending upon if the need of the person is approval or rejection as the fundamental mode of acceptance.

Remember, during these types of encounters we operate on preconceived expectations of self, which form present patterns of behavior. If we do not see the pattern at work, then it will automatically complete the cycle according to the pre-established pattern. On the other hand, if you detect the pattern by reading the symbol, therein arises an opportunity to change the attitude and subsequently, the outcome. You should then be able to pursue your goals differently, and to pursue different goals entirely.

Once you recognize destructive, non-productive patterns at work, use that window of enlightenment for positive change.

You may have a success-failure pattern, while at the same time being perceived as an achiever, a can-do person. One day, the executives at your company offer you a promotion.

That night you start thinking about how the promotion will mean a heavier workload, more hours on the job, maybe even weekend and night work. Then you realize they didn't say anything about a raise. You begin to believe that the company is going to be taking advantage of you. So, the very next day, you go to work and submit your resignation or quit outright.

With an opportunity to succeed, you chose failure instead, and an opportunity for advancement and growth was lost. Will there be a next time? Another chance? Look at the pattern--it has fulfilled itself once again.

There is no doubt in my mind that you know this person. They have a small business that they have poured their heart and soul into and it grows and grows. With the success and money in hand they began to enjoy the fruits of their labor. In addition to all of the symbols of success, they also had the opportunity to party and use drugs. There were two young guys, friends of mine, who did just that. They moved towards heavy drugs, ended up doing cocaine, lost their businesses, their homes and the last I heard one of them died from a drug overdose. They had incredible potential. They created a successful business and were creating the reality that they wanted, and yet both chose failure instead. Some will say it was the drugs that created the failure, but the desire or curiosity began in the mind before the actual partaking of the drugs. Once a person starts to do drugs, it becomes a matter of where they take that indulgence. The drugs were the vehicle used to fulfill the failure aspect of their individual patterns of behavior.

So, search for behavioral patterns in action, paying attention to where you are in the cycle of patterned responses. Then exert the necessary effort to change automatic responses, thus freeing you from life's ruts. Convert all your cycles and responses to the positive by exercising your freedom of choice based on clarity of thought and vision. As you incorporate the understandings into your life, you will begin to see change and growth almost immediately.

Remember, you can create the results you desire in life because you co-create your own reality.

5. THE MULTIPLE SELVES

Understandings

The word "understanding" is not uncommon. It peppers our daily speech and goals: Understand? I understand. We have reached an understanding. Yet, we may rarely consider the word's various definitions, so here are a few:

> ♦ *To perceive and comprehend the nature and significance of; grasp.*

♦ *To know thoroughly by close contact or long experience with.*

♦ *To grasp or comprehend the meaning intended or expressed by (another).*

♦ *To comprehend the language, sounds, form, or symbols of.*

Based on these definitions, we could say there are things we truly know and understand, but there are also many things—especially about ourselves—that we only think we know or understand.

Even within the concept of understanding, there are distinct levels. (That is why we use the plural "understandings" throughout this Work.) For instance, there are the basic, fixed understandings that affect life. A prime example is the understanding that we require food and water in order to exist.

Understandings are essential to successful living on all levels—emotional, social, physical/material, and especially spiritual. Developing the depth of your own understandings and discovering new ones will lead to mastery of your life in even greater degrees.

There is another level, the fundamental understandings, which allow for change and growth appropriate to the circumstance. A perfect example is that everything in the universe is made up of atoms. Atoms have a positive or negative electromagnetic energy. Through the process of aggregating, atoms become molecules, which in turn become something else: a cell or a piece of furniture, the combinations are countless.

Another fundamental understanding is that the brain is an electromagnetic generator, something most people haven't considered. It's important in this context because it illustrates on another level how we co-create our own reality.

When you take both understandings and work them together, you can see that your personal reality is a combination of your drawing to you, electromagnetically, those atoms and molecules that manifest not only as objects and places, but also the people you encounter. The Universal Teaching, "ask and you shall receive" is a reflection of this understanding. Conversely, you can also repel that same energy. Two questions arise: What am I attracting to me? What am I keeping away from me?

I prefer the words "keeping away" because they imply more than "repelling." There are some energy manifestations that you want in your life but don't have. An example would be discretionary income, for instance. Through the process of understanding, you can attract to you or keep away specific energies.

The mechanism that runs the electromagnetic bio-generator (the brain) is the mind. The mind is influenced by concepts, and concepts affect the flow of the magnetic energy.

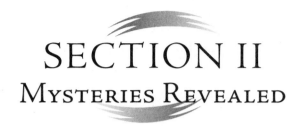

SECTION II
MYSTERIES REVEALED

1. SYMBOLS: THE LIVING LANGUAGE

Symbolic Reflections

Symbology is a universal language of the Creative Continuum based on the understanding that all aspects of life are reflections of thought.

A symbol is a sign or icon that represents a concept or pattern of behavior at work. Symbols also represent an attitude to embrace or consider changing. The term "symbolic" as used in this Work means that every situation—from accidents to diseases—is a reflection in tangible form of thoughts in action.

Your mind records situations and experiences in the form of pictures, not words. That is why it is so necessary to understand symbols, to convert them from mental pictures, events, and feelings to thoughts that will lead to actions. These actions will, in turn, lead to further understandings.

Diseases, conditions, events, and occurrences are reflections of thoughts that reside in our conscious and subconscious. Diseases are the direct result of conflict between two opposing ideas or concepts being simultaneously considered, each with its own set of guidelines. When the two collide, illness is the result. A sore throat, for example, would be the manifestation of the conflict between self-expectations and self-expression to the rest of the world. The conscious mind knows you must give a report at school or work. The subconscious mind, on the other hand, may feel inadequate at public speaking or may believe that it does not have the right or authority to produce the report. The conflict between the "must speak" and "can't perform" concepts results in emotional turmoil. This turmoil is converted in the brain into electrically charged energy that sends a message to the throat to swell up and close down. A fever could also accompany this bioelectrical transaction because of the anger of being in conflict.

There is nothing in our physical world that has come about without the beginning seeds of thought. Before a word can be uttered, it first takes form in the thought realm. Sometimes, it originates deep within the Inner Self. At other times, it comes because of events going on in the Outer Self. Once a thought has enough intent behind it, the personal willpower goes to work to make it happen. Then it can be acted upon, and the energy forces that create the reality of the thought are put into motion.

Every idea, action, or feeling was first conceived in thought, thus, the term "metaphysical" applies. All things represent a thought beyond the physical. That is why everything is a symbolic reflection of thought in action.

Healing and the "Cure"

The key to mastering life—a situation, or in this case, a disease—is the ability to read your inner-thoughts. Through understanding them, you gain control over them. Conscious control leads to mastery and the path to a "cure." Yet, when we speak of curable versus incurable diseases—and one's ability to consciously cure conditions deemed "incurable"—we must consider two issues.

First, there are recorded incidents of miraculous recoveries and cures, occurring almost instantaneously. These recoveries can occur primarily when the disease has not debilitated the body's biochemical-health integrity beyond the 50 percent mark, because once that point has been crossed, more often than not, death will occur.

When less than 50 percent of the biochemical integrity remains and even though the disease may be classified as incurable, there is still an opportunity for recovery and healing. This results through the power of faith, the second issue. Usually this is a form of blind faith because it is attributed to God, Lord or Buddha—whatever Higher Power in which the person believes.

The truth is that the power of the God Force resides within you; therefore, the healing is the result of a working faith and can bring about a true cure. Founded in your past successes, working faith means you can accomplish whatever you set out to do. The Universal Teaching that applies to this technique is, "draw on your past successes."

In everyday terms, the difference between curable and incurable comes down to levels of understanding. On a nutritional level, the best that one might be able to do is arrest a disease, to halt its further progression. Once understanding is brought into the picture, you are on a path toward a true cure. All diseases are the result of conflict between the spiritual directive from deep within the self and the ego's desire or belief, in terms of what self can or cannot do. The conflict between spirit and ego creates disease and disharmony.

With the manifestation of the conflict and disharmony comes its transmutation from the thought realm to physical reality. Through the process of understanding the physical areas affected, a clear picture emerges of what is happening at the internal levels. "What is within will manifest without" is another Universal Teaching found within Mark 4:22 in the *Bible*, where it is written a little differently: "For there is nothing hid, which shall not be manifested; neither was any thing kept secret, but that it should come abroad."

Working with this spiritual teaching offers the distinct advantage of gaining control over the disease that plagues you. As you understand, you begin to gain control, which causes the brain to adjust, accordingly. Once your level of understanding reaches the root cause of the problem and insight is applied, a cure can begin to take place. If these understandings are consistently applied, the probabilities for relapse become remote.

Now, another aspect—and a much more subtle one—is that disease will always seek to manifest because the ego always seeks to exist at all levels at all times. In understanding your belief system, your ego is dismantled, bit by bit, thus threatening what the ego perceives as its life. Therefore, it will always seek to manifest its concepts and its patterns of behavior, regardless of how enlightened your belief in yourself.

Much like water in a sieve, a concept and pattern will seek to manifest through whatever openings are presented to it. This is why a continuous, conscientious effort must be made to deal with anything presented in life, especially when it is related to health.

If a soul begins to understand the nature of its discomfort and conflict and begins to gain control over them, the disease can be cured. This control is the result of first understanding and identifying the concepts that are causing the conflict. Once you understand the concepts, the next task is to see how the concepts have created self-fulfilling patterns of behavior and how they have manifested. Finally, comes the understanding of cycles and how symbols can tell you where you are in a particular pattern of behavior. It is at this point that you begin to exercise control over the pattern's outcome.

To clearly understand the significance of a symbol, you must examine it from different perspectives: How does it function? What is its purpose? And, most importantly, when was this thing, event, or person present in my life in the past? What was I going through at the time?

When we glean answers to these questions, we begin to get clearer insight into the events or conditions with which we are dealing with and why we have created them. These questions lead to the development of a personal emotional association (PEA) with the thing/event/person. Remember this term, and always look for the personal emotional association of any symbol. This is the most important understanding of any symbol, overriding the Universal Perspective.

I use the term "Universal Perspective" because it is how I look at symbols when I am counseling someone. This point of view is based on three aspects of the symbol in question. The aspects are: What is its purpose? How does this thing function? What does it do? My interpretation will be general in nature, while your emotional connection/association with the symbol will take precedence because of your PEA.

In this Work, I present the symbolic interpretations of nutrients, the body, and diseases from a Universal perspective. Nutrients, the body, and diseases are something with which we generally do not have a PEA; if a particular nutrient saved your life, however, it would gain a personal emotional association, based on that event. To fully understand this association, review all of the circumstances taking place at the time of the illness, accident, etc.

Whenever I feel that tickle in my throat I know a cold is about to start. I always rely on one of my products to stop the cold in its tracks. This defense is based on vitamin A, one of the key components, and nourishes the thymus gland, and stimulates and nurtures antibody production. That, in turn, gives me more ammunition to fight the invading force of the germs. It is noteworthy that vitamin A is symbolic of introspection and seeing doubt at work.

Symbology of Numbers

Man as master of self, being in balance and harmony will master the material plane. In keeping with the Universal Teachings numbers are examined from that perspective. A brief overview of the numbers will prove helpful. One equals unity. Two equals balance and harmony between the Spiritual/Material or Male/Female. Three represents Understanding. Four is an advancement or block. Five represents the connection to the material plane through our five senses. Six represents man (man was created on the sixth day). Seven equals a cycle (heaven and earth were created in seven days). Eight represents material mastery. Nine represents cleansing; it is through the nine openings in the body that old material is eliminated and new material is introduced. Ten is handling (we have ten fingers and ten toes).

2. Symbology of the Body

The body is the physical manifestation of the energies of both the Inner Self (spirit) and the Outer Self (ego/mind). It is the symbolic picture of one's deepest spiritual and man-made thoughts in action.

Let us look at the symbolic significance of the individual aspects of the body. Doing so will assist you in appreciating your body's role in the communication between you and spirit. Such insight will help you to become one with the Creative Continuum.

Right and Left Sides. Certain accidents and ailments occur more often on one side or the other of the body. In the Universal Teachings' realm of metaphysical terms, the right side symbolizes spiritual thoughts and actions, our faith in self as it relates to a situation, and the future. The right side is considered the female aspect of the self, the intuitive.

The left side represents the male aspect of the self and deals with material considerations. It reflects the past and how you draw on that past in dealing with the present.

Here is an example of how an accident can have different meanings depending on the side of the body affected. If you broke your right leg, you should look for the circumstances in your life that make you question your faith in yourself. Wherein rests the doubt? What is happening now or in the immediate future that you fear you will not be able to stand up to?

If you broke your left leg, you would ask yourself what is attacking your ability to continue to support yourself. Which self-concept from the past is creating fear and doubt in your present ability to support yourself? What are you going through that is attacking your ability to continue to support yourself? Is there a financial situation brewing that you believe might create money problems?

Male and Female Aspects. The male aspect of self is your outward expression of who you are. It is that part you draw on when you need courage and confidence to face external situations. It is your ambition and motivation to grow and go forward in life.

The female aspect of the self is the inner connection that allows for the insights, perceptions, and intuitive "knowings" that you need to make decisions and choices on a daily basis. It enables you to be receptive about everyone and everything around you. It also is that part of you that draws from the Creative Continuum.

Drawing from the Continuum, your female aspect gives to your male aspect, which in turn gives it back to the All—the Creative Continuum that is the Creator, the Father/Mother.

In a channeled session with the Alpha Group, they once said, "man is whole, but not complete, while woman is complete, but not whole." This is the indication that the two are necessary to become one, as is written in Genesis: "Therefore shall a man leave his father and his mother, and shall cleave unto his wife; and they shall be one flesh."

The Head—Spiritual Plane. The head is considered symbolic of the spiritual plane because your thinking is done there in the realm of thought and creativity. This is the dwelling place of the mind, which is both the Inner and Outer Selves.

Headaches are symbolic of self-doubt. If you are experiencing headaches, look around to see what may be causing you to doubt your ability to deal with current situations. Once the elements are identified, you have the opportunity to change the nature of the situation and bring about your desired result.

It is important to remember that doubt does have an opposite side: confidence. In every situation, you will exude one of these two energies. Choose confidence, have faith in your self. Know that you are never placed in a situation that you cannot master.

Hair—Strength. From the *Bible*, we have the lesson of Samson. While Samson had his long hair, he had great strength, yet when it was cut short, he lost his strength. Hair is a symbol of strength, and that image plays a major part in acceptance for both sexes. It is an integral part of how people see you as well as how you see yourself.

For example, if your hair is dry or lack-luster, it could mean your self image lacks vitality. Oily hair may mean you are heavily burdened or overly concerned with your image, while dandruff could indicate your cleansing processes are blocked from within… and that you are holding on to old ideas of self-image or strength. Baldness can be another sign of a weak self-image at work.

Keep in mind that the interpretations of symbols given herein reflect universal perceptions of these symbols. What is going on in your body is a reflection based on man-made concepts of how you think life should be. Those concepts nurtured conditions within your body to create baldness, dandruff or dull hair. So, if you are bald, it does not mean that you are weak, it means that you think you are weak.

Only when you learn the truths of life based on the laws and principles of the Creator's Universal Teachings will you understand you have the power to choose and master outcomes.

Eyes—Perception. Through your eyes you view the world, your immediate situation, your family, friends, and yourself. "For those who have eyes to see" is a Universal Teaching that explains that clear vision is the goal of true perception.

How do you see yourself? Your future? What belief system do you use to view the world? As Jesus discussed in the second chapter of Matthew, "what is the beam in your eye that must be removed for you to see clearly the speck in your brother's eye?"

When you get something in your eye, reflect on what specifically is affecting your perception and distorting your ability to see clearly. What concept is impacting your vision? What is it that you do not want to see?

Additionally, conditions such as nearsightedness, farsightedness, glaucoma, and astigmatism all have different causative factors and one similarity: all involve the manner in which eye muscles respond, or not, to visual contact with an object. An inadequate response leads to an inability to focus the eyes.

Farsightedness, an inability to focus on close objects, stems from fear or self-doubt resulting in an inability or unwillingness to look closely at the self. Looking at self is of paramount importance, for through this process comes the insights that lead to understanding, and ultimately, control over emotional responses and mastery. The reality of nearsightedness, an inability to focus on distant objects, is created by our uncertainty about the future and arises from our doubts and fears. Symbolically, it means we cannot see with clarity or certainty into the future.

Conceivably, as we age, the fear of death distorts vision because we do not want to see it coming, and we do not want to deal with it.

Nose—Spiritual Intake. Through your nose, you draw into the body the "breath of life." Your nose is another part of your defense system, telling you when something is offensive or unhealthy and when something should be avoided, literally and figuratively.

Since everything is a symbolic reflection of thought, detrimental thoughts often pass through this defense mechanism because of the use of artificial aromas, which are really man-made concepts that give thoughts the appearance and smell of being wholesome and worthwhile, even when they are not.

Television portrays misconceptions as true and wonderful things with virtually every new image beamed out of the box, and fast-food advertising does it best of all. Just eat their food, and you will be happy and successful. In reality, should you eat most of these foods, their high fat and salt content will work against your health. Thus, TV can circumvent the body's natural, intuitive self-defense mechanism.

If you are prone to getting a stuffy nose, you may want to consider this in relation to the ideas of concepts that may be blocking your ability to receive spiritual sustenance.

Mouth—Communication, Material Consumption. The mouth is used to voice positions and thoughts about particular things or situations. You might do this by making calm, declarative statements or by screaming, allowing your emotions to be known. Digestion also begins in the mouth with the production of enzymes in the salivary glands. It is here that you begin to break down your food, which is symbolic of your material thoughts.

Generally speaking, problems within the mouth indicate either difficulty in expressing yourself or an inability to digest something going on in your life. There are other considerations and interpretations as well. If you are missing teeth, for example, image comes into play. Your teeth are used to break down your food. Symbolically, they grind your thoughts into an acceptable form. If they are missing or weakened by decay or gum disease, it symbolizes how you deal with external thoughts. You can "chew" the thoughts up properly and gain their full insights, or you can chew them halfway and swallow, causing "indigestion" and poor utilization of your thoughts.

If you have a cleft lip, then communication and image are more closely tied together. An inability to produce saliva is yet another aspect of being unable to digest new thoughts. When present, each of these conditions must be examined thoroughly to achieve a clear understanding.

Tongue—Defenses, Discernment. A part of the communication system, the tongue is another defense mechanism. Using its taste buds, the tongue alerts you to that which is harmful or certainly to things that do not suit your tastes; if the food (thought) has been treated in order to mask the real taste, however, then that defense system has been bypassed. The overabundance of sugar and salt in foods is there to try to convince you that they taste good.

This is symbolic of how distasteful ideas or toxic concepts are presented with aromatic or taste enhancement to make them more acceptable, or palatable. Just as the tongue protects you from ingesting a toxic substance, it also allows you to at least taste (discern) the flavor of everything being presented.

The tongue is also involved with communication. So, if there is a difficulty in a given situation it may be hard to articulate your objections.

Ears—Defenses, Discernment. Ears are your antennae. They discern, hear, and feel the thoughts, vibrations, and sounds coming at you moment by moment. These stimuli trigger reactions designed to fulfill self-expectations.

The ears also allow us to hear everything in relation to other people, places, and situations. They are part of the guidance system that allows you to hear the truth from within as well as from without; sometimes, however, the sounds are converted so that we hear what we want to hear.

Often, we are in situations where we overhear someone talking about us, or someone speaks directly to us about ourselves, affording an opportunity to hear another side of your own story. When we learn to listen, we gain great insights into ourselves and others.

From another perspective, you draw people to you as well as the things they say about you. You draw it out of them so that you can fulfill certain expectations about yourself. There are no accidents, happenings, or fated events and circumstances.

When there are problems with your ears, consider what it is that you do not want to hear or listen to, and why these things are issues in your life.

Beard—Image, Defenses. This can be a symbol of strength in your self-image, or it can be a defensive disguise behind which you can hide, protecting you from exposure to others.

Face—Image. Your face is the image that you present to the world, a reflection of your concepts and how you see yourself. On some levels it is also how you expect others to see you.

Often, teenagers develop acne at the very point in time when they are establishing their own identity. This is a very difficult period, filled with doubt and uncertainty. Acne is the result of a doubt-based conflict within, and that is the image projected. Similarly, when you have the energy of doubt and uncertainty at work in your life, you set up conditions to cause problems, which can take many forms, such as acne.

Neck—Balance, Communication. Within the neck are the voice box and the thyroid gland. The voice box, or larynx, is one of your main modes of communication with others. Through the expression of your thoughts, insights and understandings, you are able to maintain balance and harmony within your life. Accordingly, you are able to communicate with others in a non-aggressive, non-defensive way. This, in turn, creates better communication with all concerned.

Your thyroid helps regulate the metabolism of your body, keeping everything running smoothly. Once again, we see how the neck relates to balance, both internally and externally. Your neck supports your head, connecting the head, which is symbolic of the spiritual plane, to the body, which is symbolic of the material plane; therefore, the neck represents the need for balance between the two, spiritual and material.

A "pain in the neck" usually stems from an individual or situation that upsets your equilibrium.

Trunk—Material Plane. The trunk or torso is the realm of material absorption and utilization. It is here that all food and drink are digested and converted into fuel and building material. This is also the realm of all the supporting systems.

In the body, all of your thoughts (food stuff), and the thoughts presented by others are digested and assimilated. Each and every system, organ, and gland participates in this process. This participation ranges from the actions that the thoughts create to the reactions you will employ to handle a situation.

To help you gain a better understanding of the completeness and thoroughness of the symbology of the trunk, we will examine the individual systems.

Systems within the Trunk

RESPIRATORY SYSTEM—UTILIZATION OF SPIRIT (AIR)

The entire respiratory system feeds the body with life-giving energies. At the same time it eliminates used and potentially harmful gaseous matter. The respiratory system feeds the blood with fresh, live food, oxygen, and all of the hidden elements/foods that are part of the air, and the air is symbolic of spirit.

As you are discovering in this Work, there is more than one symbol for spirit. Here we have the air, while elsewhere we will use the head, the nose, the sinuses and the lungs as all being symbolic of spirit in some manner. Spirit is also interchangeable with faith in self.

Lungs—Spiritual Assimilation, Cleansing. It is through the lungs' action that you receive the breath of life, which nourishes and sustains you. You exhale that which is used and no longer beneficial. If retained within the body, the used air would cause damage and possibly death.

The same can be said for misconceptions about truth or man-made concepts. When you continue to rely upon these conventions and do not purge them from your system through understanding their source, they can result in accidents, sickness, disease, allergies, and sometimes even death.

Because most of us are exposed to man-made, polluted air 24 hours a day, the lungs may not provide enough oxygen to nourish the body.

When you have congestion, regardless of the source, it is symbolic of an attack on your confidence in dealing with a particular situation, one that requires self-confidence at a deep, inner level.

CIRCULATORY SYSTEM—UTILIZATION OF SPIRITUAL THOUGHTS

The circulatory system is present throughout every part of the body, with the blood that flows through it nourishing every cell. The blood also removes waste material from the cells, keeping them clean. This process prevents bacteria from gaining a foothold in the body, which in turn prevents diseases.

Blood is symbolic of the spiritual life that exists within all living things. That is why the *Bible* tells us, in Deuteronomy 12:16, to remove the blood before eating any animal.

The blood gathers nutrients, which are symbolic of thought energies, from your lungs and intestines, carrying them throughout the body. Your food—thoughts in the form of vegetables, fruit, fowl, meat, or junk food—can nourish, cleanse, and heal, or they can clog and destroy you.

A clogged, sluggish system often results from retaining debilitating and self-defeating thoughts, ideas, and concepts. They "choke off" the spiritual energy preventing it from reaching all parts of the body. When this begins to happen, it is only a matter of time before the body also chokes to death.

Heart—Emotions, Forces upon the Material Plane. We all know the heart is an essential organ. Without one, you could not live, just as without love you are emotionally and spiritually dead.

In addition to its physical attributes and functions, the heart is considered the body's love or emotional center. Emotions are difficult to control because the force they exert sometimes is so subtle that it is overlooked as an energy that can cause damage to the body. A prime example is when a police car pulls up behind you with its lights on and siren blaring. In a heartbeat you have an emotional reaction of fear/guilt. This, in turn, creates a chemical change in your system as adrenaline is secreted, and chemical changes can cause harm.

By getting involved with a particular emotion, you create biochemical and physiological changes, stresses and strains upon the body. All emotional stresses are caused by multiple concepts and these concepts can be in conflict with one another. Those that reinforce subconscious self-expectations and adherence to man-made concepts that are limiting or imposing will lead to great disharmony within.

Because the heart is the love/emotional center, it is the area most often seen affected by emotional stress. Not having enough control over your emotions in life will cause a breakdown—a heart attack. The way to gain control over your emotions is to understand which concepts are at work in causing stress and conflict in your life.

Each organ, being symbolic of a particular kind of thought and concept, draws its energy from the thoughts pertaining to that specific area of a person's life. When there is a physical problem, it symbolically mirrors the body, revealing which concepts are causing conflict.

Digestive System—Utilization of Material, Man-Made Concepts

Everything within food and drink—the good, the bad, and the ugly—is digested. With all of its various parts, the digestive system is designed to take the foods you eat and break them down into molecules, which become building material for the body.

This building material, chosen carefully and thoughtfully, can be used to ensure healthy new cells, which are then used to build the new tissue that makes up the body. "You are what you eat." Based on physiological fact, that is true, and it is also true that what you eat is symbolic of what you think. Every food to which you are attracted has an emotional association within your subconscious. Some foods are traditionally or culturally favored because they give a sense of belonging. Other foods provide deep emotional gratification because one of your parents may have loved this particular food.

Every food has meaning to you beyond eye and taste appeal. Every food is uniquely symbolic to you. There are many different reasons why you may not like something, as underlying food associations reside deep within your Ego Self.

Your dislikes may be the result of past events. For instance, imagine that as a child, you were sitting at the kitchen table with your parents when they had a fight, and imagine that one of them threw mashed potatoes at the other, and some landed on you. Had this happened, you may have made the emotional association that mashed potatoes equal rejection, anger or dissatisfaction. Today you might be allergic to potatoes.

You will be attracted to foods that first satisfy emotional needs and self-expectations, even though some of these choices may actually stress the body to the point of causing damage. The result of that choice could create and maintain weakness, illness, and even diseases. All of this would be in keeping with your self-image. Familial tendencies in health are also passed down in food tradition.

Comfort foods are a great example. They may be fried, starchy or sweet treats. My favorite is chocolate ice cream. I know that if I consistently indulged, to feel good, I would end up obese and possibly with diabetes and a cardiovascular disease.

Stomach—Digesting Thoughts and Emotions. Here, your foods (thoughts) are broken down into a liquid (material life) so that it can be further digested and used to nourish and rebuild the body. The opposite is true of toxins in food, which harm the body.

It is through this mental process that you evaluate the things you hear, see, and experience. You digest the situation and react accordingly, based on concepts and patterns of behavior. You will either assimilate it or reject it. Some situations and thoughts are so unacceptable that you literally cannot stomach them.

When you find yourself with an upset stomach or indigestion, reflect on what you have recently seen, heard or experienced that is disturbing you.

Pancreas—Regulator, Facilitator. This organ aids the digestive system by secreting enzymes into the stomach. Enzymes are living entities that fuel the living process by assisting in the transformation of one substance to another, one compound to another.

When foods are cooked or frozen, the enzymes within the food generally are killed. The food requires more effort to digest it, as a result. Put another way, by consuming foods that are cooked and processed, you are depriving yourself of life. These substances that are difficult, if not impossible, to utilize also tax the digestive system, in addition to depriving your body from nutrition.

The pancreas also regulates the amount of insulin the body needs to control sugar levels. As a regulator, it helps you deal with the sweets of life.

Many people suffer from pancreatic disorders because they cannot handle or accept the sweet or finer things in life, or they overindulge in them. By consuming man-made concepts, you accept non-nourishing and useless thoughts that do not enrich or enhance your personal growth and development.

Intestinal Tract—Absorption, Protection. The intestinal tract receives in semi-liquid form the food prepared by the stomach. Nutrients as well as toxins are broken down to molecular size, and the material is then absorbed through the intestinal wall.

Malfunctions occur when someone chooses at a subconscious level not to accept or utilize the nutrients. This rejection is related to the symbolic value of the nutrient. Another problem is when the person chooses to expel all material from the tract, and again, no nutritional benefit is achieved. Rapid expelling of material usually occurs when thoughts are so unacceptable that the body rejects them.

Each vitamin, mineral, enzyme, and co-enzyme has a symbolic interpretation, and each nutrient performs a specific function within the body. When a physical symbol is needed to get your undivided attention, the mind directs the brain to create the situation in the intestinal tract that will exclude from use a particular nutrient; this creates a shortage and sets up the opportunity for disease. These outcomes are in keeping with self-image concepts and are related to a current situation.

ELIMINATION SYSTEM—UTILIZATION OF THE CLEANSING ASPECTS

The body needs nourishment. It breaks down food, absorbs that which is beneficial, and seeks to eliminate that which is harmful, destructive, or poisonous. Of course, this is the ideal process. Our concepts of self, when not completely understood, lead us to incorporate into our diet that which is not nourishing.

We consume food and drink, as well as thoughts, ideas, and opinions that we are not able to fully digest. We take them in and are not able to fully eliminate the bad. We end up holding on to it until it corrupts us. Put simply: constipation kills. If you have this problem, look within to determine what it is that you accept or are holding on to that may be stifling personal growth.

One focal area may center on the roles of the sexes. How do you believe a man or woman should behave? How should a brother treat a sister, or vice versa? How do you think the role of husband or wife should be fulfilled? What about male/female roles, in general? These questions will bring many answers, and as you work with them you will begin to see the truth that is masked by man-made teachings.

Remember that man-made teachings are designed to give dominance to one sex over the other. In most current societies, it is the male who enjoys the dominant role. Females have been dominant in other eras and continue to be in some cultures.

Both sexes are of equal stature in the eyes of the Creator because they are two halves of one whole, a complete life force. Both are endowed with equal powers.

The trick to mastery regarding the roles of the sexes is learning to let go of the man-made misconceptions and to incorporate Universal Teachings into your life.

This takes us to the next question: why can't you eliminate the man-made concepts holding you back?

Kidneys—Cleansing, Balance. The kidneys remove liquid waste from your bloodstream. Obviously, if this system did not function properly, you would die from toxicity.

Kidney disorders are indicative of an emotional conflict. Some concept or idea about material life and self-expression is not being understood; therefore, it cannot be eliminated from the mind. Concepts and ideas that pollute your body/life have the potential to kill.

The kidneys help to balance the water levels in the body as well as the blood's acidity and alkalinity, also called the pH level. Thus, kidney problems can also mean an imbalance in your life, indicative of a breakdown in the cleansing process. There are two types of cleansings to consider: the physical and, more importantly, the emotional/spiritual.

Spiritual cleansing is the process of eliminating man-made ideas, values, and standards that are based on misconceptions and wrongful interpretations of the truth. Man is always striving to enslave his fellow man in ways, such as creating roles for the sexes that makes one more dominant over the other or by acquiring money, which gives one perceived power over others. In truth, from the Universal Teaching perspective, everyone is equal.

When the kidneys malfunction, the place to look is in the inability to cleanse the misconceptions of truth from the belief system.

Liver—Converter, Protector. The liver is the largest internal organ, and its main function is to produce glycogen (sugar) for the body. It also cleanses the blood and acts as a chemical converter.

Cleansing is what the material plane is all about. The liver seeks to nullify the potential harm of toxins through conversion to harmless substances, and then they can be eliminated. Entering the body in solid, gaseous or liquid form, toxins are carried by the blood to the liver. There, they are converted into harmless substances for nullification and elimination. Of course, when there is a constant source of toxins coming into the system, the liver protects the body by encasing the overflow within fat cells. What cannot be eliminated or stored continues to float in the bloodstream. Finally, the toxins are incorporated into the building of new cells; thus, disease is born.

If not properly processed and eliminated, certain thoughts generated from within as well as food waste have the potential to cause great stress, disharmony, disease, and death.

A regulator and a converter, the liver is part of the digestive and immunological systems. The organ performs over 500 different transactions and produces more than 1,000 different enzymes that aid in chemical transactions, among them digestion and removal of toxins. If your liver is malfunctioning, many probable causes (concepts) could be at the root of the disharmony. Determining which one requires careful analysis.

The liver stores and converts one substance to another. It stores glycogen, which is changed to glucose and released into circulation as needed by the body for energy. Other major functions include bile production; the processing of proteins, vitamins, and fats; and converting poisonous ammonia to urea.

It is possible that the liver can become loaded, or too heavy, with fatty deposits. When this happens, the liver begins to lose its efficiency and disease can set in.

Liver problems usually denote a difficulty in the cleansing operation within the mind as well as the body.

Bladder—Storage, Control. The bladder is a holding sac, designed to retain the wastes filtered out of the bloodstream by the kidneys. Upon command, the bladder will empty. Those suffering bladder problems might consider which concepts are being retained that might create the problem. For example, what ideas about the material or physical life are you finding it hard to surrender?

Remember that the bladder also symbolizes control and maturity. When you learned how to control your bladder, you step into a new realm of growth and personal responsibility.

ENDOCRINE SYSTEM—THE REGULATORS

Pituitary Gland—Growth, Expression. This gland plays a major role in the body's growth and sexual development and is also involved in the production of hormones and enzymes. The sexual act is tied to the concepts of expression, creation, and creativity. These concepts would also relate to your views of the role of your own sex. In addition to those thoughts, the role you play and your interaction with the opposite sex are reflected within the development.

Thyroid Gland—Growth, Balance. The thyroid regulates the body's metabolic rate and deals with physical and mental growth. Situated in the neck in front of and on each side of the trachea, it is also close to the larynx. Because it is situated in the neck, it plays a part in your balance between material and spiritual considerations. Symbolically, it is affected by attitudes stemming from concepts dealing with image and expression.

Interestingly, people with sluggish thyroids are generally overweight. From a symbolic interpretation, it may indicate that the person is imbalanced, stemming from doubt or fear in their dealings with life. The weight is protection. Of course, there are other symbolically valid definitions for putting on excess weight.

On the other hand, those with a hyperactive thyroid may have a hard time maintaining weight…weight that would give them the strength to deal with life. The lack of weight gain and the corresponding psychological feelings of weakness also come from doubt or fear.

In both instances, the root concept needs to be understood to determine which forces are at work in creating the imbalances.

Parathyroid—Balance. This gland maintains normal blood levels and regulates the metabolism of calcium and phosphorus, ensuring there is a steady, stable supply of these minerals. Blood is symbolic of spiritual life, calcium is symbolic of strength, and phosphorus is symbolic of inspiration and courage. By affecting the metabolism of these two minerals, the parathyroid provides the body (self) with the courage to continue, regardless of that person's situation. Without courage and inspiration, any strength a person has does not contribute to their growth.

Adrenals—Courage, Strength, Inspiration. The adrenal glands can make or break you. They perform many important functions within your body, including the secretion and manufacture of corticosteroids, androgens, epinephrine, and norepinephrine—hormones that control key bodily functions such as carbohydrate and protein synthesis and functions influencing the cardiovascular system, the muscular system, and other organs.

When stressed and depressed, this gland also allows the immune system to falter, likewise becoming depressed. When that occurs, everything that the immune system normally suppresses has an opportunity to flourish. This is when conditions such as acne, herpes, shingles, chronic fatigue, fibromyalgia, allergies, menopause, and hypoglycemia are at their worst.

Symbolically, you can see that many different scenarios are unleashed when this gland is under stress or attack. For complete understanding, each separate condition that manifests would need to be seen and analyzed independently.

Pineal Gland—the Third Eye. Because of its physical location, deep within the brain, it is often considered the "third eye" in esoteric circles. This implies it can provide you with the ability to view the Material and the Spiritual Plane at the same time. Many clairvoyant psychics have learned how to use this gland to channel energy into a more spiritual perception of life.

Thymus—Immortality, Defenses. The thymus gland is considered the seat of the immune system. It is here that T-cells and certain antibodies mature before moving on to carry out their roles in protecting the body from invasion and harm. Based on that understanding, the thymus is also symbolic of the defenses.

The down side of a defensive position in life is the fact that it can limit, hamper, and isolate you. Defenses prevent you from expressing your True Self. This is why Jesus said, in Matthew 18:3, "except ye be converted, and become as little children, ye shall not enter into the kingdom of heaven." This is because children are usually non-defensive. They have not hardened themselves against the world or one another and are still open and receptive.

Pancreas—Digestive Abilities, Converter. This gland produces enzymes for digestion of food and produces insulin. The pancreas is symbolic of your ability to take certain thoughts and ideas and make them work. They can provide you with the fuel (courage and strength) to carry on.

Prostate—Aid in Reproductive Process, Control. The prostate gland helps regulate urine flow and also plays a part in the reproductive system. Because it is tied into these systems, it is affected by concepts that deal with expression of manhood and self-image. When prostate problems occur, look for what has dampened your enthusiasm or made you sluggish.

Skin—Sensitivity, Protection, Cleansing. The skin is your point of physical contact and experience with the surrounding material world. The largest organ, it also acts as a protective device against the millions of infinitesimally small microbes that cover the body at all times. Skin also acts as a ventilator for moisture and toxins.

Your sensitivities to life are expressed here. The way you think influences how you are "touched" by certain situations and how you react to them.

When you have problems with your skin, it might prove helpful to reflect on your sensitive areas. What kinds of skin reactions do you experience; i.e. rashes, blotches, sores, bites, pimples, etc.? Equally important is their location.

Through understanding the symbology of each affected area, you can begin to have a clear picture of the particular concept that is causing you disharmony, not to mention unclear skin!

Reproductive Organs—Expression. These are symbolic of how you unconsciously view yourself. More than any other set of glands or organs, they "speak" the loudest from one point of view: they influence your ability to express yourself as a person, and they even influence how you look and act.

If you are well developed, people look at and react differently to you than if you were underweight or overweight. You, in turn, respond according to the energy of their reaction. What this means is that life is a cyclic process of reciprocal actions and reactions. You react to people based on their reaction to you. In all situations, remember two things: you are the center point, and it is from within you that all things manifest, especially attitudes that come from other people.

Reproductive organs also reflect faith in yourself, as well as the role you have chosen to portray. Recall the roles of males and females in your life and your beliefs about them. Examine them closely and see how they relate to where you are emotionally at this point in time. What expectations are you seeking to fulfill regarding your sexuality and its expression?

Difficulties in this area usually stem from concepts of physical image, personal expression, and the acceptance of man-made roles for the manifestation of masculinity or femininity.

Ovaries and Testes—Expression, Self-Image. These glands deal with the body's maturation process. They stimulate, prepare, and maintain the body for participation in the reproduction process.

The symbology for both glands involves self-image and expression. The way you see yourself at a subconscious level is how you project yourself outwardly. Your thoughts truly shape your body as well as your personality.

For women, an inability to have children is often tied up in concepts surrounding immaturity, lack of authority, fear of responsibility, and lack of self-expression or self-worth. It may also result from denial of one's gender.

A man with testicular problems may believe that he cannot express himself or that he has no authority to bring forth new ideas or create new things. The testes may be small or oversized, based on basic self-image and concepts surrounding expression of manhood.

NERVOUS SYSTEM—COMMUNICATIONS

The skin and nervous system work together, hand in hand, to gather and transmit data of what is being experienced. The data is then transmitted to the brain where it is processed according to the most prevalent concept currently at work. Other bits of information are stored for later use. This is why people sometimes have fights over seemingly small issues. The truth is these little things are triggering devices that release all the other bits of stored data, the material and emotional experiences filed according to concepts and patterns.

All incoming data, regardless of the source and type, are compared to your personal and environmental conceptual precepts.

Once evaluation takes place, the data are converted from mental thought energies into action energies that are transmitted throughout the nervous system. The parts of the body that must act will do so in a manner that is necessary for the situation. The evaluation also sets in motion actions that ultimately lead to other transactions or manifestations.

The nervous system is symbolic of communication on an internal level. It is the "telephone line" of the inner system. Problems dealing with the nervous system result from the inability to carry out needed messages or transactions. People have these types of problems for various reasons. They may believe they cannot handle a situation or stand up to life, or they may believe they do not have the strength to deal with certain levels of stress.

This constant onslaught of doubt can lead to a nervous breakdown, which is any mental condition that disrupts normal functioning due to an inability to deal with the amount of incoming data at a particular time.

Doubt in your ability to make effective decisions based on incoming data would lead to a feeling of being overloaded, and this overloaded feeling creates a breakdown of problem solving capabilities. As you shut down and refuse to move forward to resolve problems, you become totally dependent on an outside source of guidance.

MUSCULAR SYSTEM—THOUGHTS IN MOTION

Your muscles move almost everything in your body. When you think certain thoughts, they are converted into electrical energy. That energy flows through the nervous system to receptor sites on the cells that make up the muscles, and the action is then carried out instantly, unconsciously. The muscular system converts thought energy from one type of muscular movement to another, such as pulling power to pumping power. This is especially important when you consider the extension and retraction of the limbs and the beating of the heart. From digestion to circulation, your muscles play a great part in the proper functioning of these important systems.

How you think is how you act. Are you flexible or inflexible in either thoughts or movements or both? What ties you up in knots? Do you feel overpowered and helpless, or are you compelled to control everything around you?

SKELETAL SYSTEM—SUPPORT SYSTEM

Your body's inner framework is the skeletal system. It is the foundation you use to support yourself. Through muscular movement, it affords the ability to move about in an upright and controlled fashion. You can literally get yourself from place to place.

Reflect for a moment on the type of thought framework that you use as your foundation, your support system. For instance, are you deeply religious? Do you come from a strict or a particular religious, moral, ethical, economic, or social background? Each one of these areas plays a role in how you think and react to every stimulus that comes your way.

Bones also produce blood, symbolic of the spiritual life of the self. Your blood feeds your body in its material form. Your body feeds your bones with the nourishment that you feed your body, and your nourished bones and personal concepts combine to produce your blood which, in turn, nourishes, feeds, and cleanses the body, your temple of the Creator.

Broken bones indicate a deep, working doubt in a particular area of your life at the time of the break.

Spine and Spinal Cord—Expression, Communication, Action, Support. The spine is also a part of the support system, and as such, it deals with image, self-confidence, courage, and stamina. When there are inner feelings of weakness, this may cause a spinal problem because you would not have sufficient faith in self to support yourself in the current situation. To determine the symbology of the concept at work, look at the type of problem or injury affecting the spine.

The spinal cord is the power line of the total system. Much like a major telephone line that carries all calls to a central point for dissemination through local and regional lines (nerves), the spinal cord receives impulses through the nerve endings in the skin and transmits them back to the control center, the brain, which makes evaluations based on concepts and patterns. Decisions are then made to fulfill the expectation of how to handle that type of situation. The spinal cord receives the electrical energy messages from the brain and transmits them to the areas that have been designated as receivers.

Difficulties within the spinal cord are indicative of breakdowns in communication, because the spinal cord has "telephone lines" that go throughout the body.

To understand the concepts at work, look at the symbology of the afflicted area.

Arms and Legs—Strength, Support, and Mobility. Both sets of extremities are symbolic of strength. The arms add strength to those things you handle. They provide flexibility by bringing things closer or keeping them away. The legs add strength to the support system. They allow you to follow the path of your choices. They also allow you to aspire. The legs can help you climb above the situation and get a different perspective.

Problems with the arms indicate doubt or fear regarding your ability to be strong in a situation that requires your handling. Legs support and transport your body, the material vehicle. Problems here indicate doubt or fear in your ability to move forward and support yourself, to aspire to your highest potential, and to be independent in reaching your goals.

Hands—Handling life, Expression. Your hands, along with your fingers, give you the opportunity to get a firm grip; therefore, they are symbolic of handling. Problems with the hands indicate self-doubt in your ability to handle a specific situation.

The hands are also symbolic of self-expression and are used for artistic endeavors such as writing or painting. They might be used for more practical expression, such as mechanical work or woodworking; even using your hands to make a point while talking is symbolic of expression.

Fingers—Indicators. Each finger has its own meaning.

The thumb relates to control and will power. Without the use of your thumbs, you could not fully control or grasp objects (or situations) at hand. The strength of your will is necessary to accomplish a task, and the thumb is symbolic of the strength of your will.

The index finger relates to the emotions. With this finger, you point at others for your problems. It is interesting to note that when you point at someone with your index finger to place blame, your hand is held in such a position that three of your own fingers are pointing back at you! In truth, we are the cause of our own reality, whatever it may be.

The middle finger relates to spirituality and spiritual or material aspirations. This is why it is the longest finger.

The ring finger relates to social relationships. The left one relates to unity and the right one relates to others in a general social way. Many social statements are expressed through rings worn on this finger, including friendship, marriage, school, or financial status.

The little finger relates to the ego, which is of little use to us. You do not really use the little finger, and the loss of it would not hamper your ability to handle a situation. It is the smallest finger, just as the ego is the least important reflection of your self.

Feet—Direction. Guided by your mind, your feet take you where you want to go. You choose the direction or goal and proceed. Difficulties here always signal doubt in regard to your direction. When foot problems arise, you need to examine your direction and what you stand for in life, both spiritually and materially.

The basis for a form of body therapy called foot reflexology, for example, is that all parts of the body are connected to nerve endings in the feet. Isn't it interesting that the term for the bottoms of the foot, sole, is a homonym for soul? It is easy to see that the feet reflect the direction of your path or journey.

Toes—Balance. It is a medical fact that without toes, you would have a hard time maintaining an upright position or balance. Toe problems warrant a look at any involvements in your life that might be causing you to lose your balance.

Ankles, Knees, Elbows and Wrists—Flexibility. The ankles and knees demonstrate the ability to be flexible in your direction. Without flexibility, you would have great difficulty in pursuing your plans, hopes, desires, and aspirations.

Stiffness in the joints is indicative of having an unyielding or unbending attitude. This is in keeping with concepts that promote a narrow viewpoint about whatever is taking place.

Flexibility of the elbows and wrists alludes to how you deal with situations. Inflexibility can and does prevent you from realizing the most positive outcomes or potential.

The need for flexibility in life is extremely evident in today's world. Changes happen on a daily basis, and you must adapt yourself if you are going to prosper. Flexibility is a great asset.

Tell Me Where It Hurts

Aches, pains, and ailments are symbolic of current hassles. You need to look around and examine all of the different activities that you are involved in to understand your aches and pains. Some activities or people with whom you deal may be more than you are willing to handle or believe you can handle.

Remember that all current problems are merely points on a cycle of a pattern you are going through. The specific cycle that you are in establishes the way a particular aspect of a pattern of behavior will manifest. The end result of the pattern is in keeping with your expectations.

Stimuli trigger particular concepts that support the belief system. This, in turn, determines how you respond, based on how you have dealt with this event or situation in the past.

If the situation does not seem familiar, in the sense that you have done it before, it is because you are not looking at it from the perspective of your past history. History does repeat itself, and although it may take a different form, the energy will be similar to that of the past.

3. SYMBOLOGY OF COMMON AILMENTS

Before we begin examining the symbolic interpretations, a few issues must be discussed in order to avoid debate or denial about a person's condition.

Drugs as Causes

Drugs as causes of conditions within the body do not negate the symbolic interpretation of the condition. If a condition exists because of a particular drug, then an examination of the reason the drug is being prescribed is in order.

In examining the original condition, we will invariably find the commonality of both conditions on a symbolic level. The same underlying subconscious concepts and patterns of behavior are present.

Autoimmune Diseases

Under normal conditions, the body's immune mechanisms tolerate their own tissues and molecules. At times, however, self-tolerance breaks down and this leads to an autoimmune disease, when the immune system fails to recognize its own antigens and produces an attack against them.

Among the diseases classified as autoimmune are rheumatoid arthritis, lupus, rheumatic fever, insulin-dependent (Type I) diabetes, multiple sclerosis, thyroiditis, and Crohn's disease.

Medical science is not 100 percent sure why autoimmune diseases occur. From a symbology standpoint, we might approach autoimmune diseases from the fundamental premise that strong emotions alter the body's biochemistry and physiology.

The reason such changes occur is illustrated in two universal examples. All parents will relate to the first scenario. It's evening, and it's dark outside. The children are out playing, and the phone rings. Almost invariably, the parents' response is to think something has happened to one of the children. Immediately, the body secretes hormones from the adrenal gland, the old "flight or fight" response. This puts the body into a high state of alertness, the heart begins to beat faster, and there may be a queasy feeling in the stomach. It is not uncommon for someone to actually pass out upon hearing terrible news about a relative.

Any driver who has ever driven past a police car parked by the side of the road will relate to the second example. The driver's immediate reaction is to check the speedometer or seat belt.

Seeing a police car behind you with its lights flashing and siren blaring can cause yet another, more intense physical biochemical reaction. Once again the body goes into biochemical change out of fear. Again, there is that rapid heartbeat and queasiness, and the mental questions: What did I do wrong? Why are they coming after me?

These and all stimuli, and the way you react to them, create reactions within. What you see and hear evokes actions based on your subconscious concepts. The way you respond creates the biochemical changes.

Since autoimmune diseases are essentially self attacking the self, then we must look symbolically at concepts relating to self-image. Based on feelings of resentment, guilt, or unworthiness, the person with an autoimmune disease is literally beating up on himself or herself. The body part or function under attack in an autoimmune disease gives clues as to some of the concepts involved.

In Crohn's disease, for instance, a portion of the intestinal tract and the colon are attacked. In addition to the autoimmune component of this particular disease, stress and fatigue play a part. The person may feel a lack of strength or capacity to deal with everything, perhaps based on existing subconscious concepts regarding a need to be dependent on others to handle life. Those with the disease have been led to believe they lack the fortitude to move forward without help.

All concepts are introduced and become conditioned during the first three years of life. Thereafter, experiences, attitudes, and observations continually reinforce these concepts. Personal weakness, a need for external support and an inability for self-expression are a few of these man-made concepts.

The truths of life are different. One truth is in knowing that no matter what situation confronts you, you have the power and ability to deal with it successfully and from a position of strength.

Defenses

People begin constructing defenses on an emotional level at an incredibly young age, and the body develops physical defense systems that help protect it from internal and external damage. The ego also creates a set of defenses that protects it from damage. The unfortunate aspect of defenses is that while they protect the ego, they also suppress the spirit.

We are spiritual beings in a material body, all seeking a return to the harmony of the Creative Continuum. Once that is achieved, we can enjoy not only the tranquility of being in that harmonious state, we will also be able to manifest the spiritual power of that energy in the material plane. We will be able to create any reality desired.

Our defenses curtail that; they suppress that true expression of self. One of life's key objectives is to understand who you are. Only through understanding the concepts that create and support the defense structure can you dismantle it, and only through the process of identifying and learning about the patterns of behavior and the defenses they set in motion can you gain control over their effects in your life.

Herein is one of the most valuable reasons why you should learn how to identify the symbols in your life. Symbols will help you to understand where you are at any given moment. Of course, this also implies that you are aware of factors such as some of the concepts at work, some patterns of behavior, and some personal expectations. I say "some" because the process of self-awareness is always ongoing. Often, we are not able to see ourselves clearly; therefore, we must keep seeking the truth of what we think we are in order to become who we really are. That is achieved through the dismantling of the defenses.

Giving up defenses literally allows your ego to disappear so that you can confront and handle life from a position of strength, knowing that whatever is before you is your own doing. This is your opportunity to learn something about yourself and your personal power. Because it is your own creation, you will be able to master and control it. Remember, you will never be placed in a situation that you cannot handle and master.

Since all physical problems begin within, you must look within for the cure or solution. Presented below are some common ailments and questions you might ask yourself, should you suffer from one of these conditions.

Common Ailments and Their Symbolology

Backache. Backaches usually deal with support issues. Generally, it is advisable to look first to finances (material plane).

What is happening that makes you feel you cannot support yourself? What is making you feel personally weak, as if you do not have the strength to handle your responsibilities? What do you consider a burden? What is threatening your finances?

Broken Bone. Breaking a bone signifies a break in your strength and support system, and the symbology is related to which bone is broken. When this happens, look at the system affected. Should you break a finger, for example, look at your ability to handle something going on in your life as well as the symbology of the particular finger.

Colds and Allergies. Colds and allergies are often the physical result of a direct emotional attack. Sometimes they are brought about by a need, as when colds are used as a means of soliciting love in the form of attention, or to avoid certain situations. The same is largely true for allergies, with the difference that allergies are an overreaction to the irritant.

In all cases dealing with allergies, the irritant (idea) is the item you seek to understand symbolically. The type of side effects you suffer—watery eyes, a stuffed nose, itchy skin—give insight into your reactions to the irritant.

Another dimension of allergies is that they are the result of past emotional situations. For example, an adult who has an allergy to animals as a child had a negative emotional experience with or in the presence of the animal triggering the allergic reaction. The animal did not necessarily have to be directly involved in the experience, only closely enough in some way to be the symbol or picture the mind used to record the experience.

Your mind records situations and experiences in the form of pictures, not words, which is why it is so necessary to understand symbols. Understanding is the term used for converting symbols from mental images and feelings to thoughts that will lead to actions and, in turn, to further understandings.

Congestion and Stuffy Nose. Congestion is a lack of faith in self, indicating a feeling of being overwhelmed. The nose is a port of entry for the spirit that infuses one with power and life. When nasal passages are stuffed up, doubt is at work.

Reflect on who or what might be weighing you down, slowing you up or blocking your renewal of inner-strength.

Constipation, Diarrhea, and Hemorrhoids. Constipation is the result of holding on to the past. If we do not remove the toxins from our body, they will poison us to death. If we do not let go of old ideas and concepts, they, too, will poison us to death.

Diarrhea is another form of constipation in which ideas are expelled as quickly as possible. This leads to depletion of vital nutrients and fluids and can create conditions leading to disease.

Hemorrhoids also signify difficulty in letting go of the past and are a frequent companion of constipation. They can also be brought on through muscular weakness, exhaustion, and lethargy, all of which can allow the vein to "pop out." (Varicose veins are similar in this respect.) Muscular weakness can also lead to a sluggish intestinal tract.

To understand the causative factors behind these conditions, find the thoughts or situations that have been difficult for you to cleanse from your mind. What are you holding onto? What is your belief system? What is blocking your natural cleansing process? And, at the other end of the spectrum, what is so distasteful that you must expel it immediately?

Earache. The quick and easy understanding of this problem is to look at what is being said that you do not want to hear or accept. The question you must answer is why.

Eye Problems. Shaded by our belief system and concepts, vision is a two-fold tool allowing us to see our self and others. Our expectations create our vantage point.

Not seeing clearly? What concepts are affecting your vision? What about the present or future do you not wish or fear to see?

Fever. Fever indicates anger. The anger can stem from resentment, frustration, guilt, or disappointment; forces that can "burn you up." What is the source of your emotional turmoil, and why does a situation or a person trigger such a response?

Headaches. Because the head is the spiritual center, all head afflictions and trauma reflect self-doubt or a lack of self-confidence. What situation or relationship in your life is causing your faith in yourself to be strained or attacked?

Heart Attack. The heart is symbolic of the emotions. Heart attacks are the result of emotional stress, strain, and rejection. Dying from a heart attack is one way of avoiding a highly charged emotional situation.

What concepts and attitudes do you feel are debilitating? Are you being subjected to these situations and thoughts? Is it possible that not dealing with them will lead to your death? Death is another aspect of rejection.

Indigestion, Stomach Ache, and Vomiting. Stomach distress is a sign that a thought is being presented or imposed that is not in keeping with your belief system; therefore, thoughts and situations are hard to digest and accept.

Ideas can be indigestible in the sense that although you have partaken of them (by choice or not), their consumption is not satisfying. Should you have had a choice, you would have rejected them at the outset. If the thoughts or events were intensely repulsive to your belief system, you might also have rejected them by "throwing them up," thus, eliminating them from your system.

If you are bothered by such symptoms, explore your life for adverse ideas, events, and people who are so disagreeable to you that you simply cannot stomach them. What about them evokes this response?

Be mindful, also, of the Universal Teaching: "Excess leads to rejection."

Obesity. Being obese may have its roots in a number of places, including the need for protection or authority (the need to throw one's weight around). Obesity can be a source of artificial power.

What concepts make your think and feel that material things will make you feel secure? From what or whom are you protecting yourself?

Sore Throat. Although the throat represents both balance and expression, problems usually lie within the realm of expression. Either you are compelled to express but believe you should not, or you want to express something but cannot. Is something "hard to swallow" in your life? Look for doubts, fears, and imbalances that may be creating communication problems.

Stubbed Toe. Toes represent balance, and they are a part of the foot. So, when stubbed toes become a symbol, it is wise to question where you are going. What thoughts or situations are making your path unsure?

4. "ACCIDENTS"

Accidents don't just happen. Like ailments, accidents are symbolic forms of communication that begin within the mind. All accidents are a form of guidance.

Understanding Symbols: Seeking the Creator

Remember from the first section how life works: concepts create patterned forms of behavior, forms that are triggered by certain stimuli. The pattern starts a chain reaction of events that ends in a particular fashion as it completes its cyclic flow. All patterns of behavior flow in cycles. The outcome or end result of the pattern is preprogrammed to have a specific conclusion designed to fulfill a particular expectation that a person maintains about the self. This, in turn, validates the original concept that supported the particular pattern of behavior.

By being able to identify a symbol and interpret it correctly, you will be able to determine which concepts and patterns of behavior are at work and where you are in a particular concept or pattern. With understanding comes the ability to gain control over emotional responses within the pattern. By gaining control, it is possible to direct the outcome of both energetic and emotional responses, ultimately manifesting your life's desires.

In summary, all diseases begin within the self. Diseases are a reflection of the conflict between the Inner/Spiritual Self and the Outer/Ego Self. The Ego Self seeks to live pursuing fulfillment of expectations, while the Spiritual Self seeks to live in harmony with the Creative Continuum. Your spirit, on its upward journey of unification with the Creator, gives your mind guidance in the form of symbols and spiritual energy to aid in its quest for peace and tranquility with the Creator.

Your mind translates energy into thoughts within your brain, which transfers the thoughts to your body so that you can "see" what you are thinking, and your body moves through the material plane, in accordance with your thoughts. This process brings you into all of your experiences, and by knowing your experience for the symbolic guidance that it is, you can move closer to mastery over your ego and mastery over your man-made concepts.

It is through knowing, understanding, and gaining control that you aspire and master the material plane. You may have heard the expression, "for those who have eyes to see and ears to hear." My purpose in writing this book is to provide you with the information necessary to develop the ability to truly see and hear.

Once you learn to have eyes that see and ears that hear, you will never be without true guidance from the Creator that dwells within you. You must always remember that no one knows your life better than you; therefore, you are the source of the best, most correct answers for yourself. And yes, you will be able to tell the difference between what you want to hear and the truth. You will always know the truth of yourself if you are honest with yourself.

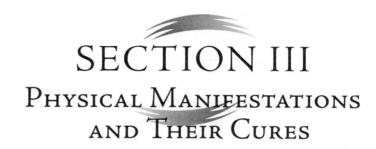

SECTION III
Physical Manifestations and Their Cures

1. Understanding Physical manifestations and Their Cures

The term "symbolic" means that everything, including situations from accidents to diseases, is a reflection of tangible, dimensional forms of thought in action. When conditions or diseases manifest, it indicates thoughts are in conflict with each other. You may want to do or be something while at a deep, subconscious level, you do not believe you have the right or authority to do so. Therein resides the conflict.

Nothing in our physical world has come about without originating in the realm of thought. Even the creation of the universe resulted from thoughts generated by the Creator.

Before a word can be uttered, it must first take form in thought. Before it can be acted upon, forces of energy are put into motion to create the reality that was first conceived in thought. That is why everything is symbolic of thought.

The key to mastery of a situation, or in this case a disease, is the ability to read inner-thoughts and understand them, thereby gaining control, mastery and cure.

In this section, we look at the symbolic associations for some common ailments and conditions as well as for the nutrients, minerals, vitamins and amino acids helpful to these conditions. As a metaphysical counselor, I also use and recommend herbs as part of a healing program. Herbs have chemical constituents that have toning, stimulating and immune-performing properties.

(For additional information on symbology of specific body parts and common ailments, see Section II: Mysteries Revealed. For additional information about the symbology of nutrients, see Section IV: Basic Nutrition.)

2. SYMBOLOGY OF CONDITIONS AND DISEASES

Acne and Skin Problems

Understanding the root causes of acne and eliminating the contributing factors is important to teens and adults. Doing so provides the necessary confidence to get a handle on life and turn negative situations around. If you catch it early enough, you will be able to positively influence the outcome and may be able to avoid the scarring that accompanies many cases of acne.

Acne is defined as a breakout of pimples, usually occurring in or near the oil glands of the face, neck, shoulders, or upper back. While the exact medical cause is unknown, a bacterium does exacerbate the condition.

The first consideration in dealing with acne is to eliminate the contributing factors. What elements combine to create acne?

Let's look at that old adage, "you are what you eat." The typical American diet centers on fried foods, meat, and meat by-products—guaranteeing a large intake of saturated fatty acids. Saturated fatty acids are fats found mainly in beef, lamb, pork, veal, and whole milk products, such as cheese, ice cream, and milk. Other sources are plant oils like cocoa butter, coconut oil, and palm oil. Margarine and hydrogenated shortenings also contain high amounts of saturated fatty acids. It is wise to avoid all products with hydrogenated oils.

When the body is laden with fats and other types of consumed toxins, it tries to remove them. This process involves the blood, lungs, kidneys, bowels, and, of course, the skin. The blood carries the fats and toxins to every part of the body for elimination. The skin eliminates whatever it can, via the drops of perspiration that ooze from the skin's pores.

During times of stress and uncertainty, acne can become aggravated.

Skin. Perspiration consists of water with salt (sodium chloride), phosphate, urea, ammonia, and other waste products. These wastes, removed from the body's interior can become food for the millions of microbes that live on the skin's surface. When the wastes are laden with impurities from the diet the pores become clogged, microbes flourish, and acne can set in. Consequently, the pores must be kept clean and open. This means that the body must also have a clean diet and a regular supply of nutrients in order to manufacture healthy replacement cells for the skin.

Blood. In addition to supplying the body with life-sustaining nutrients, the bloodstream is also involved in waste removal. As old cells die or are destroyed by various natural processes within the body, they must be removed, along with organic waste that cells generate. If these wastes remain, problems can result, including acne and other types of skin eruptions; the skin is the body's largest organ of elimination, after all!

Liver. Liver cells seek to render harmless substances such as alcohol, nicotine, other toxins, and various substances introduced into the bloodstream via the intestines. What cannot be rendered harmless is then stored in fat.

Dietary Changes. The logical starting point for cleaning the body's interiors and preventing most incoming toxins is the diet. Eat as many living, organic foods as possible: fresh fruits and vegetables, such as celery, garlic, carrots, and spinach; freshly sprouted seeds; and whole grain products like millet and brown rice.

Water is an important nutrient so drink plenty, preferably distilled or very deep spring water with some freshly squeezed organic lemon juice. This is good for the liver, helping to keep it clean from fatty deposits, plus it has alkalinizing effects.

Nutrients and Herbs for Acne and Skin Concerns

The following will assist the body in cleansing the blood, skin, and liver, and will speed healing of acne conditions.

Nutrients	Herbs
Niacinamide	Burdock Root
Vitamin A	
Zinc	

Niacinamide. A buffered form of niacin, this B-complex nutrient helps promote growth and repair. It participates in maintaining skin health by facilitating reactions that dilate the arteries and capillaries that carry blood to cells that construct skin. Cells are kept healthy by the blood being able to bring in fresh building material and carry away toxins.

Vitamin A. Important for the skin and for maintenance of the outer layer of tissues and organs. Good for healthy hair and the growth and repair of body tissues. Used successfully in the treatment of acne[1].

Zinc. Plays a fundamental role in normal tissue development, including cell division, protein synthesis and collagen formation.[2]

Burdock Root. An all-around blood purifier, strongly diuretic and diaphoretic. Cleanses the body of toxins; markedly enhances liver and gall-bile functions.

Symbology of Acne

By going back to acne's medical definition as being pimples on the skin of the face, neck, shoulders, or upper back, it is easier to examine the condition from a symbolic perspective. Pimples are the first sign something is out of balance internally. If everything were okay within, there would not be an external change to the skin.

In fact, if an individual's internal thoughts were okay, this balance and harmony would be reflected in health, wealth, and happiness. This would be in keeping with several Universal Teachings found throughout the *Bible*. Here is one that is rarely understood, yet it occurs everyday without conscious control: "Ask, and you shall receive."

Unfortunately, most people never realize it is their stronger, subconscious mind doing all of the asking, rather than the conscious. This is why people continually repeat events in their life. Biblical authors understood this truth, writing of it in Ecclesiastes 3:15: "That which hath been is now; and that which is to be hath already been."

The task is to understand which thoughts are creating conflict in your self-image; in this case, the result is acne. We can begin by examining the symbolic reflections of acne's physical manifestation on the skin of the face.

Symbology of the Skin - Face

The skin is your physical contact point with the material world. A sensory organ, the skin acts as a protective device against millions of microbes as well as the sun's light rays and radiation.

Your sensitivities to life are expressed here; the way you think influences how you are touched by and react to certain situations. If you are experiencing skin eruptions or problems, look inward to identify your particular sensitivities. The location of skin eruptions—face, arms, legs, back, shoulders, or chest—is also crucial. Through understanding the symbology of each affected area, you can begin to have a clear picture of which concept is causing you disharmony.

Based my counseling experiences, the face usually is the primary area affected by acne. Here is why: your face is a reflection of how you see yourself and how you expect others to see you. This is all based on the concepts that you were taught about yourself.

Often, teenagers develop acne at the same time they are establishing their own identity. This is a difficult, painful stage of life, one filled with doubt and uncertainty. Teens have doubts about what they want to be, what they are supposed to be, and whether or not they can achieve their goals. And let's not forget peer pressure.

When these energies are at work in your life, many problems can result, including acne. Acne is the result of the doubt both within you and with the image that you project to the world.

Symology of the Skin - Back and Neck

In addition to the face, the upper back and neck are prime targets for acne. Within the neck are the voice box and the thyroid gland, key structures for communication with others. Through the expression of your thoughts, insights and understandings, you are able to maintain balance and harmony within your life. Of course, this is predicated on the understanding that you are aware of who and what you are about. At this level of understanding, you are able to communicate with others in a non-defensive way, which creates better communication overall.

The thyroid helps regulate the body's metabolism and helps to keep everything running smoothly. Once again, we see how the neck relates to balance—within and without.

Your neck supports your head. It also connects the head, which is symbolic of the spiritual plane, to the body, which is symbolic of the material plane; therefore, it represents the need for balance between the two.

A "pain in the neck" usually refers to an individual or situation that upsets your equilibrium.

Your upper back and shoulders reflect your thinking about how well you are able to shoulder responsibility and how well you can support yourself during tough times. Tough times can result from schoolwork for teens, professional work for adults, or other emotional conditions.

With acne, there is an underlying need to examine your concepts and belief system. (For more insight on the way you think, see Section I: From the Inside Out.)

Symology of the Nutrients

Niacin/Niacinamide. Represents openness and receptivity. Receptivity is associated with niacinamide because of how it relates to growth, nerve function, and metabolism as well as how it affects the cardiovascular system, which is responsible for the delivery of the blood throughout the body.

Blood, the body's lifeline, represents spirit within the material realm. Blood carries nutrients to every cell within the body, and cleans and carries away the toxins that would destroy the body if left to collect. Poisonous thoughts left within the mind to operate freely will ultimately kill a person. All toxins, both of the thought and physical realms, must be eliminated from the system if there is to be true growth.

Spirit (blood) also symbolizes courage and confidence. This is why every disease that requires niacin as part of the healing program is a condition that requires faith in one's ability to handle the situation.

Vitamin A. Essential for healthy night vision. Symbolically, with proper vision, especially during periods of preparation (nighttime), you can avoid all of the doubt and frustration that accompanies aspects of preparing for a situation. Vitamin A strengthens vision, giving you greater insight.

When you can go into a situation totally prepared, courageously and confidently, then the question of your image is not at risk. Without doubt and fear, your reflection of your confidence will show in an improved complexion.

Vitamin A is instrumental in protecting you from invasion from outside forces, because it feeds the thymus gland, which is an immune center. From here, T-cells rush out to do battle with invading forces. The forces can be allergens, germs, bacteria, viruses, fungus, or toxins from the environment. Forces can also be thoughts from others that are projected onto you.

Zinc. Important to many functions, including taste, smell, and reproduction, zinc is symbolic of the thoughts that contribute to courage, confidence, and expression. With acne, a lack of zinc would denote that an inability for adequate self-expression has led to a poor self-image, as reflected in the breakout.

Allergies

An allergy is an exaggerated or abnormal reaction to something in the environment. Triggers can be substances, situations or physical states; in medical terms, these triggers are called allergens.

The allergens in foods are somewhat of a mystery to medical science. According to an article about them in Modern Nutrition in Health and Disease, it is largely unknown why some food proteins are more allergenic than others.[3] This aspect becomes clear when the symbolic reflections of foods are examined.

Allergies are labeled, identified, and classified by the degree to which and how the body's cells react to specific allergens. They are further divided based on how soon the body responds to the allergen, either a quick or a delayed response. An example of the delayed type of allergic reaction can be seen in contact with poison ivy. After being exposed, it normally takes a day or two for the rashes to appear.

Rashes are a common symptom of allergic reactions. Other symptoms include watery, swollen eyes, lung or nasal congestion, itching, fever, and even vomiting. For some people, the reactions can be fatal.

Allergy sufferers tend to have imbalances in their biochemistry, and in almost every instance, this can be traced back to an immune problem.

Symptoms manifest once the immune system fails to eradicate the allergen that has entered into the body. The immune system identifies everything that enters the body as either friend or foe. Allergies flourish when the immune system is not functioning at optimum levels. Even food allergies are believed to be an adverse reaction involving an immune response.

NUTRIENTS, HERBS AND OTHER SUBSTANCES FOR ALLERGIES

For support in eliminating common symptoms of allergies, including watery eyes, runny nose, and sneezing, incorporate the following elements into your nutritional program.

Nutrients	Herbs and Other Substances
Manganese	Bee Pollen
Pantothenic Acid	Dandelion Root
Potassium	MSM
Vitamin A	N-A-C (N-Acetyl-Cysteine)
Vitamin B-6	Stinging Nettle Leaf
Vitamin C	
Zinc	

Manganese. Is involved in a wide variety of metabolic functions and helps certain white blood cells carry out the process of phagocytosis, the ingestion and destruction of toxins or other invaders.

Pantothenic Acid. Helps to nourish the adrenal glands; the stress centers of the body which are tied directly to the proper functioning of the immune system.

Potassium and Vitamin B-6. Reduce inflammation that may accompany allergies. Potassium is wonderful for stimulating the kidneys into eliminating toxins from the bloodstream.

Vitamin A. Essential for the immune system.

Vitamin B-6. Reduces inflammation that may accompany allergies.

Vitamin C. Stimulates immune response[4,5] and is essential for the proper functioning of the immune system. Large concentrations of vitamin C are found in the adrenal glands and are necessary for the formation of adrenalin. During physical stress, and allergies definitely create stress, the level of adrenal ascorbic acid (vitamin C) is rapidly depleted.

Zinc. Necessary for proper immune system function.

Bee Pollen. Often used by people with allergies, especially those with airborne allergies. Introducing small amounts of bee pollen into the body is equal to what a physician does by introducing a small amount of an allergen into the body so that it builds a tolerance and, thus, helps get the allergies under control.

Dandelion Root. Wonderful for the liver, which helps in the detoxification process. Most allergens are alien proteins that the body has not identified; the liver protects your body from these allergens.

MSM (Methylsulfonylmethane). A source of sulfur. Excellent for the immune system.

NAC (N-Acetyl Cysteine). For detoxification.

Stinging Nettle Leaf. Traditionally used by herbalists for hay fever and as an expectorant to help loosen a cough.

SYMBOLOGY OF ALLERGIES

In tackling allergies, it is essential to understand the significance of the symptoms because they are the outward manifestation of an internal condition. Because allergies are exaggerated reactions to triggers that would not harm most other people, it is safe to say that people with allergies are overly sensitive.

Being sensitive has many different definitions. When you hear that another person is sensitive, let alone overly sensitive, you may avoid offending them, understanding that if you upset someone's sensitivities, there may be an adverse, usually outward, reaction.

But what happens internally? Certain enzymes or hormones are released, altering the current health state, at least temporarily. Adrenalin is a prime example. Think back to a time when you experienced an event that changed your state of mind and altered your body's bio-chemistry.

People can be offended by what they see or hear, and some are offended by what they eat (food allergies) or by what others eat. People can even become offended when someone else tries to feed them something that they believe is not good for them.

To gain insights and understandings into allergies, look closely at your symptoms and the allergens that trigger them. An allergen is any foreign substance that enters or comes into contact with the body, causing an allergic reaction. The interest here is primarily with what enters the body. If you are paying attention (are conscious and aware), you likely will not come into contact with an external source that you know will offend your sensibilities, be it a substance, situation, action, attitude, thought, or person.

We must also look within for understanding. "What is within will manifest without" applies here, as does this passage from the Gospel According to Thomas: "For there is nothing hidden which will not manifest." Both are Universal Teachings.

Everything that we do, think, or experience on an emotional level will ultimately be made public. The "public" here is not referring to broadcast news, but to actual physical results, like an allergic reaction to a substance.

Because not every allergen affects every person, it is important to understand the symbolism of common allergens.

Pollen. Technically defined as the "fecundating element" in seed plants, pollen is the fine powder substance that forms within a plant's anther, part of the stamen of a flowering plant. Symbolically, "fecundating element" says it all. It means fertilizing or impregnating. How true it is that some thoughts offered or imposed by others can be so impregnating as to induce an immediate reaction—doubt, fear, or even anger.

Other thoughts can create situations that germinate within and slowly manifest outward, such as resentment. Pollen equates to thoughts that conflict with our belief system so strongly as to elicit a physical reaction. These thoughts or substances do not affect everyone, in fact, they are harmless to most people.

That is both a positive and a negative. In the positive sense, it may be that your sensitivity, once mastered, will guide you to great heights and accomplishments. The down side of being overly sensitive is that your reactions can cause you great stress and discomfort, even death.

Be aware of thoughts that are being directed at you and listen carefully to what is being said in order to understand implications and attitudes that will cause you to react in a negative way and trigger a pattern of behavior that you will find disharmonious or destructive to a relationship or to yourself.

Feathers. The protective covering of birds. Feathers symbolize protection. Once used as writing instruments, they are also symbolic of expression, the ability to communicate personal thoughts.

The type of bird causing an allergic reaction should be examined because every bird has its own symbolic meaning. For example, the American Bald Eagle stands for freedom and independence.

Birds, in general, are symbolic of lofty, spiritual thoughts. Birds live and operate in the air, which is symbolic of spirit because the Creator lives in heaven (air/sky).

Animal Dander. This substance from the animal kingdom may trigger strong allergic reactions. Dander is the term given to the dried scales of skin or hair that are shed by animals. Feathers from birds can also produce dander, and the symbology is much the same with animals and birds, with one important twist: with animal dander, it is important to understand the habits and functions of the specific animal as well as whatever emotional relationship exists between person and creature. Every animal has a function and a lesson to teach man.

House Dust. House dust is a true sensitivity to the place you call home, or to people, animals, or things in the home. There is some type of imposition that may be at work in this environment. Keep in mind that dust is a conglomeration of dead skin cells, yours and every other member of the family as well as animal dander and pollen from the outside air. Other allergens in the home can come from new paint, carpet, flooring or wallpaper.

Cigarette/Tobacco Smoke. The physical presence of smoke is an obvious allergen, yet there may be other associations at work. For instance, if as a child you were burned by a parent's cigarette, your allergy could stem from fear, resentment, or anger. Today, the odor of smoke may reignite fear in your subconscious because of the past burn, and you may create an allergy to reflect the feelings of imposition, resentment, abuse or neglect.

Smoking diminishes the amount of oxygen available to the cells, and as we have discussed, oxygen is symbolic of spirit. You could also say that oxygen is symbolic of faith. Smokers rely on an outside device to deal with stress, which means they lack faith in self on some levels.

Food Allergies. Although medical science has not connected all the dots regarding what makes some substances more allergenic than others, your mind is capable of working with your body and the Universal Teachings to keep you informed about how to stay on the narrow path that leads to a healthy and balanced life, as is written in Matthew 7:14: "Narrow is the way, which leadeth unto life."

Your mind is constantly receiving guidance on how to handle every situation. It then takes that guidance and converts the energy of thought into the energy of action by converting the energy into electrical impulses that flow through your nerves and stimulate, direct, and manipulate your glands, organs, and muscles.

Every food to which you are attracted has an emotional attachment. If you are allergic to a particular food, you are really allergic to the thought that it represents. Foods are recorded as thoughts as well as by taste, touch, sight, and smell.

Looking back into childhood and recalling the first association with the food can reveal the thought behind a particular food. For instance, children are often told that if they eat spinach, they will grow up to be strong, like Popeye. A child's parents may even have forced him or her to eat it, so, over the years, this child will develop an attachment between resentment of the authoritative imposition used and the vegetable itself, thus, spinach becomes an allergen.

Look closely at your food triggers to discover how to control and cure your allergies. Through understanding, you will eliminate your sensitivity to the substance and the thought behind it.

One important, overall observation about food allergies: some researchers believe food allergies are an adverse reaction involving an immune response. Allergens are thoughts that attack, and depending on your belief system, you will either handle them from a position of strength, or you will have a reaction because of your sensitivities.

QUICK AND DELAYED ALLERGIC RESPONSES

Every situation generates some response, and some allergic responses can be quick or delayed. An allergen evoking a quick response is symbolic of the level of doubt, fear, or anger generated by the situation, substances, or person involved. The type and degree of your reactions depends on the concepts that you maintain about yourself, and the expectations that you are trying to live up to.

With a delayed response, you stew over something, consciously or subconsciously, and then you react. Someone might make a comment to you that is not immediately taken as offensive, yet it becomes so once you have the time to reflect. With that realization comes the reaction.

There are times when, because of defenses, you suppress your feelings to the point that you no longer realize when you are bothered by something. This is when an allergic reaction tells you, symbolically, that you are reacting to a given stimuli. Seek to identify what it is that stimulates your reactions. To gain a clearer picture, examine the symptoms of your allergy as well as the triggers.

Rashes. Why are rashes one of the most common signs of an allergic reaction? People who are overly sensitive often show their defensive reactions on the most visible physical defense system they have: their skin. Pay attention to the location of skin rashes and study the symbology of the affected body part for deepest understanding.

Watery, Swollen Eyes. It is through your eyes that you view the world, your immediate situation, family, friends, and yourself. If your vision is impacted, look inward for what is affecting your perceptions and abilities to see.

Emotions such as love and rage can both create tearing reactions that blur vision. When your eyes are watery, your clarity is distorted and the truth may be blurred.

Nasal, Lung Congestion. Through your nose, you draw into the body the "breath of life." Congested breathing is another common allergy symptom. The nose is also part of your defense system, alerting you to what is potentially offensive or unhealthy, and what should be avoided, literally and figuratively.

Because everything is a symbolic reflection of thought, detrimental thoughts often pass through the defense mechanism of the nose. This happens due to the use of "artificial aromas," which are really man-made concepts that give off the appearance and smell of being wholesome and worthwhile.

One of the most abundant sources of misconceptions in our time is television. Through it, we are exposed to many messages, particularly through advertising. Fast-food restaurants are a frequent sponsor, portraying in their commercial the thought that if you will eat their food, you will be happy, have a great family life, and be successful, when in reality the high fat content and excessive salt in their products actually work against your health. In this way, TV can circumvent your natural defense mechanisms. If you suffer frequently from a stuffy nose, look for the issues that are blocking your ability to receive spiritual strength.

The lungs work to help you receive the breath of life. You inhale that which nourishes and sustains you; you exhale what is used and no longer beneficial, something that would cause harm and possibly even death were it to be retained within the body.

Breathing spent or polluted air (a man-made hazard) is no different from taking in fouled concepts of the truth; both hurt if you attempt to hold onto them. Just as you inhale fresh air to sustain your body, look for understanding regarding man-made concepts and misconceptions before they lead to accidents, sickness, allergies, or even death.

When you have congestion, regardless of the source, it is symbolic of an attack on your faith in dealing with a particular situation, one that requires self-confidence at the spiritual level.

Itching. This symptom denotes the need to handle an irritating situation as quickly as possible, lest the person be driven crazy by the itching. This occurs when your reaction to a stimulus is such that immediate awareness and understanding are essential and is symbolic of feelings of being unable to cope.

Fever. Fever is symbolic of anger, resentment, and frustration. A person becomes so angry because of a situation that he or she literally begins to "burn up." These feelings can be brought about by doubt and fear. Look inward to determine what is causing this emotional turmoil.

Vomiting. Vomiting happens when the intensity of the thought or situation is so difficult to stomach that rejection begins immediately. Examine the environment for people, activities, words, or thoughts unpalatable enough to cause this type of forceful rejection.

Death. Some people have allergic reactions so severe that they can lead to death. Death is the greatest rejection symbol a person can have; it also signifies a new beginning.

Symbology of the Nutrients

Manganese. Represents protection by helping the process of phagocytosis, which destroys invading toxins. By being constantly aware of what is being said and implied, you have the opportunity to control a situation so that none of the toxic implications and suggestions will have an effect.

Pantothenic Acid. In its role as nourishment for the adrenal glands, pantothenic acid represents inspiration. The adrenals produce hormones that help the body deal with making quick movements or actions based upon quick decisions, as reflected in the "flight or fight" concept.

When most people face an intense force, they go into a state of fear, and each person's reaction to fear stems from how well-equipped he or she feels to deal with the situation. The part of the body that reacts to the fear impulse, translated into electrical energy, is the adrenal system, which sends hormonal signals to body parts telling them how to react.

Pantothenic acid, from a nutritional point of view, is the nutrient that represents inspiration, courage and confidence because of its role in growth, energy, and overall health. If your adrenals are exhausted, you will lack energy, and energy is directly related to enthusiasm, inspiration, and confidence.

Potassium. Represents balance and harmony, combating allergens and toxic thoughts that create imbalances. Potassium stimulates the kidneys to eliminate poisonous body wastes, demonstrating that balance and harmony in your thinking are essential for eliminating obsolete, detrimental thoughts.

Vitamin A. Excellent for the immune system as well as improving night vision. The symbolic importance of vitamin A is the ability to see into the doubt that causes reactions to thoughts and situations. When you engage in self-examination, you improve your internal vision and strengthen your defenses against invading thoughts (allergens).

Vitamin B-6. Represents regulation as well as protection. Both are demonstrated by how the vitamin helps maintain adequate numbers of white blood cells, the body's main defense against invaders that could cause harm or disease.

Thoughts are much the same; they are forces that can invade the personal belief system. Some ideas require regulation by emotional response while others require a protective mode so as not to destroy a current position or stand on issues or concepts. These regulating, protective thoughts are necessary to keep the body in a state of good health because thoughts change biochemistry in response to external stimuli or emotional responses to a given event.

Vitamin C. Plays a supportive role in the defenses of the body, and ensures that the ability to maintain faith and courage is intact. When your courage and faith in self are compromised, doubt and fear set in, opening the door for frustration, anger, and resentment. Allergies are only one of the many different conditions and diseases that can result.

Zinc. Plays an important role in nourishing the thymus gland, the power seat of the immune system, and it liberates vitamin A from the liver. As we have seen before, vitamin A is essential in our defense against invading forces.

Symbolically, zinc represents those thoughts that contribute to supportive or fundamental expression and a working faith. When you have true self-confidence, you have a working faith, and you can handle anything that comes your way.

Alzheimer's Disease

See Memory Problems.

Arthritis and Inflammatory Diseases

One of many different types of inflammatory conditions classified as degenerative diseases, arthritis has two main forms: rheumatoid and osteoarthritis.

Rheumatoid arthritis is considered an autoimmune disease, causing chronic inflammation of the joints, and it can also cause inflammation of the tissue around the joints as well as other organs in the body. In some people with rheumatoid arthritis, chronic inflammation leads to the destruction of the cartilage, bone, and ligaments, causing deformity of the joints.

Occurring mostly in older people, osteoarthritis is caused by the breakdown and eventual loss of the cartilage, which can occur in joints throughout the body. In the aging process, the water content of the cartilage increases, while at the same time, the protein makeup of cartilage degenerates.

Repetitive use of the joints over the years also plays a part. The constant movement combined with inadequate nutrition irritates and inflames the cartilage, causing joint pain and swelling, and eventually degeneration.

Most diseases that are classified as degenerative have no known cause, according to The Merck Manual, a physician's reference that describes causes, symptoms and recommended drug therapy for every known ailment in humans.

In working with arthritis from a natural healing perspective, we must first examine the medical knowledge, looking first at the symptoms and then at the probable causes.

Inflammation. Joints are affected, primarily the knuckles, wrists, fingers, toes, ankles, and knees. Arthritis can also affect the spine, neck, and hips. Since inflammation of these various joints causes pain, an immediate goal would be to reduce the inflammation as quickly as possible, thereby lessening the pain caused by the joints rubbing together. There are various ways to reduce the inflammation.

Since we are taking a natural approach to healing this condition, we need to understand the nutritional influences of arthritis, which reflects a state of nutritional imbalance in the body. Interestingly, people with arthritis are generally deficient in potassium, which is used by the body to help regulate the balance of fluids within the cells. When there is a decreased amount of potassium, there is generally an increase in sodium. Sodium forces the body to retain fluids and this retention, in part, causes the cells to swell with fluids, thus, creating an inflamed condition.

Sodium also has an important role in the preservation of normal muscle excitability and contractibility and in the permeability of the cells.

There are many different herbs that can also speed up the removal of water from the body, such as the diuretic herbs: corn silk, parsley, watermelon seeds, uva ursi, and hydrangea.

Calcium Deposits. Another aspect of arthritis is the calcium deposits, or spurs, that form at the joint sites. Spurs may develop because the proper nutrients, enzymes, and other biochemical factors are not available in adequate amounts for proper absorption of calcium. Thus, calcium deposits accumulate in inappropriate places, including the arteries.

The other goal is to dissolve these spurs and have the body re-assimilate the calcium into the cells and bloodstream where it is needed.

Probable Causes. Research has demonstrated that arthritis sufferers are deficient in the amino acid histadine as well as the mineral potassium, and have an increased need for other nutrients such as vitamin B-6, pantothenic acid, and magnesium.

In some medical circles, arthritis is being examined as a viral disease that has been able to flourish because of the body's lowered defenses, brought on by a compromised immune system. As research on this aspect of the disease continues, it seems clear that stress is a major factor in the lowering of the immune system's overall function.

Stress taxes the adrenal glands, which secrete hormones that carry messages to other glands on how to perform or what to manufacture. All of the glands of the body are tied together in a complicated system. Each and every aspect of life within the body is dependent on every other aspect, and that is why it is important to maintain a proper nutritional balance.

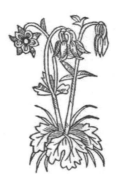

Nutrients, Amino Acids and Herbs for Arthritis and Inflammatory Diseases

Nutrients	Amino Acids	Herbs
Calcium	DL- Phenylalanine	Alfalfa
Magnesium	L-Histidine	Celery Seeds
Niacinamide		Chaparral
Pantothenic Acid	*Enzymes*	Corn Silk
Potassium	Bromelain	Fennel Seeds
Vitamin B-6		Hydrangea
Vitamin D		Uva Ursi
		White Willow Bark
		Yucca

For support in regaining nutritional balance to assist with reducing inflammation in the joints, dissolving calcium deposits, neutralizing the acidity of the blood, improving circulation, increasing the body's threshold for pain, and improving resistance to stress and infection incorporate the following elements into your nutritional program.

Calcium. Wonderful for helping the body to maintain an alkaline base because with arthritis you have high amounts of uric acid in the bloodstream.

Magnesium. Aids in calcium assimilation; helps regulate the body's acid-alkaline balance.

Niacin/Niacinamide. Opens arteries and improves blood flow, promotes growth, and the proper functioning of the nervous system. One of niacin's actions is to dilate blood vessels, allowing the blood freer access to the extremities.

Pantothenic Acid. Serves as a part of co-enzyme A, which is essential for the production of energy.

Potassium. Regulates water balance and acid-alkaline balance in the blood.

Vitamin B-6. Helps maintain the balance of sodium and potassium, which help regulate the distribution of fluids through the cell membranes and help reduce inflammation.

Vitamin D. Assists the body in assimilating calcium from the intestinal tract. It also assists in the breakdown and assimilation of phosphorus, which is required for bone formation.

DL-Phenylalanine and White Willow Bark. Great for pain relief.

L-Histidine. An amino acid that all arthritics are deficient in. Histidine chelates heavy metals, and may act as a neurotransmitter and vasodilator. Necessary for maintenance of myelin sheath of nerves.

Bromelaine. Functions as an anti-inflammatory.

Alfalfa and Celery Seeds. Reduce acidity and inflammation; rich in micronutrients.

Chaparral and Yucca. Contain saponins, which act as a joint lubricant.

Corn Silk , Hydrangea, and Uva Ursi. Excellent diuretic herbs that help reduce inflammation.

SYMBOLOGY OF ARTHRITIS AND INFLAMMATORY DISEASES

In seeking to understand the symbolic implications of arthritis, I refer back to The Merck Manual where we get the perception that the cause of arthritis is unknown. When something is unknown, it is usually because it is not understood. With that concept in mind, new questions arise: From what frame of reference have we historically looked at this condition? What guidelines and points of reference did we use? Did we ask all the right questions?

Let us look at how a disease grows. What causes a healthy body to move to a state of ill health? The answer is simple—it has to be as a result of something the person brings into the body.

There are five primary avenues of introduction: thought, food, water, air, and light. The abundance or lack of each of these elements leaves its own distinctive mark on health. For example, the fluorescent lighting to which most of us are exposed daily during our working lives has cumulative, detrimental effects. Over time, the skin becomes yellow and heavily creased.

Sunshine therapy, as outlined in Vitalogy,[6] was practiced as a healing art long before the start of chemical drugs. Sunshine is known to stimulate vitamin D production from cholesterol; unlike all other vitamins, vitamin D acts like a hormone. Other vitamins become parts of enzymes and are co-enzymes.

The physical and biochemical actions and reactions within the body are enzymatic processes, in other words, enzymes run the body, and vitamins are integral parts of these enzymatic transactions. Without the proper amounts and availability of vitamins, there is a breakdown in the processes. This breakdown is what allows diseases and other physical problems to manifest. Without vitamins, the body would come to a standstill, with death the ultimate result.

In every area of the world, we have air pollution to some degree. In many metropolitan areas, there frequently are smog or pollution alerts, ozone alerts, high particulate matter warnings, or poor air-quality days when residents are cautioned to remain indoors. There are even recorded deaths related to air pollution.

Every day, you and I breathe air that contains some type of chemical pollutant, and the same is true for the water we drink. At any given time, we are eating, drinking, or breathing minute pieces of toxic pollution, which alter the systems within the body. This creates conditions of weakness or vulnerability, compromising the integrity of certain systems and leading to many health issues.

Importance of Dietary Choices

Let us go back to the concept of unknown causes. We can begin to see that substances, food, and pollutants play a role in affecting our health, but diet plays the major role. For arthritis sufferers, the first step is to drop acid-producing foods, such as meats, fowl, seafood and dairy as well as most nuts and grains which exacerbate the condition. At the same time, the intake of fresh, organic vegetables and fruits should be increased as they increase alkalinity. However, avoid the nightshade family of vegetables and fruits such as bell peppers, eggplants and tomatoes (these are known to aggravate arthritis). Fresh foods are full of energies that are closer to promoting vitality than cooked, frozen, or canned foods; cooked foods produce a lifeless type of energy in the body because heat destroys the vitamins and enzymes that make life happen.

If you knew that certain foods were bad for you, would you continue to eat them? For most people, the answer is no, yet some people continue to eat the foods they know may be detrimental to their health. Why? The answer is in the thinking process, wherein can be found the true cause of arthritis as well as other diseases. Every action and reaction that people have begins within the mind. There is not one interaction that you can think of that is not directly related to a particular thought.

Every choice that you make, including your foods, is the result of emotional associations and desires buried deep within your subconscious mind. Advertising messages use this psychological tendency to their advantage in their commercial messages. The beef industry, for example, puts out a strong message that eating beef make males "real men," a misconception that even appeals to the masculine side of women. And the dairy industry wants you to grow up "big and strong" by drinking plenty of milk.

The truth behind some of these foods is frightening. If you realized everything that went on in their production, you would not eat them. You desire certain foods because they fulfill certain emotional needs, even when they poison your system.

Emotional needs are based on the ideas that people maintain about themselves, and they can be detrimental, even poisonous, to true self-growth. When people feel emotionally empty in some aspect, they seek to fill the void however they can, but it is often with food.

Your deepest thoughts motivate every action, including eating and drinking. Your thought processes are trying to accomplish some very specific goals. Unfortunately, not everything flows according to your desires.

Arthritis is a disease born out of conflict between the innermost self and the ego. The innermost, Spiritual Self desires to create a particular kind of life, while the ego has ideas of its own. This also sets up the ultimate cause of arthritis: inflexible thinking, an unwillingness to go beyond what has always been.

Your Spiritual Self has a connection to the infinite God; the Ego Self is a construct brought about by living. You are the result of what your parents have taught you, and on some levels, you are trying to be what they expect you to be. You have either accepted them whole-heartedly and tried to be like them, or you have chosen to go in the opposite direction. The latter happens with individuals who seek approval through rejections. (See Section I: From the Inside Out for more about rejection as a form of acceptance and love.)

In all things, it is wise to be clear about which self rules your choices.

Symbology of the Joints Afflicted by Arthritis

Arthritis is symbolic of stubbornness and inflexible, rigid thinking, and the symptoms reflect these very qualities. Individuals with arthritis have a tendency to allow people and events to eat at them, particularly when something falls outside their acceptable frame of reference—this is the beginning of inflexible thinking.

Every individual operates within a personal framework, with boundaries that stem from their upbringing as to what is acceptable. Everything that falls outside that framework is un-acceptable. If you cannot stretch your framework, over time you will become rigid. Physically, this rigidity can manifest in the joints, which are the body's flexible parts.

Arthritis attacks different joints, and each carries its own symbology. Understanding this symbology will help you to understand limitations in your thinking and areas of your inflex-ibility. At that point, you can begin to make the changes that will open up your thinking, cre-ating a different reality. As you work with these concepts and understand them, the healing process speeds up; rigid thinking and inflexibility are now mobile, open. The limitations once imposed by the ego will disappear.

The following is the symbology attached to joints commonly impacted by arthritis.

Fingers. The joints of the fingers give you a great degree of flexibility in being able to grasp and hold on firmly to material objects. From another point of view, they provide you with the ability to manipulate and control events. Arthritis in the finger joints shows a person's inability to be flexible in what they can grasp. For the meaning of each finger, see *Section II: Mysteries Revealed.*

Wrist. Arthritis restricts the ability to make circulation movements with the wrist. This translates to an inability to bend as needed to handle situations. Often, people find themselves losing their grasp on a situation because the situation turns to a direction or degree outside their realm of mobility.

When arthritis afflicts the finger joints, it is difficult or impossible to grab hold of anything. When it attacks the wrist, it is possible to grasp or hold objects only to a limited degree. The degree is equal to the amount of flexibility in the wrist, which reflects a rigidity of thought.

Toes. In all my years as a counselor, I have rarely encountered anyone with arthritis in the toes. When examining the symbolism of their function, however, you find that the toes are tied into balance and the ability to maintain a straight, erect position. The toes prevent a person from rolling forward and falling face down. Arthritis in the toes would show that the areas of thought that help maintain balance and equilibrium in life are limited in scope.

With the toes, you are also dealing with direction, because your feet are vehicles by which you move in the direction of your choice. If you begin to "point" to a certain area of your mind and move toward it, and your Ego Self says no, then you must examine and work through those limitations. As you come to see the truth, those limitations will dissolve and you will move forward.

Ankles. Like the wrists, ankles give degrees of mobility in directional thinking. The term "directional" is used because the ankles connect to the feet, which take a person the direction in which they want to go. The mind chooses the direction.

The ankles allow the necessary flexibility to accomplish the goal of getting the body where the mind wants it to go. Goals or directions do not always entail physical destinations—they can be areas of thoughts and desires. When the ankles are arthritic, the ability to move forward is hindered greatly.

Knees. By making it possible for our legs to bend, the knees help us to get where we want to go, allowing for movement and flexibility in all directions. They also represent support of your thinking.

Legs and Back. We never think about arthritis in the leg because the only place it occurs is in the knee. Your legs are a means of support and to that end, everything that happens from the hips down deals with your direction and your support of thinking.

Legs are symbolic of the support of faith in self, especially when you are standing up to life's challenges and responsibilities. Leg problems often indicate doubt in your ability to deal with a current or upcoming situation, and may be limited, symbolically, to one side of the body.

In metaphysics, the right side of the body is symbolic of spiritual thoughts and actions, representing the future as well as our self-confidence. The right side reflects the female aspect of the self. The left side, male aspect, deals with material considerations, reflecting your past and how you draw upon it in dealing with the present.

Back concepts are also built upon self-confidence in accomplishing goals. When there are back problems, it is usually in connection with support of either material or spiritual issues, or both.

With regard to flexibility in both the legs and back, we are talking about flexibility in terms of how you get to your destination. It is a cold reality that life's destinations are not always sitting at the end of a straight and easy path. Our goals and journeys often take us down narrow, rocky paths fraught with bends and hairpin turns; therefore, keep your thinking flexible, and you will remain in a position of control as you adapt to change. With flexibility of thought comes flexibility in physical mobility.

Hips. Here we have another set of joints tied into direction and support, yet in a more complex sense. Like the wrists and ankles, the hips allow for degrees of mobility in many directions, and they are also a part of the support system.

Often the ability to support the self in life requires the need to make quick changes in direction and means of sustenance—sustenance in this case means not only food, but can also mean income or expression. Through personal expression, people move forward in their lives; for some, it is the means to earning their living.

Neck and Vertebrae. The neck connects your head, the dwelling place of your mind, and to your body; therefore, it is a symbol of balance between two aspects of the self, material and spiritual. These terms are used because the body processes all the material substances that enter it, while the head/mind processes the spiritual considerations, such as setting goals, thinking and providing direction.

If you are dealing with arthritis in the neck, look to any areas of imbalance in your life: Do you lean more toward the material or the spiritual? Is your thinking too rigid?

The vertebrae in your neck are also part of the spine—the back. As you explore your concepts, review how you support yourself and meet your responsibilities. What are your values and guidelines for living in a turbulent world?

Remember that even the mightiest oak bends in the storm to avoid breaking, so, too, must the mind and body.

Shoulders. The shoulders afford the mobility you need for directional grip, allowing you to maneuver your arms to hold objects or situations at different levels. If you have arthritis in your shoulders and cannot reach up, hold down, or maintain control over the different levels of situations in your life, what does that say?

Your shoulders give flexibility in many different areas, even allowing us to swing our arms around to scratch our own back. This tells you that flexibility at that level of thinking can accomplish a great deal. If you lose that flexibility, your life becomes very limited because you believe yourself limited in what you can handle.

When arthritis attacks the shoulder, reflect on what it is you feel you cannot "carry off" well or what it is you are unwilling to "pick up" and allow into your life. To what degree can you be flexible about what you handle in life?

Elbows. How flexible are your elbows? Will they bend up and close to cross over your chest, like a protective shield? Or are they rigid, making your arms into long, stiff rods that push people away, keeping them at arm's length?

If you suffer from arthritic elbows, reflect on what would make you believe that you need to defend yourself or push people and situations away from you. Examine your boundaries, your frame of reference. What situations are you willing to be drawn into? Why do you reject others? Look carefully at your willingness to give and receive.

SYMBOLOGY OF THE NUTRIENTS AND VARIOUS HERBS

Calcium. Another aspect of arthritis symbolically involves calcium deposits in the joints, when calcium, which is symbolic of strength, is not assimilated. On a symbolic level, calcium represents strength because it helps build bone, and, therefore, helps build strength and flexibility.

If calcium is not assimilated into the tissues and cells where it is needed, it is a clear sign that the person does not believe they have the strength to deal with certain situations, when in truth, they can do and handle anything. If the belief is that they do not have the strength to flow with situations, then calcium begins to gather in the area of weakness, in this case, gathering in the joints. It concerns flexibility of thinking, adapting and changing.

A Universal Teaching from Matthew 25:29 dealing with strength: "For unto every one that hath shall be given, and he shall have abundance: but from him that hath not shall be taken away even that which he hath." Translated to modern day English, this means that if you use what you have, more will be given. That which you do not use, will be taken from you. The lesson is clear—if you have a faculty or a way of thinking and you choose not to use it, you will no longer have access to it, and at that point, it can and will begin to work against you.

Magnesium. A facilitator, it assists in the assimilation of thoughts that lead to strength. From a position of strength, all actions taken lead to a positive conclusion. When you act out of fear, doubt, a lack of self-confidence, or uncertainty the seeds for failure are sown.

Niacin/Niacinamide. Represents openness and receptivity. The receptivity associated with niacinamide denotes its relationship to growth, nerve function, metabolism, and the circulatory system.

Blood is the lifeline of the body, representing spirit within the material realm. It carries nutrients to each cell, feeds, cleanses, and carries away the toxins that will destroy the body if left to collect. Toxins, like poisonous thoughts that are left within the mind to operate freely, will ultimately kill. All toxins, of both the thought and physical realms, must be eliminated from the system if there is to be true growth.

Pantothenic Acid. On one level, represents inspiration. I use this definition because pantothenic acid nourishes the adrenal glands, which produce hormones that help the body deal with making quick actions based upon quick decisions. This is reflected in the "flight or fight" concept.

When you face a vast force or feel overwhelmed, you may go into a state of fear, in keeping with your degree of self-confidence. The part of the body that reacts to the impulse of fear translated into electrical energy, is the adrenals, which send out hormonal messengers to signal other body parts on how to respond. When the adrenals are exhausted, the person lacks enthusiasm, inspiration, and confidence.

Pantothenic acid represents inspiration, courage, and confidence. This is because of its role not only in growth and energy, but also for its support of skin health. The skin is a protective shield, literally and symbolically, protecting the inner workings of the body and protecting the self from attack. This is another reason why some people are obese as they fill their skin with additional padding to protect them from the harshness of other people.

Potassium. Represents proper balance and harmony, the keys to flexible thinking. When there is balance within, it allows you to bend in many areas or directions, without fear of loss of balance or falling.

Another aspect of balance is seen in the fact that persons with arthritis tend to have high levels of acid in their blood. When the physical manifestation of thoughts becomes acidic, it eats up all possibilities for movement in any direction.

Remember that an overly acidic internal body is a factor in arthritis and its complications. By its very definition, acid is a substance that eats away at other materials. When the body becomes predominately acidic, the internal state is highly conducive to illness. It is significant, symbolically and physically, that meats, fish, and fowl are among the biggest dietary sources of acidic conditions within the blood. Meat remains a top American food favorite.

Vitamin B-6. Represents balance due to its many roles in balancing systems within the body. Balanced thinking is crucial with regard to gaining strength. Without strength, you may believe yourself helpless in dealing with the forces or energies of life. The truth of this perception is seen in the way a lack of B-6 leads to muscle weakness.

Vitamin B-6 functions to balance the water levels within the cells. Balance is something arthritis sufferers need in order to make flexible decisions. It is the imbalance in thinking that creates the rigidity.

Vitamin D. Its role in calcium assimilation tells us that vitamin D represents insight, and to a degree, understanding. This interpretation relates to the fact that calcium represents strength, helping to build the bones of the body that provide support. Without insight and understanding it would be virtually impossible to achieve true strength. To be manufactured by the body, vitamin D requires sunlight, which is symbolic of insight and clear vision. Nothing is hidden in the light if you have the eyes to see.

Arthritics need to see the truth from a Universal perspective. This is closer to the truth of God's laws than the teachings of man. As human beings, most live according to the teachings of man, while at the same time, we are supposed to follow the ways of God. If you look with clear vision, you will see that as a civilization, we have strayed far from the Universal Teachings of how to live and love one another. From a religious perspective, there is no justification for the wrongs that proliferate in today's world. Religion is supposedly teaching us to love one another; the truth of the matter is that we are killing one another.

Alfalfa. What an interesting specimen to examine! First, its roots grow to a depth of thirty feet, significant because of the numeral 3, which represents understanding; 1 equals unity and

2 equals balance. When unity and balance are represented in any situation, there will always be an understanding; obviously, the opposite is also true. For our purposes, we shall stick to the positive aspects of these symbols.

With alfalfa we can see that deep understanding will provide food for thought and promote growth. Growth is the result of flexibility in one's ability to think, accept, and expand. Alfalfa represents nourishing thoughts that lead to flexible thinking.

Yucca. It works on removing waste material. Wastes generated by the body are equal to thoughts that are no longer viable in the sense that the individual has outgrown them, or they were never functional to begin with.

Native Americans have used roots as a poultice to reduce inflammation for hundreds of years.

The yucca plant grows in dry, sandy soil. Symbolically, it is interesting to know that even an arid environment can sustain life. If you live in a place of dry and lifeless thoughts, this is no excuse for being unable to grow—life always seeks to manifest. By reducing the wasteful and inflamed thoughts of confinement and restriction, you will have greater versatility and mobility.

Asthma

See Conditions That Restrict Breathing: Congestion, Asthma, and Emphysema.

Backaches

Several factors contribute to backaches, for example, stress, strain, and injury. When there is stress, whether it is emotional or physical, it is going to create a nutritional demand upon the body. In most instances, the body is already at maximum output based on dietary intake. This often causes an imbalance, and muscle fatigue or cramping can be the result.

Another set of causes can be strictly nutritional. In this case, it is a matter of inadequate amounts of minerals and B-complex vitamins, both of which are essential because of their roles in electrical message conduction.

NUTRIENTS FOR BACKACHES

Here are the nutrients that ease backaches and help the muscles return to balance and harmony.

Nutrients
B-complex Vitamins
Calcium
Magnesium
Potassium

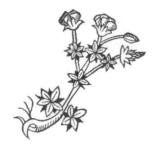

B-complex Vitamins. Essential for proper nerve function and communication; they participate in the communication necessary for the muscles to relax as well as to contract.

Calcium, Magnesium, and Potassium. Minerals that help the electricity of communication flow between the nerve endings and the receptor sites on the cells. This allows the cells to get the message of how to perform, facilitating all of the cells to work in harmony, in this case to relax the back muscles.

The real issue is the communication that takes place between the nerve endings and the receptor sites on the cells that make up muscle, and that requires calcium and magnesium for the transmission of the electrical current of impulses.

SYMBOLOGY OF BACKACHES

In general, backaches and back problems usually deal with support issues. It is advisable to look at finances first. Through this expression of manhood, we deal with support. This refers to those acts, attitudes, and emotions—often in a material sense—that make us who we are. Manhood, therefore, applies to males and females.

If you are plagued by backaches, reflect on what is happening in your life to make you believe you cannot support yourself. Why do you feel weak? What burdens or threatens you, particularly with regard to your income and finances?

SYMBOLOGY OF THE NUTRIENTS

B-complex Vitamins. This family of nutrients represents courage and confidence. It is easy to see how they would eliminate backaches and all muscular discomfort. Remember backaches symbolize doubt in your ability to support the self in current matters. When a person has courage and confidence, doubt and fear cannot operate.

Calcium, Magnesium. The calcium represents strength while magnesium represents inspiration. Backaches denote doubt about support, again, generally of a financial nature. There is a question in the individual's mind about being able to support him or herself in this particular cycle or endeavor.

By taking in the necessary nutrients, the body's chemistry will change, and so will the energy. This, in turn, sparks other subtle changes that can help the person become inspired. Subconsciously, the individual will recognize that he or she has the strength to confront whatever it is they must.

Once a person comes to that understanding, bolstered by positive affirmations and physical supplementation, confidence levels should return, allowing the backache to subside.

Potassium. Symbolically represents balance and harmony. Backaches may be the result of an imbalance among three minerals: calcium, magnesium and potassium, which is one of the reasons why all three are necessary. Keep in mind that calcium represents strength and magnesium represents inspiration. You can see how having the trio together is not only conducive to electrical flow, energetic flow, but it is also conducive to a relaxed approach to every given situation because you know you are coming from a position of strength and you are in balance and harmony.

Blood Toxicity

Blood is the life stream of the body, affecting every cell and system. The bloodstream is a conglomeration of different elements, each working in a specific way to keep us alive.

The blood system is composed of plasma, a sticky substance made up of 95 percent water and 5 percent nutrients, proteins, hormones, and waste products, among other components. The cleansing process of the blood is carried out by the body's detoxification system. Without such a system, the body would become toxic and unable to support itself.

Three main examples of the body's detoxification systems are the respiratory, defacatory, and urinary systems. The respiratory system expels wastes in the form of carbon dioxide, which is exhaled from the lungs. Solid organic wastes and dead blood cells are expunged by the defecatory system, and the remaining waste products, transported by plasma, are expelled by the urinary system.

The main waste product in plasma is urea, a mixture of old blood cells and metabolic waste, which is transported to the kidneys to be eliminated. The kidneys receive their blood supply directly from the aorta through the renal arteries, which branch off many times in the kidneys, forming small capillary tufts called glomeruli. There are over one million glomeruli in the kidneys, combining as the filtering system for cleaning the blood.

Blood cells and big molecules are kept within the glomeruli, while small molecules and water pass through their walls. Over 140 liters of fluid pass out of the glomeruli each day, back through the renal tubules, where 99 percent of it is reabsorbed back into the blood. At the end of the tubules, the waste products, excess salt, and some of the water remain unabsorbed. These form urine that drains down the ureters and into the bladder.

Both old blood cells and waste products in the body are toxic—so, it is essential that the detoxification systems work properly. As old blood cells die or are destroyed by the various processes in the body, they must be removed. If the dead cells and other organic waste are not removed from the bloodstream, they will create a homeostatic imbalance in the body with the potential to negatively impact health.

Nutrients and Herbs to Support Blood Detoxification

For the complex operation of the body, the blood requires a constant source of nutrients. Nutrients are essential for the feeding of cells that comprise tissues and the sustaining of their intricate functions as they constantly reproduce new cells. Each cell requires nutrients for their formation and specific function, and when each cell within the body functions properly, homeostasis is achieved.

The following will support your body in the elimination of toxins:

Nutrients	Herbs
Iron	Burdock Root
Manganese	Echinacea
Molybdenum	Gotu Kola
Zinc	Red Clover
	Yellow Dock

Iron. Essential to transportation of oxygen in the body; permits cellular respiration to occur.

Manganese. Necessary for the synthesis of glutathione synthetase, an enzyme needed for the body to make the detox conjugator glutathione from glycine. Glutathione functions in the destruction of peroxides and free radicals and in the detoxification of harmful compounds.

Molybdenum. An essential trace-mineral that functions as an enzyme co-factor. Certain molybdenum metalloenzymes detoxify various compounds that play a role in uric acid metabolism and sulfate toxicity.

Zinc. A constituent of at least 25 enzymes involved in tissue respiration, digestion, and metabolism, including the one needed to breakdown alcohol.

Burdock Root. An all-around blood purifier, strongly diuretic and diaphoretic. It assists in cleansing the body of toxins; markedly enhances liver and gall/bile functions.

Echinacea. Significantly stimulates the body's own blood-cleaning system. It destroys the germs of infection directly and bolsters the body's defenses by magnifying the white blood cell count. Echinacin, the active constituent of echinacea, has an interferon-like action, protecting cells against virus-related diseases, such as herpes, influenza, canker sores, etc. This herb is also good for lymphatic cleansing.

Gotu Kola. A blood purifier, glandular tonic, and diuretic as well as an oxygen carrier.

Red Clover. An herb that acts as a wonderful blood detoxifier/purifier.

Yellow Dock. Primarily affects liver function and the health of related organs, increasing their ability to strain and purify the blood. In addition, the herb has antibacterial properties. It also possesses a high iron and high thiamine content.

SYMBOLOGY OF BLOOD CLEANSING

Everything in the body lives to preserve and serve the brain. The mind/brain interface runs the body, and the brain is fed through the bloodstream, even though blood does not come in contact with it. The nutrients, especially oxygen (spirit), pass through the blood-brain barrier, which protects the brain from poisonous toxins that may be present in the bloodstream.

As the transport system of the body, the blood distributes nutrients, symbolic of thought energies, and carries these energies to all the parts of the body. When there are toxins in the bloodstream that have not been detoxified or filtered out through biological channels, they sometimes become part of biological transactions.

This changes the biochemistry of certain cells, and over time, of the whole body. Disease originates here, through this cellular fusion with unnatural chemicals. The bloodstream provides a medium for this process.

The process holds true for the mind, which must constantly detoxify or nullify negative, nonproductive thoughts. Your positive thoughts (food) and those directed toward you, can nourish, cleanse, or heal you, if you allow it, while negative thoughts can defeat, corrupt, poison, and ultimately destroy.

Blood is symbolic of the spiritual life that exists within all living things. That is why the *Bible*, in Deuteronomy 12:16, tells us to remove the blood before eating any animal, "only ye shall not eat the blood."

Toxins are symbolic of man-made concepts and thoughts that are not in keeping with Universal Teachings. Such thoughts lead to disharmony and imbalances, resulting ultimately in disease.

Blood detoxification is symbolic of the natural process of shedding the old and bringing in the new and nourishing. Through the process of detoxifying and eliminating man-made concepts, the spirit within grows.

Symbology of the Nutrients

Iron. Represents emotional control. If the emotions get out of control because of a lack of faith (anemia), all kinds of repercussions can occur, including a lack of energy. On the other hand, if the emotions are controlled beyond a balanced perspective, then they create feelings of anger. This is one of the causative factors in the development of cancer. A physical manifestation is when men retain too much iron and get colon cancer.

When emotions are low and imbalanced, the individual is exposed to outside forces (negative suggestions, thoughts, put-downs) that could lead to illness. This is demonstrated by the role iron plays in support of the immune system.

Low iron results in a decreased amount of oxygen available to the cells, translating into lack of faith and inspiration—in other words, energy. It takes oxygen to make fire (also symbolic of emotions). Fire, or combustion, symbolic of rapid oxidation, is essential for all living transactions in the sense that oxygen is necessary for life. Spirit is involved in everything that we do, and emotions give us the "juice" to utilize the spirit within.

Manganese. Represents will, in combination with iodine's intent. These are the two fundamental aspects of self that are required to master the material plane.

If you are clear about your intent and can visualize it as reality, then your will makes it happen. We already operate under the influence of will and intent on a subconscious level;

this is how we create our reality. By gaining control over will and intent, you will manifest your vision, your ideal situation at the time.

Zinc. As a symbol of a working faith, you can see the role that it would play in the detoxification process. It takes courage and confidence to give up past ideas that no longer support the person in the true sense of expression.

Cancer

Besides AIDS, cancer is one of the most devastating diseases plaguing mankind today, claiming millions of lives each year. The most frightening thing is that the numbers are growing, and cancer is getting progressively worse. In some medical reports cancer is now the number one cause of death for people under the age of 85.

Medical science tells us that researchers have absolutely no idea what causes this disease. From a physiological perspective, it can be seen that cancer is mutated or uncontrolled cellular growth. So, the medical community does know what causes cancer but is reluctant to admit it. This reluctance is based on economic and political considerations.

The doctors who say that cancer can be cured through dietary changes and increased nutritional supplementation are drummed out of the medical community. To cure cancer or to admit its cause would create financial havoc in the world economy because we would not be able to change quickly enough to a non-cancer-causing system of economics. Everything we are currently doing would become invalid. Therefore, the truth of the situation is played down, rebutted, and ignored, and the people who bring up the truth are generally disgraced or eliminated.

The truth is easy to see when you examine the facts of cancer. There really is no mystery. Cancer is a general term for forms of new tissues that have no controlled growth patterns. These tissues, at a cellular level, are due to a growth of mutated cells. Mutated cells are generated within the body when certain cells are affected by mutagens. Mutagens are any chemical or physical agents that cause a gene change (mutation) or speed up the rate of mutation.

Chemicals are identified as a major source of mutagens. What are all of the sources of these chemicals? Unfortunately, chemicals are everywhere—in our food, the water we drink, the air we breathe and the substances we rub on our skin. It is virtually impossible to eliminate them from our world at this stage. In fact, the amount of chemicals in use is so staggering that we may have created a cancerous situation for the earth as well, which—if we do not correct our ways quickly—will kill the planet. Earth is a living entity, too, and can only take so much abuse and neglect.

In addition to polluting the planet, we have disrupted its own natural feeding and replenishing cycle. We have depleted the soil of nutrients and contaminated it, so that it no longer supports life in the same abundance it once did. The vegetables, grains, and fruit produced using these soils are nutritionally depleted, as are the animals that graze on the grass growing in it. All living things that require the soils as a source of nutrients are undernourished because the soil is sick, and so are we.

Why doesn't the government regulate the harmful chemicals and ban them from human consumption? As for government involvement, or the lack thereof, could it be that commerce in the pursuit of profits and dollars is more important than the conservation of life—the planet's and ours?

Cancer Is...

In essence, cancer is a disease born out of a man-made chemical occurrence at a cellular level. The chemicals enter the body through the food chain as well as the air we breathe and the drinks we consume. In an internal atmosphere, a chemical "fire" is ignited. As it burns and smolders, the "smoke" or cells of it spread, and as it spreads it consumes or infects everything in its path. Eventually, if left unchecked, the "fire" will destroy the body.

Cancer does not require oxygen to thrive and grow, an illness of this type is called an anaerobic infection. The opposite of an aerobic organism or process that thrives only in oxygen, an anaerobe is a microorganism that can live without oxygen.

In seeking to understand the symbolic implications of cancer, just as we did with arthritis, we need to go back to definitions of cancer contained in medical textbooks and references, such as The Merck Manual, where we get the perception that the cause of cancer is "unknown." When something is unknown in life, it is usually because it is not understood. With that concept in mind, new questions arise: From what frame of reference have we historically looked at this condition? What guidelines and points of reference did we use? Did we ask all the right questions?

Let us look at how a disease grows within the body. What causes a healthy body to move to a state of ill health? The answer is simple, it is a result of something the person brings into the body. There are four primary avenues of introduction: food, water, air, and light.

The abundance or lack of each of these elements leaves its own distinctive mark on health. For example, the fluorescent lighting to which most of us are exposed daily during our working lives has cumulative, detrimental effects. Over time, the skin becomes yellow and heavily creased.

When natural sunlight is concerned, there are two distinct outcomes. Some people have health problems because they don't get enough natural sunlight, on the other hand, we are told that too much exposure to the sun increases skin cancers. Maybe it is not the sun at all, but the pollution in the air and food. Maybe the pollutants in these substances, once in our bodies, are reacting with the sunlight and creating a chemical reaction we call cancer. (For more insights regarding sunlight, see also Arthritis.)

Other vitamins differ in that they become parts of enzymes and are, therefore, considered co-enzymes within the body. Without vitamins, the body would come to a standstill, with death the ultimate result.

Every day, you and I breathe air and drink water that contains some type of chemical pollutant. At any given time, we are eating, drinking, or breathing minute pieces of toxic pollution that alter the systems within the body, and create conditions that cause weakness or vulnerability, compromising the integrity of certain systems and leading to many health problems, including cancer.

By the time an individual is seventy years old, he or she may have had a form of cancer up to six times. One difference between those who manifest it and those who do not is the immune system, your body's first line of defense.

If you understand symbology, you are constantly aware and in prime defensive mode. Even though there is not a defensive attitude, you know that you need to be in control. You know everything you are dealing with and can make the proper decisions, because you see it clearly and deal with it from a position of strength. This leaves no room for failure, which can lead to feelings of guilt, resentment, or possibly even blame, and this continual barrage of strong emotions contributes to the development of cancer.

Warning signs for cancer may be a change in bowel or bladder habits, a non-healing sore, unusual bleeding or discharge, a thickening or lump in the breast or elsewhere, indigestion or difficulty in swallowing, an obvious change in a wart or mole, a nagging cough or continuing hoarseness.

THE FIRST STEP

The first step in physically dealing with cancer is to modify your diet. Look at the foods that you eat on a daily basis, and if yours is the typical American diet, the need for dietary change is obvious. Begin immediately to increase your regular intake of fresh, organically grown raw vegetables and fruits.

Fresh foods are full of energies that are closer to promoting vitality than cooked, frozen, or canned foods. Organic farming methods also mean that fewer chemicals will ultimately be introduced into the body. Cooked foods, on the other hand, produce a lifeless type of energy in the body. Heat destroys the vitamins and enzymes within foods that make life happen within the body.

Let us go back to the concept of "unknown" causes again. We can begin to see that the substances, foods, and pollutants that enter the body play a role in affecting our health; our diet plays the major role.

If you knew that certain foods were bad for you, would you continue to eat them? For most people, the answer would be an immediate and resounding no. But some people will continue to eat the foods they know may be detrimental to their health. Why?

The answer is in the human thinking process, wherein can be found the true cause of cancer as well as other diseases. Every action and reaction that you have begins within your mind and there is not one interaction that you can think of that is not directly related to a particular thought.

Every choice that you make, including your food selection, is the result of emotional associations and desires buried deep within your subconscious mind. Advertising messages use this psychological tendency to their advantage in crafting their commercial messages.

NEW THEORIES

In some medical circles, cancer is being examined as a viral disease that has been able to flourish because the body has lowered defenses. This is brought on by an improperly functioning immune system and stress. As research continues to focus on this aspect of the disease, it is becoming very clear that stress is a major factor in lowering the body's immune system.

Stress taxes the adrenal glands, which secrete hormones that carry messages to the other glands on how to perform or what to manufacture. When the adrenal glands are stressed and begin to falter, the immune system also falters. All the body's glands are tied together in a complex system, and each and every aspect of life within the body is interdependent. This is why it is so important to maintain a proper nutritional balance. In this way, you are providing the system with the ingredients it requires to function properly in a state of optimum health, thus, eliminating opportunities for disease to take hold.

NUTRIENTS, AMINO ACIDS AND HERBS TO SUPPORT THE IMMUNE SYSTEM

In regard to the nutrients for cancer, suffice it to say that every nutrient is absolutely essential in battling cancer. There are some that are especially important, such as selenium, astragalus and the Chinese mushrooms: reishi, shiitake, maitake, and cordyceps, all of these are wonderful for strengthening the immune system, and that is one of the things you must do with cancer.

The best nutritional approach to prevent or combat cancer is a comprehensive daily, foundational program that includes all nutrients available today. To strengthen immune response and increase adrenal stamina, include the following nutrients, amino acids and herbs:

Nutrients	Amino Acids	Herbs
Beta-carotene (Vitamin A)	L-Cysteine	Astragulas
Folic Acid		Codonopis
Magnesium		Echinacea
Pantothenic Acid		Ligustrum
Vitamin B-6		Reishi Mushroom
Vitamin C		
Zinc		

Beta-carotene (Vitamin A) and Vitamin C. These should always be included in any formula designed to fight disease/infections.

Nothing is more stimulating and nourishing for the thymus gland than vitamin A, which affects cell-mediated immunity.

Vitamin A and beta-carotene have been found to protect against cancer in humans.[7] Higher intakes of beta-carotene[8] and vitamin A[9] are associated with a lower risk of cancer, and beta-carotene has been found to have specific anti-tumor activity in animal studies.[10] Synthetic forms of vitamin A have been used to correct pre-cancerous conditions[11] and to treat cancer itself.[12]

Vitamin C, or ascorbic acid, has its own history when it comes to fighting disease and infections. It has prophylactic and therapeutic effects in pathologic conditions. Studies indicate vitamin C modulates cyclic nucleotide levels in B-cells and T-cells, a process that may mediate immune reactions.[13]

Pantothenic Acid. Nourishes the adrenal glands, which in a weakened state can allow the immune system to become lowered. It is also involved in energy production.

Vitamin B-6. Vital because of the role it plays in antibody and red blood cell production. The presence of vitamin B-6 also increases the number of T-cells. T-cells are phagocytes, white blood cells that are matured by the thymus gland.

Zinc. Plays an important role in nourishing the thymus gland as well as liberating vitamin A from the liver. Zinc deficiency impairs phagocyte function, cellular immunity, humeral immunity, and their inter-communication.[14,15]

L-Cysteine. An amino acid active in the production of antibodies.

Echinacea. A very powerful immune booster that stimulates interferon production and helps to cleanse the lymphatic system thoroughly. Echinacea normalizes the white blood cell count and stimulates intracellular processes that destroy pathogens such as viruses and bacteria.[16]

SYMBOLOGY OF CANCER

By its very nature and impact on the human body, cancer is a disease of great symbolic implications. It implies that man is consumed by a multitude of thoughts on many levels that are inherently unbalanced and consuming in their nature.

Like all diseases, cancer can play a major role in our lives as it helps us to understand what we as a civilization, and as individuals, are involved in at any given time.

Each moment of our lives is flowing into the next, and it is through this process that all change takes place. How things will change depends solely upon you, and only you are in control of your own destiny and health.

All diseases have had their "day in the sun." They have gone through the cycle of rising to prominence and then falling into remission or "cure." This is easily seen in such diseases as polio, typhoid fever, tuberculosis, and leprosy—even though some of these diseases are making a comeback. In truth, the appearance of a particular bacterial/virus strain or a disease can only be reflective, symbolically, of a level of thinking that is predominant at that particular point in time.

When cancer occurs, it typically starts in one area of the body and then spreads. The site of origin is symbolic of the prevailing thoughts of the time, which can be personal, global, or environmental. Even the moods of the country and its political climate have symbolic significance.

In today's ever-changing world, when countries receive new names and geographical boundaries, their significance changes as well. The dissolution of the former Soviet Union is a prime example. While it once reflected aggression, confinement, and loss of freedom, it is now beginning to carry new symbolic significance, as will each of the new republics formed after the fall. Time will determine the meaning of each, although each entity's pre-Soviet history will likely again be part of the present for some.

Symbolically, the United States stands for liberty, justice, independence, strength, and unity. The U.S. is a land of opportunity and freedom. The same thing should be said of the human body because it is a reflection of the mind, which is also a thing of freedom and independence, and within it there should be no rebellion, although sometimes there is. Some people live daily with the energies of disharmony, dissatisfaction, and anger, to name a few.

CAUSES OF CANCER

There are four energies that can manifest physically as cancer: anger, resentment, frustration, and guilt. Each of them influences thoughts, feelings, actions, and reactions within the mind. The real significance of these energies and cancer is how those particular concepts operate in your life.

All of the different energies that make up life operate in specific areas of your personal life and expression. For instance, the energy of enthusiasm, which may be a prominent energy for you, operates in one area of your life, such as in your work, while the energy of despair operates in another, maybe in relationships or finances. There are multiple energies at work all the time in every area and on every level of each person's life.

Learning to identify the energies that influence you begins to give you a degree of control over them. From that position you can begin to effect change that will lead to balance and harmony. This will manifest in every area of your life in the course of time, and this change will be relevant to the depth of your understanding and the degree of control you exercise.

How can you identify those aspects and energies that you need to change? Let us examine the different types of cancers and where they affect the body. More than one form may be at work in a cancerous condition; to better understand the true significance of the concepts involved, examine the body part affected.

Recall that medical science defines cancer as a tumor or various forms of new tissue cells that lack a controlled growth pattern. Cancer cells are mutated cells with uncontrolled growth that usually invade and destroy normal tissue cells. A cancer tends to spread to other parts of the body by releasing cells into the lymph system or bloodstream. In this way, cancer cells can be carried to a place in the body that may be far from the first site or tumor.

The first site of cancer is sometimes called a primary cancer, and the tumor that grows as a result of the cancer spreading is called a secondary cancer. A secondary cancer is often detected before the primary cancer can be found.

Cancer has many different causes, including viruses, too much exposure to the sunlight or X-rays, smoking, and chemicals in the environment. Cancer is also a broad term describing any of a large group of diseases in which malignant cells are present anywhere in the body. The most common sites for the growth of cancerous tumors are the lung, breast, colon, uterus, mouth, and bone marrow. Many cancerous tumors or lesions are curable if found in their early stages.

Strong Emotions. Looking at cancer as a tumor or forms of new tissue cells that lack a controlled growth pattern makes you wonder what that means symbolically. Stop and think about anger, guilt, resentment, and frustration. If an individual allows those thoughts to permeate in the mind, they will influence thought patterns. When you have no control over your emotions and thought processes, these aberrant thought patterns have an uncontrolled growth pattern. They will begin to infiltrate every area of your life, affecting or corrupting your perception, and alter the way you look at things, ultimately impacting your evaluations, interpretations, actions, and reactions to people and the things they say and do.

Once you look at things from a shaded perspective, you begin to react differently. Emotionally, you may begin to lose control and draw upon malignant thought patterns that can take you so far out of control that there is no telling how they will influence your actions, nor is there any way to determine how they will manifest within your body.

Normally, when we think about lack of control, we think of ending up in anger-producing situations, which often involve an element of retaliation; if you attack or offend others, they, in turn, will ultimately attack and offend you. On the other hand, if you internalize your anger, it will attack and consume you, and you may end up with a cancerous situation.

Another characteristic of cancer cells is that they usually invade and destroy normal tissue cells. The symbolic parallel is seen when you begin to lose control over your thoughts and your thinking process. You begin to scan around, and you mentally start looking for all the reasons that justify the anger, resentment, or guilt to manifest in your life.

In the areas where there is harmony, you look to find disharmony; in areas where there is acceptance, you look for the rejection; and where there is completion and success, you look to find incompletion and failure. In everything you do, you allow your uncontrolled thoughts to infiltrate everything that is already well-established.

By definition, a cancer also tends to spread to other parts of the body, either through the lymph system or the bloodstream. Consider the symbology of the lymphatic system, a system designed for cleansing. The body has an ongoing cleansing process designed to keep it free of accumulated toxins, too many of which will sicken and possibly kill you. Toxins will interfere with the normal function of cells and systems, infecting, polluting, corrupting, and even destroying your body. Ergo, that which we do not cleanse from our system kills us, be it physical toxins from the physical body or toxic, man-made thoughts from the spiritual one.

The material body is a direct reflection of our deepest inner-thoughts, as shown in the Universal Teaching that "whatever is within us will manifest without." Put another way, you become what you eat and think. Using this framework, it is not too difficult to see cancer as a direct result of toxic thinking.

Continuing with our definition of cancer, let us consider how the disease spreads through the bloodstream, which nourishes every part of the body. Thus, it is easy to understand how cancer cells could spread everywhere. The symbology of the bloodstream is in the blood cells, which carry oxygen throughout the body and are one of many symbols of spirit. You will recall that oxygen (air) is symbolic of spirit because it is where God dwells (heaven).

While the first site of cancer is called the primary cancer, the tumors that grow are usually at a secondary cancer site that is often detected before the primary cancer can be found. So, what you may be seeing in your life when you are reacting to something is only the superficial side of it or that which is most apparent, much like the secondary cancer site. What you may not be seeing is the root cause of the anger, resentment, or frustration that is stimulating your reaction. You are not finding the primary concept, the primary source of antagonism or aggravation.

The basic concept that makes you believe you are guilty, unworthy, inadequate, etc., is the primary cause of the disharmony. In all diseases there is a primary cause that sets the stage for disharmony and disease.

To bring about a cure or to arrest a condition and stop it dead in its tracts from spreading, you must understand what supports, nourishes, and promotes it. All of those things that contribute to its uncontrolled growth and rage must be identified, dealt with, and—most certainly—controlled.

Viruses. Of all the different causes of cancer, viruses are the most interesting. A virus is a lifeform that comes into our system and affects the body. From another point of view, life-forms are symbolic of thoughts, and just as chemicals are symbolic of thoughts, viruses symbolize a specific kind of thought.

A virus is a thought that is presented to you from an outside source, a thought that has power and a life of its own. If you allow someone else's thoughts to dominate your life, then it is easy to see where anger and frustration are born. It is also easy to see where the guilt begins, when you do not follow what you are told. Listen to the words of people and how they communicate with each other, especially in a family setting, and how guilt is used as a tool to control and dominate.

Anger and frustration also result from constantly being put down and humiliated: "He is not bright enough." "She is not pretty enough." These negatives can produce incredible resentment. Is it any wonder we grow sick based on the things that we hear and on the viral thoughts implanted into our belief systems?

Overexposure to Sunlight. Another suggested cause of cancer is over exposure to sunlight, X-rays, or microwaves. While it has been proven cancer results from X-rays, or radiation, I do not personally subscribe to the belief that sunlight causes cancer. I believe that is more of a man-made construct and a way of keeping people in ill health because sunlight is essential to the manufacturing of vitamin D. Keep in mind moderation in all things.

Vitamin D is a fat-soluble vitamin, meaning that excess amounts of it can be stored in the body's fat tissue. It is known as the "sunshine" vitamin because the action of the sun's ultraviolet rays converts a form of cholesterol present in the skin into vitamin D, which aids the body in assimilating calcium. This is important symbolically because calcium is symbolic of strength.

Let us look at all of the other functions of vitamin D. It aids in the absorption of calcium from the intestinal tract and also helps with the breakdown and assimilation of phosphorus, which is required for bone formation. Vitamin D helps synthesize those enzymes in the mucous membranes that are involved in the active transport of available calcium. It is particularly important for the normal growth of children and also helps the body maintain a stable nervous system, normal heart action and normal blood clotting—functions related to the body's supply and use of calcium and phosphorus. Vitamin D is most effective when used in conjunction with vitamin A.

Tobacco Use. Smoking is a very specific act that causes cancer. It poses a threat for both smokers and non-smokers, alike.

The smoker is trying to fulfill two driving forces: the need to present a particular image and the need for nicotine. Each brand of cigarette paints a different picture designed to appeal to a different aspect of ego or personality type, for example, the Marlboro man is portrayed as rough, rugged, and manly. Other brands may stir feelings from a different aspect of personality, for example, Virginia Slims portrays those who smoke their cigarettes as sleek and elegant.

Marketers know that most people are insecure and lacking in self-acceptance to some degree. To capitalize on these emotions, marketing messages present many pictures that demonstrate how to be happy, fulfilled, and successful.

Advertisers play upon people's weaknesses and perceived needs, which in truth do not exist. People are whole and complete because they are part of the Creative Force that is God. Nonetheless, we don't believe that, we don't accept that, and, therefore, we have this emptiness within that we try to fill with external things: gold, money, cars, sex, drugs, wine, whiskey, or cigarettes.

It is our own frustrations in life that drive us to any one of the "pleasures" that we seek to make us feel whole and complete. Smoking is one of them. It paints a picture that we want to be a part of because we want to be happy. Many people are angry, however, and frustrated that they are not happy, content, or successful, so they become open to the energies that produce cancers in the body on different levels.

There is a Universal Teaching that says: "Excess leads to rejection." This does not imply that you can smoke tobacco in moderation without causing harm. Smoking has been shown to be detrimental to the lungs. This means that the more you attempt to attain something by a certain means but do not reach the goal, the more you will continue to do it. The more you do it, the more imbalances you create. How often have you heard someone talk about how they loved a particular food as a child but can't stand it now?

Chemicals. Chemicals are believed to be a major contributing factor to cancer. Just look at the chemicals in the environment! The environment is comprised essentially of three things: water, air, and land. These substances represent three different elemental states of matter.

THE BREATH OF LIFE

Let us begin with air. To survive, we need to breathe air—oxygen. Without air, we are physically dead. Air is symbolic of spirit, the heaven in which God dwells, and without spirit, we are also dead from the inside…empty shells. What is the symbolic significance of the fact that our air is loaded with chemical toxins?

We will start by defining chemicals. Chemical in the sense that we use the term means a substance made by man. These substances are either ingredients in manufactured products or they are by-products of the manufacturing process.

Man creates all manner of products, ostensibly to make our lives better. But what kind of better are we talking about? Do we mean emotionally better? On some levels, yes. We think if we have a bigger, better, brighter car, our lives will be better. True? Not at all. A car is just a vehicle we use to get from one place to the next. The type of car you drive is purchased to satisfy a particular ego need, regardless of the sales presentations about engineering.

The bottom line is this: you buy something that tells the rest of the world who you think you are and where you are financially. In that process we have created chemicals that are, in truth, toxins that pollute not only the air, but also the water and the land. Through our own needs and emptiness within, we have created toxins as by-products that destroy every part of our lives.

Spiritually, we have multiple religions in the world telling us how to live. Not all religions or the people who follow them live in accordance with true Universal Teachings. As a way of understanding and seeing the truth in that, look around at how much murder and mayhem is going on in the world. You can see how many different religious factions are fighting one another every day (each of them full of anger and hatred). You can see that there is no understanding, love or acceptance. There is only greed and attempted domination. These attitudes and outcomes also generate by-products that create chemicals that create toxins in our system.

ESSENCE OF LIFE

Water, like air, is essential for our existence. Water is symbolic of our material life, without it, we would dehydrate and die of thirst. In viewing the symbology of air and water, we can see that we are in reality both material and spiritual beings: two in one house. We are all part spiritual being and part ego persona, each half with its own set of directives. You might say man is a house divided.

SUBSTANCE OF LIFE

Another aspect vital to our existence is the land upon which we grow our foods. The foods that are cultivated by major commercial farms use chemicals for the growing of the plants. These chemicals are drawn into the plant and become part of its structure, we then consume these additional chemicals from the land.

The symbology involved here is that the land represents our body and the physical plane. All of the chemicals are symbolic of man's erroneous thinking, they corrupt the natural process of growth and development. This is especially true of our spiritual and mental capabilities. When people lack both understanding of the Inner Self and emotional control, it can create a familiar situation, underwritten by uncontrolled patterns of behavior, and because we live daily with man-made misconceptions, there is the potential for anger, resentment, guilt, and frustration: all factors that cause cancer.

What you must do is take inventory of your own life, identify those situations that produce anger, and then seek to understand why. Only within you will you find your answers, for your concepts, expectations, and memories are unique unto you.

Most others can offer you only man-made theories in the way of guidance. Of course, there are those who do counsel from the Universal Teachings based on Universal Laws, but they are rare and hard to find.

SYMBOLOGY OF MALIGNANCY AT VARIOUS LOCATIONS IN THE BODY

Another characteristic of cancers is that there are malignant cells present, which means the tumor or condition could get worse, may be spreading, and could cause death. No matter how you look at it, you are in deep trouble if you are dealing with malignant cells. Symbolically, you are dealing with malignant thoughts, thoughts that will ultimately kill you if not brought into check, and if they are not identified, understood, and controlled, they will spread.

Based on findings reported in medical journals, the most common sites for the cancerous tumors are the lung, breast, colon, uterus, mouth, and bone marrow. Let us look at each one of these areas from a symbolic perspective.

Lungs. The lungs are the organs with which you process air (spirit). They take the oxygen out of the air and draw it into the bloodstream, so from another perspective, your lungs are symbolic of your faith and courage in self. A working faith is the foundation for courage, and these are but two basic elements of true, spiritual power. They are what serve you when you must act upon the truth of a situation. A working faith comes from the knowledge that you are a part of God; therefore, you would never be placed in a situation that you could not master or overcome.

Because of the nature of the material plane, our lives are loaded with misconceptions. These man-made ideas of how things should be were presented to us from birth, and we absorbed them as truth and built our lives on them. We draw upon those beliefs when confronted with an event, situation, or person.

Problems arise when what you need to do is in conflict with what you think (believe) you can do. Often when these two directives are in conflict, the result is physical disharmony. Therefore, all diseases of the lungs revolve around a lack of faith and self-doubt.

Symbolically, the lungs deal with faith in self because they deal with drawing in spirit. This is another situation where doubt and fear allow anger, resentment, and frustration to manifest. Since there is self-doubt in one's ability to deal with the forces and situations of life, the person becomes frustrated, and the thought or situation eats at and literally consumes the person, just as cancer does.

Breasts. This is a site of high incidence of cancer in women; men develop breast cancer as well.

There are many concepts of female self-expression tied into the breasts; the breasts are a key symbol of womanhood. Breasts are also considered by most cultures as one gauge of a woman's attractiveness as well as her potential to be a mate and mother.

Many women are prone to breast cancer because they may feel guilty—or angry—about the role that they are living. Perhaps the woman's position in life is subservient, leaving her frustrated because she has no freedom to speak or express herself. Some women may feel that they were supposed to have been male, but are born female instead. While there are many areas to be explored when a woman develops breast cancer, in the end the symbolism goes back to self-expression, or how one expresses one's self as a female in the material plane.

Colon. The colon is really the "bottom line" for all of us, on many levels. It is an integral part of the elimination/cleansing process. The body must constantly cleanse and eliminate harmful wastes, before it becomes toxic.

To advance emotionally, spiritually, and materially in life, one must cleanse and eliminate toxic thoughts. As with any material held internally, if you hang on to that which no longer serves or works for you, you will ultimately compromise and destroy yourself through auto-intoxication.

This is analogous to what happens in the colon. Most people have one, maybe two, bowel movements a day, a holdover from our potty-training days. Being in the workplace is also not conducive to evacuating our bowels as frequently as we need to, so we suppress the urge and hold on to that fecal matter for release at a more convenient time. From a physiological standpoint, the body is reabsorbing toxins from this matter as it sits in the colon waiting to be evacuated. It is no wonder that there is cancer in the colon because of all of the additives, colorants, preservatives, and other chemicals in our diet.

Wastes that are not eliminated become toxic and poison the body. Thoughts that are not in keeping with Divine Truth but are maintained as a way of living life are also wastes, and these wastes must also be eliminated before they become toxic to the self. In both instances, the toxins will destroy the person on every level.

Symbolically, we know that our thought "diet" is poisonous to us because it is a diet of falsehoods, a diet lacking true Universal Teachings based on Divine Truth, truth that is applicable to everybody because everybody is a part of God.

When we fail to eliminate the man-made misconceptions from our belief system, they are at work all the time, polluting our true Inner Self, and they are killing us.

Uterus. The uterus relates to female expression. It is where children are nurtured before they are brought into the world. This is also where thoughts are nurtured before they are expressed.

If a woman has cancer of the uterus or any part of the reproductive system, there is a tremendous amount of anger, frustration, resentment, or guilt present in her ability to create. Either she feels denied, is suppressed, or is rejected because of it. This also applies to breast cancer, where rejection and fear definitely play a part in developing the disease.

Remember that every single source, every single energy that creates a reaction in one area has a reaction in other areas as well. Rejection can bring about anger, guilt, or resentment, and once feelings of rejection are experienced, there can be an overcompensation to avoid it. That, in turn, sends out the energy of obligation to someone else that, in turn, reacts from an anger/resentment point of view, and the anger is returned. Thus, develops a destructive cycle between any two human beings who are working at things from patterned reaction points. Patterns flow in a very specific cyclic fashion, and every action has a reaction. Cancer of the reproductive system deals with another aspect of self-expression, an aspect of creativity.

Again, there is a possibility of a woman feeling guilty about being a woman and guilty about bringing forth personal expression (life) into the world.

Remember that it is vital to understand each area of the body affected by the cancer because cancer needs to be more specifically understood. Your perceptions should be fine-tuned in order to get back to the root cause, the primary concept, and the physical site.

Mouth. Through your mouth, you express yourself, communicate. Additionally, you take nourishment for the body in through the mouth. Another way of putting it is that you provide for yourself through your mouth.

When there is cancer in the mouth, there is a tremendous amount of guilt and frustration in one's ability for self-expression. There could be anger and resentment about what one is forced to consume through the mouth. Essentially, the individual is dealing with a forced or imposed consumption as well as difficulty in expression. It is interesting how many people, males and females, have difficulty in truly expressing themselves. The amount of doubt and fear that permeates our society today is staggering.

That identical fear and doubt permeates religious teachings. Teachings that should be giving us faith and hope do nothing to give us courage and confidence in dealing with the day-to-day issues of living. Of course, it is also taught that you are unable to effectively deal with your life on your own. Therefore, you need an outside force greater than yourself to help you cope. If anything, man-made religions instill guilt, doubt, and fear.

In truth, when you understand the concepts and forces affecting your life and exercise control over your emotional reactions, then you are in harmony, within and without, and this harmony is reflected by excellent health. Whatever your life is about, it is a reflection of what you are going through internally on both conscious and subconscious levels.

Bone Marrow. Bone marrow produces antibodies, T-cells and B-cells, for the immune system. Your bones also represent inner-strength and your ability to support yourself.

When people feel that they cannot defend themselves, cancer of the bone marrow occurs. This is true on both the emotional and material levels. When people feel that they cannot defend themselves, they are helpless in the world, and that alone is enough to generate anger, resentment, and frustration. Caught in such a belief system, they feel inadequate to the task at hand, and that is enough to eat them up alive. Once again, we can see how cancer can develop and consume a person.

One must also remember that God would never place an individual in a situation that he or she could not master. Never! The understanding here is that no matter what you are involved in, you are 100 percent capable of mastering it. All you need to do is understand what concepts you are working with that are shading your perception. These same concepts are motivating you to act in certain ways, which creates reactions from other people, and their reactions cause you to respond and act in yet another way.

Life is really about you reacting to people reacting to you. This perception and understanding brings everything back to the self, as it should. It takes you to the Doctrine of Personal Responsibility, which in essence means that you are totally responsible for everything that happens to you, including the diseases with which you live.

Interestingly, many doctors say that some cancers are curable if found in the early stages. What could be a better determination or a better validation of awareness, not only on a physical level, but catching something on the thought level as well. If you can identify what you are going through and what you are about early on, then you have an opportunity to begin to control that energy as it manifests in your life. Through that control mechanism, you can begin to alter your own personal reality.

Learning to have eyes to see the things you and others do, and ears to hear what is said will lead to a heightened awareness. Remember that symbols come in many different forms of sight, sound, and physical contact. They also tell you which part of the cyclic expression of your particular pattern of behavior you are drawing on to deal with the symbolic stimuli.

Look around, and pay attention to what is going on in your life. That way you can realize where you are in the cycle. What kind of result, based on subconscious expectations, is it that you are creating with your energy? What energies of expectation are you sending out, and what energies are you magnetically drawing back to yourself?

Nothing stands alone in the universe. Everything and everyone is interconnected, and this is something that you must bear in mind. It is essential for healing resolutions to take effect that you understand that the nature of your disease is of your own doing, and that it is based on concepts that you have brought with you or accepted from others, concepts you must understand to gain control over and resolve them in this life cycle.

SYMBOLOGY OF CANCER'S WARNING SIGNS

Change in Bowel or Bladder Habits. The warning signs of cancer are also symbolically interesting because the first one doctors list is a change in bowel or bladder habits. It is interesting because both your bowels and bladder are both part of your cleansing and elimination systems. This tells you if you do not take the time or make the effort to eliminate the toxins from your thinking and from your body, they will accumulate. In their accumulation are the seeds of physical disharmony—the thought seeds of frustration, anger, and resentment.

It is amazing how often we keep coming back to the same causative factors. The unwillingness to eliminate toxins from the body will cause serious consequences in the elimination system first, and then as the toxins accumulate and progress, they create mutagens at a cellular level, thus, cancer is born.

It is no wonder that with everything going on in life—from the physical level to the man-made thought level—that one out of three people will end up with cancer. This is because of the way we have been taught, based on man-made teachings, about how to act in and react to certain situations of life. Life can produce frustration, anger, and resentment, and on top of that are the situations other people create to make you feel guilty.

The other side of all of these energies is the positive manifestations, based on courage and confidence, and having excellent health is one example. The flip side of anger is acceptance and love, and the opposite of frustration is easy going, flowing smoothly, ease of accomplishment, and ease of understanding. The opposite of resentment is acceptance, forgiveness, and embrace. Embrace people for where they are and what they are. Why resent the situation? Look at it as opportunities for growth.

What is guilt? It is a device to make you feel bad about doing something that you wanted to do, kind of like sin. What is sin? Sin is an action that you take based on the need to fulfill a perceived need within yourself, yet the action you take is viewed as sinful to others because it is not in keeping with their laws, rules, and regulations. It may well be that all of their rules and regulations are so far from the truth that we live in total disharmony because of them. The truth of that perception can be found as we look at the world around us, which is full of anger, war, violence, hatred, disease, corruption, and pollution. These are all reflections of who we are in our thinking.

If you are dealing with cancer on a personal level, you now have an insight as to where you are and what must be done. If you catch it now, you may be at a point that you will be able to turn it around and eliminate it from your life. The very first areas to begin in are in bowel and bladder habits—cleansing habits. Remove the toxic thoughts from your system, and eliminate the toxic situations from your life. The only way to eliminate anything is to understand it, and understanding is the key to self-mastery, expression, and emotional control. It is also the only key leading to true cure.

Non-Healing Sore. That is a great symbol in itself. A sore is an area of great sensitivity within. You would have to look at the body part where the sore exists to know where your greatest sensitivity is, and obviously something is going on where you are so sensitive to the situation that no matter what is said or done, you are beyond the point of healing.

A non-healing sore is a sign that you can no longer deal with life from a position of strength, and your immune system cannot even begin to function at any level of strength. Your whole modus operendi, your whole way of dealing with things, is from a position of weakness. You have an area in your life that from your perception is not healable.

The truth is that there is nothing that cannot be healed. All that is required is understanding. Everything in life can be brought back into balance and harmony with the proper amount of understanding and control.

Unusual Bleeding or Discharge. Doubt and fear have opened up the release of energy and faith from within. Symbolically speaking, we must remember that blood is the lifeline of the body. It is the spiritual aspect of the self made material (physical).

If there is unusual bleeding that will not stop, regardless of the location, it reflects an area of weakness and great doubt, and the doubt will lead down the path toward anger and resentment. To understand the reason for the loss of faith, look symbolically at the area of bleeding or discharge.

Thickening or Lump in the Breast or Elsewhere. If a thickening or lump has formed at a certain location in the body, it is an indication that this is where the conflict between concepts on a subconscious level is the greatest, and is beginning to show itself symbolically. It is not necessarily the primary spot of where the cancer is being generated, but the secondary area of difficulty within the person.

An example of this is when one of the causes of cancer is not expressed and the area affected is symbolic of the area of conflict, but the cause still remains in the subconscious until it is dealt with through understanding the concepts involved.

Indigestion or Difficulty in Swallowing. This deals with the mouth, esophagus, and stomach. Difficulty in swallowing can relate to forced consumption. What is it that you are being forced to ingest? What is it that you cannot stomach anymore, that you really do not want to swallow anymore? Is there a lot of anger about being forced into it?

Warts and Moles. A change in the appearance of a wart or mole is another sign of trouble.

Warts are little viral enclaves on the body where a virus has taken up residence and rooted itself, seeking to penetrate into the system. Where did the wart come from, and where is it on your body? What thoughts does this area symbolize?

A mole is a birthmark, and again, this indicates sensitivity in a particular area. Examine the area symbolically.

Nagging Cough or Hoarseness. These symptoms tie into our faith in self. If you are constantly coughing, you are not able to bring in the full amount of spirit/oxygen that you need, and this creates a situation in which you are not able to draw on the totality of your strength, the totality of your inner power.

Hoarseness takes us back to our inability to communicate clearly from a position of courage and confidence. The hoarseness would be indicative of the fear to clearly express one's feelings and thoughts. Some people operate from anger, even when they talk with authority, so power may be based on anger. The true power—spiritual power—is a soft voice that does not need to yell or shout in order to be heard.

SYMBOLOGY OF CANCER TREATMENTS

Surgery. Often, the very first approach to treating cancer is surgery, which reflects how we are in life. If we do not understand something, we want to cut it out and try to eliminate it completely.

You cannot eliminate any kind of a thought process unless you understand it, so to cut something out of a body is useless from that perspective. If you have not dealt with the primary site, you have not dealt with the root cause of the guilt, anger, or frustration, so it remains there.

Maybe this is one reason why the survival rate for people who have gone through cancer with surgery and radiation is only five years. Because, no matter what you do, if you do not identify and understand the true cause, it will re-manifest in the next area of weakness within yourself.

Radiation and Chemotherapy. These two forms of treatment can themselves generate other problems. One would be the load placed on the liver to detoxify as much of the poison as possible. Both treatments are designed to destroy, but the belief and understanding behind these approaches is that although healthy tissue will be killed along with the cancer, the body will respond by generating new, healthy tissue.

Again, you have the same kind of survival rate and the same kind of thinking of trying to destroy something without understanding it. If you do not change the way you think and bring in new, fresh, living thoughts and truth, then you will never eliminate the disease. This is because all diseases are the result of internal conflict between the Spiritual Self and the Ego Self.

You can cut out physical parts of the self, and yet there will still be conflict between the Spiritual Self and the Ego Self. You are not changing the belief system upon which the ego is built; therefore, you have not really changed anything.

In order to bring about a cure for cancer, it is absolutely essential that you understand the cause. The primary cause is the basic concept that you believe about yourself that is in total disharmony with the truth.

The truth is that part of you that is the God within is always seeking to manifest itself in love, acceptance, compassion, harmony, and balance. Often when we try to express ourselves in those ways, we run into conflict with what we were taught. We are never taught to look within, we are not told how wonderful we really are, how divine, full of grace, full of love, or full of personal power we are and that we are able to accomplish anything we set our minds to do.

If you had cancer of the brain, it would directly affect one or more specific functions of the body, so the areas that first showed signs of deterioration would be a reflective symbol of the concepts in conflict. I use the term conflict because every time you develop a disease, it is the result of two different internal drives. On one side is your ego, motivating you into certain thoughts and actions in order to accomplish some goal. The ego houses your True Self and is the defensive cover that you use in the world. At the same time, your ego suppresses your True Self from manifesting its ideas, so you have conflict when the Ego Self and the True Self try to express themselves. The conflict creates friction, which sets the stage for a chemical "fire" to take place; cancer is one such "fire."

If you had cancer of the eye, then it would deal with the way that you look at things, with anger or guilt, for example. Maybe you feel guilty about something you have seen and have not been able to understand or deal with. Maybe you cannot bear to look at yourself because of feelings you maintain about a past action.

Perceptions in life are shaded by your belief system, which results from programming based on man-made teachings. Man-made teachings are the ideals, standards, and guides for living that help man control and dominate others, but these teachings are not in keeping with Universal Truth as expressed by the Universal Teachings.

If you had cancer in the throat and became incapacitated, no longer able to speak, then the conflict would be in concepts tied into communication. When there is conflict in this area of your body, it is a direct indication that you believe that you do not have the authority or the ability to speak up. It may be that you were raised in a house where children were to be seen but not heard, or there was a very authoritative parent who constantly shut you down.

There are thoughts/beliefs within your belief system that tell you that you do not have the ability to communicate clearly, intelligently, or effectively. They may tell you that you have nothing of value to say, and all of these types of thoughts and energies lead to suppression. As you grow older and seek to express yourself because of life's demands or requirements, there is conflict, and one result of this conflict could be cancer.

Each area of the body has its very own symbolic meaning. Therefore, each gland, organ or system requires a specific set of questions to elicit a clear understanding of the concept at work.

SYMBOLOGY OF THE NUTRIENTS

Beta-carotene (Vitamin A). Essential for healthy night vision. What is the symbolic significance of night vision? Night, itself, symbolizes a time of preparation. It is when, through your dreams, you receive proper guidance on actions to take based on your personal patterns of behavior. If you cannot clearly see which path to take, then you will proceed with doubt, so it can be said that the night is symbolic of both preparation and doubt.

Vitamin A is also instrumental in protecting you from invasion from outside forces because it feeds the thymus gland, which is the immune center. From here, T-cells rush out to do battle with invading forces. On a physical level those forces can be allergens, bacteria, viruses, fungus, or toxins from the environment. Symbolically, those external forces can be the thoughts, deeds, and actions of others projected onto you. In essence, vitamin A is an essential nutrient in the defense of the body as well as the mind.

Vitamin A is important for the outer cellular layer of many tissues and organs, such as the mucous membranes. The mucous membranes are the thin sheets of tissue cells that cover or line various parts of the body that open to the outside. Examples include linings of the mouth, digestive tube, breathing passages, and the genital and urinary tracts. The mucous membranes release mucus, which contains water, cast-off tissue cells, mucin, and white blood cells. Mucin is a carbohydrate that is the main part of mucus, and is present in most glands that release mucus.

White blood cells, also called leukocytes, function in the destruction of bacterias, fungi and viruses. They also render harmless poisonous substances that may result from allergic reactions and cellular injury. Leukocytes are produced by diverse components of the body's immune system, particularly by the bone marrow, the thymus gland, and the spleen. Vitamin A is required in that production process.

Folic Acid. Has a direct nourishing and fortifying effect on the "front line" of the body's defense system.

It is easy to see the symbology of folic acid when you look at how closely it is tied into how you live your life. Symbolically speaking, folic acid is a fortifier, a vitamin that helps in building and defending your perceptions of the truth. Truth is always a relative term, which is why you must know yourself so that you can see the truth of the Universal Teachings and look away from the teachings of man. The teachings of man instill doubt, fear and other negative attributes that affect your life in a negative way.

On a daily basis, the body requires every nutrient. The daily folate requirement hinges on the daily metabolic and cell-turnover rates, and the requirement is increased by anything that increases metabolic rate (such as infection) and anything that increases cell turnover (such as malignant tumors).

Magnesium. An essential mineral, it activates enzymes necessary for the metabolism of amino acids, which helps to make antibodies. It helps promote absorption and metabolism of other minerals, such as calcium, phosphorus, sodium, and potassium.

Magnesium is important in the conversion of blood sugar into energy. Symbolically, magnesium is a facilitator, assisting in the assimilation of thoughts that lead to strength. From a position of strength, all actions taken lead to a positive conclusion, whereas, when you act out of fear, doubt, a lack of self-confidence, or uncertainty, the seeds for failure are sown.

Pantothenic Acid. A member of the B-vitamin family, pantothenic acid nourishes the adrenal glands, and is also necessary for energy production in each cell.

The adrenals are the stress centers of the body; they go into action when the body's systems are being overtaxed. When the adrenals are weak, they allow the immune system to become lowered in its ability to function properly; this happens because of the supportive role the adrenals play in immune system health. Limited research suggests that patients with rheumatoid arthritis and hypo-adrenalism should use pantothenic acid, also known as vitamin B-5, to relieve symptoms and stimulate healing of the tissue.

Symbolically, on one level this nutrient represents inspiration, due to pantothenic acid's nourishing of the adrenals and its role in facilitating energy production. The adrenals produce hormones that help the body deal with taking quick actions based upon quick decisions. This is reflected in the "flight or fight" concept.

When you face an intense force, you may go into a state of fear, and the reaction to this fear is based upon your self-concept and self-confidence. The part of the body that reacts to the impulse of fear is the adrenal glands, which send out hormonal messages to signal body parts about how to react.

Vitamin B-6. Vital because of the role it plays in antibody and red blood cell production. The presence of vitamin B-6 also increases the number of T-cells. T-cells are phagocytes, white blood cells that are matured in the thymus gland.

Symbolically, one level vitamin B-6 represents balance. In this instance, balance is maintained through the correct amount of white blood cells necessary to keep the person in a good state of health, and vitamin B-6 acts to create balance within the system. This can be seen by how it works within the body by increasing the number of mature phagocytes.

It is interesting to realize how important balanced thinking is in regard to gaining strength, and without strength, you may believe you are helpless in dealing with the forces or energies of life. The truth of this perception is seen in the physical fact that a vitamin B-6 deficiency leads to impaired immune response and muscle weakness.

Vitamin C. Increases the absorption of iron, which symbolically deals with faith and courage. Iron is a major constituent of hemoglobin, it helps to carry oxygen to the cells, and removes carbon dioxide and carries it to the lungs for removal. Oxygen is symbolic of spirit because heaven is located in the sky, or air, and heaven is symbolic of God's home or dwelling place. Oxygen, therefore, is symbolic of spirit, and because iron is an oxygen carrier it is symbolic of faith and courage.

Vitamin C is also essential for the immune system, because it has prophylactic and therapeutic effects on pathologic conditions. These conditions include infectious diseases and immune deficiency disorders. Vitamin C plays a supportive role in the defenses of the body as well as ensures that the ability to maintain faith and courage is intact and functioning properly. It should be said that when faith and courage are present, guilt, anger, frustration, and resentment are not as predominant in your life. This translates to a diminished receptivity to cancer causing conditions.

Zinc. Nourishes the thymus gland and plays a role in liberating vitamin A from the liver, which is another source of nourishment for the thymus. Zinc has many different functions within the body, some of them deal with taste and smell—which are two defense mechanisms—and reproduction. From that perspective zinc is symbolic of those thoughts that contribute to courage, confidence, and expression, and represents protection from negative forces.

When your ability to discern spoiled or adulterated foods is compromised, you are susceptible to being poisoned. The same holds true for toxic thoughts that are presented in tasty and fragrant ways. In this instance, a lack of zinc would denote that the inability to defend and express the self leads to anger and frustration, two of the causes of cancer.

Candida Albicans (Yeast Infection)

Candida albicans is a yeast fungus that occurs naturally in the body in small quantities. However, when this organism has the chance to grow and proliferate, a yeast infection can erupt. This often happens when there is a deficiency of our "good" bacteria allowing for over growth of other bacteria and yeast. Taking antibiotics are often the culprit in allowing for this condition.

Antibiotics kill the friendly flora in the intestinal tract, creating a vacuum of sorts, and since Candida is the first flora to grow back down into the intestinal tract, it will dominate there because of its own natural ability to multiply.

Additionally, there is an opportunity for Candida and toxins to enter the bloodstream via a condition called "leaky gut." As a result of malnutrition and the ingestion of harmful substances, cells within the intestinal lining die, creating holes through which these materials can pass. Candida does not perform the same supportive function for the body as do the friendly flora, such as acidophilus, and it can actually drain the body of energy. As a by-product of metabolism, friendly floras produce B-vitamins for the body, while Candida does not.

B-complex vitamins are involved as co-enzymes in energy production as well as other enzymatic processes within the body, they help the body to develop and maintain energy, and function properly. When the body and the intestinal tract are overwhelmed by Candida, an inadequate amount of B-vitamins is produced, causing the body to go into somewhat of a dive, both on a physical and an emotional level.

Consequently, the person who has Candida throughout the intestines and bloodstream has a hard time generating and maintaining strength and energy. In order for the body to free itself of this infestation and rebalance, it must become nutritionally fit. This means establishing both a strong immune system and a hostile environment for the yeast. Creating a hostile environment means depriving the yeast colony of its food sources and attacking them full force with natural substances that will destroy them, and also means strengthening and stimulating the immune system to "clean house."

NUTRIENTS, AMINO ACIDS AND HERBS TO SUPPORT ELIMINATION OF YEAST AND BACTERIA

The following will boost your body's immune system and increase elimination of toxins, yeast, and bacteria:

Nutrients	Amino Acids	Herbs
Pantothenic Acid	L-Cysteine	Black Walnut
Vitamin A		Buckthorn Bark
Vitamin B-1		Cascara Sagrada
Vitamin B-2		Corn Silk
Vitamin B-6		Dandelion Root
Zinc		Echinacea
		Garlic
		Goldenseal Root
		Myrrh
		Pau D'Arco
		Uva Ursi

Pantothenic Acid. Nourishes the adrenal glands, which helps to support the immune system.

Vitamin A. Nourishes the thymus gland, increasing its size and antibody production.

Vitamins B-1, B-2, and B-6. Involved in nourishing the adrenal glands. When the body is sick or under attack, it places stress on the adrenals, which can, in turn, stress and deplete the immune system. By keeping the adrenals well nourished, it should help to prevent illness or hasten recovery time.

Zinc. Essential for natural antibody production.

L-Cysteine. Involved in natural antibody production.

Black Walnut, Goldenseal Root, Myrrh, and Pau D'arco. These herbs are known to contain natural properties that kill fungus and bacteria.

Buckthorn Bark, Cascara Sagrada, Corn Silk, and Uva Ursi. Help in cleansing the system of toxic and waste material.

Dandelion Root. Improves liver function. Bile and certain enzymes produced in the liver aid in maintaining proper intestinal flora.

Echinacea. Cleanses lymph system and improves antibody production.

Garlic. A wonderful anti-bacterial, anti-fungal, anti-microbial agent and is great for killing Candida.

SYMBOLOGY OF CANDIDA ALBICANS

A Candida infection symbolizes thoughts imposed by others; though they sounded good at first blush and may have been accepted joyfully, they do not provide any sustenance or nourishment to the mind or body. Rather, they work against the body because they do not provide what the body requires.

When Candida enters the bloodstream, it can be truly debilitating. Blood is the lifeline of the body, and is symbolic of the spirit within the body. With polluted thoughts coming in, faith in self ultimately diminishes, and courage and confidence are undermined, leaving you to believe you cannot do what is needed.

Much like fibromyalgia, another debilitating condition, Candida symbolizes a lack of inspiration on some levels. When Candida infects the intestinal tract, it prevents friendly flora from creating B-vitamins, which help comprise enzymes that the body uses to manufacture energy.

A lack of energy is symbolic of a lack of inspiration. Therefore, by finding something that you want to do, such as a favorite hobby, you become inspired anew, gaining the impetus to overcome the debilitating effects of the Candida. Through the process of inspiration, you end up energizing your system (including the immune system) to bring the body's flora back into balance and harmony, thus, creating a more energetic involvement with life.

SYMBOLOGY OF THE NUTRIENTS

Pantothenic Acid. Represents inspiration. When you are inspired, you have an internal drive to accomplish something, whatever the endeavor may be. Someone with Candida is in dire need of exactly these types of thoughts and energy because Candida's presence saps desire and motivation.

Vitamin A. An aspect of the symbology of vitamin A is that it is instrumental in protecting you from invasion by outside forces. These forces can take the physical form of viruses, fungus, bacteria, or good old-fashioned germs. Symbolically, each type of pathogen represents a different type of attack against the body. Some attacks manifest quickly, while others build in intensity over time. The difference would depend upon the nature of the attack and the substance as well as your level of courage and confidence.

The more confidence and courage you have at the time of attack, the less likely the attack will have strong effects. Vitamin A is essential for the health of all mucus membranes, and it feeds the thymus gland from which all the different forms of T-cells rush out to do battle with invading forces.

Forces, as the term is being used in this work, represent thoughts, attitudes, and energies from others. Usually, we are apt to willingly and consciously accept them, especially when they come from loved ones. This is done to help fulfill subconscious expectations that we maintain about ourselves.

Vitamin B-1. Symbolically represents a facilitator. On one level it facilitates communication by ensuring a healthy mouth, which has multiple symbolic meanings. The mouth is the portal through which you take in material sustenance for the body, and is also a key medium for communication and self-expression.

Vitamin B-2. Represents courage. It works with vitamin B-1 in supporting eye, skin, and hair health. When looking at attributes in symbolic terms, the need for confidence and courage is apparent. Were any one of the three missing or damaged, it would not only affect the way others see you but how you see yourself as well.

Vitamin B-6. Represents regulation as well as protection. Both are demonstrated through maintaining the correct amount of white blood cells in the bloodstream, and these cells are the body's main defense mechanism against invading forces.

Thoughts are forces that can invade your belief system, creating an upset in your status quo. The invading thoughts are in conflict with subconscious expectations that you maintain about yourself.

It is noteworthy that the positive symbolic interpretation of the color white is faith. This is a working faith in self, which implies that regardless of the nature of the attack, you have the faith and ability to eliminate the threat. On the negative side, white symbolizes a lack, emptiness. Here white indicates there are not enough white blood cells available to combat the invaders, which would indicate doubt at work.

An excess of white blood cells characterizes leukemia, a form of cancer in the blood. In this case the symbology is you are eating yourself alive because of strong self-doubt.

Zinc. Represents a working faith. Zinc helps to boost the immune system which kills the invader (Candida), and that is exactly what it takes in dealing with life, a working faith to eliminate doubt and fear from taking root in your expression. Whenever you are overwhelmed with a situation and it pulls you away from your energies and vitality, doubt is at work. Here, by bringing in zinc, by bringing in a working faith, one is able to deal with the situation at hand.

Cataracts

Three-fifths of all people between the ages of sixty-five and seventy-four show the beginning signs of cataracts, and by age eighty, they cloud nearly everyone's vision to some degree. Removing and replacing eye lenses damaged by cataracts is the most common surgery in the U.S., with some 650,000 of the procedures performed annually at a whopping cost of one billion dollars!

Some experts contend that if preventive measures could be taken to delay cataract formation by an average ten years, then the number of operations could be cut in half.[17]

Various types of stressors can result in cataracts. Besides the aging process itself, illnesses like diabetes are one cause. Frequent exposure to X-rays, microwaves, the intense heat from blast furnaces or welding torches, and the sun's ultraviolet rays are among other known causes.

Protein and vitamin deficiencies can be a contributing factor as well as drugs, such as cortisone, or even a severe blow to the eye. More common causes suggested by the Journal of the American Dietetic Association[18] are insufficient levels of water and other fluids in the body, and the excessive consumption of milk in later adulthood.

A study published in the New England Journal of Medicine[19] reports minerals and vitamins can prevent diabetic cataracts. Chief among those recommended are calcium and magnesium, plus all vitamins from the B-complex group. Additionally, vitamin A is very important in preventing the eyes from drying out.[20] Finally, vitamin C, especially its bioflavonoids, can prevent cataracts.[21] At least one study also reports that the sulfur amino acid glutathione likewise protects against cataracts.[22]

There is yet another natural approach to eliminating cataracts. One of the older European approaches is to place eight to ten drops of raw, unfiltered, uncooked honey in the eyes at bedtime. The honey's enzymes will eat away at the cataract. In the morning, one simply washes the eye with warm water.

NUTRIENTS, AMINO ACIDS AND HERBS FOR EYE AND VISION SUPPORT

The following will assist the body in creating healthy eye lenses, improving eyesight, and protecting against damage caused by free radicals:

Nutrients		*Amino Acids*
Bioflavoniods	Vitamin B-2	L-Arginine
Calcium	Vitamin B-3	L-Cysteine
Folic Acid	Vitamin B-6	L-Glutachione
Inositol	Vitamin B-12	L-Glutamine
Magnesium	Vitamin C	
Niacin	Vitamin D	*Herbs*
Pantothenic Acid	Vitamin E	Chickweed
Selenium	Zinc	Eyebright
Vitamin A		Ginger
Vitamin B-1		Red Raspberry Leaves

Bioflavonoids. Contain citrin, hesperidin, rutin, flavones, and flavonals. Essential for the proper absorption and use of vitamin C.

Calcium. Needed for nerve and muscle action.

Folic Acid. Essential for cell division, and is necessary for healthy eye cells in this particular instance.

Inositol. Helps to support healthy eye membranes.

Magnesium. Activates more enzymes in the body than any other mineral.

Selenium. A component part of glutathione peroxidase, a free radical scavenger, which protects the eye from damage. One of the concepts behind the causes of cataracts is pre-radical damage to the eyes.

Vitamin A. Vital to the formation of rich blood and maintenance of good eyesight. Essential in the formation of visual purple, a substance in the eye necessary for proper night vision.

Vitamin B-1. Essential for proper nerve function.

Vitamin B-2. Cataracts can easily be produced in laboratory animals by depriving them of this vitamin, also called riboflavin. A diet low in protein has also been linked to this eye disorder. Riboflavin deficiency can also cause visual fatigue, a "sandy" feeling of the eyes, and inability to endure bright lights.

Vitamin B-3. Used in many enzymatic reactions used to promote energy and blood flow.

Vitamin C. Protects thiamine (B-1), riboflavin (B-2), folic acid, pantothenic acid (B-5), and vitamins A and E against oxidation.

Vitamin E. An antioxidant that protects against the damaging effects of many environmental poisons present in air, water, and food.

Zinc. The vascular coating of the eye; contains more zinc than any other part of the body.

L-Glutamine, Arginine, and Cysteine. Amino acids, which are basically free radical scavengers. They participate in free radical scavenging and nurture the eye lens.

L-Glutathione. Protects metabolism in the eye's lens by preserving the physicochemical equilibrium of its proteins, maintains the molecular integrity of the lens fiber membranes, and protects membranes and organelles from oxidation.

Chickweed. Useful for eye infections (glaucoma, cataracts), hemorrhoids, blood diseases (leukemia, tetanus), and eczema.

Eyebright. Useful for sore, inflamed eyes in which there is considerable stinging and irritation associated with watery-to-thick discharges, or conjunctivitis (pink eye).

Red Raspberry Leaves. Astringent for the eyes (reduces mucus in them); also reduces hyperglycemia (excess glucose levels in the blood), which may be linked to cataract development.

Symbology of Cataracts

We view the world through our eyes, making vision an incredibly powerful tool on many different levels. Not only is it a key navigational sense, but vision is also central to our perceptions of reality.

Many factors affect vision, including insufficient levels of water and other fluids in the body and excess milk consumption later in adulthood. Each fluid within the body, including water and milk, has its own symbolic interpretation. Water reflects the material plane; living things cannot exist without water.

Relative to cataracts, low water levels in the body would indicate a refusal to see the power of self and your ability to acquire material strength. This does not mean you have nothing; it means only that you are not acknowledging or appreciating what you do have or are capable of achieving. This, in turn, would create a sense of lack in your life.

Milk is symbolic of sustenance for the young and immature, and is only necessary and important for newborn and growing children. A continuous consumption of milk indicates a tendency to resist maturing, and reflects a continued attachment to mother/child dependency concepts.

Cataracts can also represent the mind's way of blocking out what it is seeing. It is similar to deafness: we come to a place in life where we are tired of "hearing it" from others. With cataracts, either we do not want to see it any longer or we are tired of looking at it.

A cataract is also symbolic of the unwillingness to examine what is going on in your life. Known causes of cataracts include frequent exposure to the intense heat from blast furnaces or welding torches, X-rays, microwaves, and the sun's ultraviolet rays.

Sunlight causes free-radical damage to occur within the lens, so the body forms a cataract on the eye to protect itself. Because the sun symbolizes inspiration and insight, it can be seen that too much of a good thing can do harm. This adage is based on two Universal Teachings, "everything in moderation," and "excess leads to rejection."

The European honey method for dissolving cataracts is symbolically interesting in that honey represents the sweets in life. Perhaps having the sweets in life and feeling self-confident results from a society wherein sweets have come to represent rewards or security. By having life's sweets, doubt and fear are eliminated at some levels because of the sense of achievement associated with its "sweet" aspects.

In reality, life's true guarantees do not rest on its sweets or on material acquisitions. True security comes from one's personal power, gained through the process of self-examination. True security and power stem from repeatedly building on insights to gain self-control and master the tasks at hand. You must turn your eyes inward, so to speak, to look within and truly see what needs to be understood in order to move forward in life.

Symbology of the Nutrients

Calcium. Represents strength. Cataracts create distorted vision, so there is no clarity of sight. The same thing can be said when doubt is at work in an individual's life, it distorts clarity. It is essential that strength be present when one is ready to move forward; therefore, calcium is necessary.

Folic acid. Represents fortification. This ties in with calcium (strength) because by fortifying the self and coming from a position of strength, a position of courage and confidence, clarity of vision becomes normal.

Inositol. Symbolic of integrity. It takes integrity to see things clearly with courage and confidence—without fear and doubt affecting one's vision.

Magnesium. Represents inspiration. Life requires inspiration, and inspiration is symbolic of coming from a place of courage and confidence, being willing to look at everything clearly to see the truth of situations, and being able to find those pearls within a given situation that will inspire the individual to want to do something more. We can begin to see how this would also work in terms of eye health.

Niacin. Represents openness and receptivity. The symbolic concept of all of these nutrients is to be able to create an environment within that allows for openness, to move forward in life sure-footed, clear-eyed, and with courage and confidence to see things as they truly are. Niacin, as a vasodilator, allows blood (symbolic of spirit) to flow more easily to the extremities. It takes spirit and faith in self to see things clearly and to move forward from a position of strength.

Pantothenic acid. Much like magnesium, is also symbolic of inspiration. It is an energizer, and that is what inspiration does for us, it energizes us. In terms of cataracts, it allows for clarity of vision.

Selenium. Symbolically represents protection and cleansing. By bringing in selenium, we are taking a preventative measure to protecting the self. At the same time, because it represents cleansing, it helps clear up the vision so one can move forward again with courage and confidence, taking sure-footed steps.

Vitamin A. Essential for healthy night vision, which symbolizes the ability to see into the doubt that exists within the self. You could even say that vitamin A aids in self-examination by its role in improving (internal) vision.

With proper vision, you can avoid all of the doubt and frustration that accompanies aspects of preparing for and dealing with a situation. Vitamin A helps you to see well, thus giving greater insight into a situation, and going into a situation totally prepared gives you courage and confidence. With these energies at work, there can be no doubt about your ability to master a situation.

B-complex Vitamins. B-1, B-2, B-6, B-12, inositol, folic acid, niacin, and pantothenic acid represent confidence and courage on multiple levels. These two attributes contribute to many other emotional feelings that we experience.

Vitamin C. Symbolic of two major aspects of the material plane: material/physical protection (much like vitamin A) and our dependency on the material plane.

Vitamin D. Represents insight and understanding, owing to its role in the assimilation of calcium, which represents strength.

People with true strength know that they can accomplish just about anything they set out to do because they have proven it to themselves time and time again, even when man-made situations appeared beyond their control and abilities. With insights and understandings, strength is easily achieved, without them, it would be virtually impossible to achieve true strength.

Look at how vitamin D is manufactured in the body—it requires sunlight, which is symbolic of insight and seeing clearly.

Vitamin E. Symbolically seen as self-confidence.

Zinc. Symbolically represents a working faith in self working towards support and expression. You have to have faith in self in order to move forward in life, in order to see things clearly and without fear, to know that you can handle whatever it is that is placed before you. It is important to see things as clearly as you possibly can so that you can take forward movements that will continue expanding your expression and allow you to grow to be the person you want to be.

Circulation Issues

The circulatory system is the lifeline of the body, carrying the oxygen and food (vitamins, minerals, fats, proteins, and sugars [fuel]) that our body requires for health and performance. A well-fed body is healthy and vibrant.

Keeping the lifelines (arteries) open and free-flowing ensures that all the organs, muscles, nerves, and skin remain well fed. Problems arise when the arteries begin to clog, causing a reduced amount of blood to be available for all functions and structures.

Clogging results from excess fats or cholesterol in the bloodstream, which can clump to-gether to form ever-larger fatty deposits. As they grow in size, these deposits capture minute particles of minerals (ions) floating in the bloodstream. This is the beginning of the condi-tions that can manifest in arteriosclerosis, commonly called "hardening of the arteries," where excess fatty deposits cling to the arterial walls.

To avoid major circulatory problems and the possible heart disease associated with them, it is important to identify the most common symptoms of poor circulation. They include:

- ◆ *Hair loss*

- ◆ *Memory loss*

- ◆ *Hearing loss*

- ◆ *Cold hands and feet*

- ◆ *Numbness in fingers and toes*

- ◆ *Arms and legs that "fall asleep" easily*

If three or more of these symptoms are present, it's time to take action to get those arter-ies open to their maximum again.

One step should be to reduce the intake of those foods that contribute to excess fats or cholesterol in our blood such as refined carbohydrates and hard fats. Remember the fat/cho-lesterol is the "cement" that binds the minerals in our blood to the arterial walls. Cholesterol also has the positive function of cementing up or "patching" weak spots in the vessels, this is where the "cementing" begins.

A second step would be to start a nutritional program that will dissolve existing excess fat/cholesterol deposits, which should improve blood flow to the heart, head, and extremities.

NUTRIENTS, AMINO ACIDS, HERBS AND DIGESTIVE ENZYMES FOR CIRCULATORY SUPPORT

The following will assist the body in opening arteries, dissolving cholesterol and triglycerides, reducing water content, re-assimilating calcium from arterial walls, regulating cholesterol, equalizing blood pressure, and toning the heart.

Nutrients	Amino Acids	Herbs
Calcium	L-Methionine	Apple Pectin
Choline		Capsicum
Inositol		Garlic
Magnesium		Ginger
Niacin/Niacinamide		Hawthorne Berry
Pantothenic Acid		
Vitamin B-6		*Digestive Enzymes*
Vitamin D (from Fish Liver Oil)		Betaine Hydrochloride
Vitamin F		

Choline and Inositol. Lipotropic nutrients that work as "fat burners," dissolving excess fat and cholesterol.

Magnesium and Betaine Hydrochloride. A mineral and digestive aide, respectively, that both support calcium assimilation.

Niacinamide. Excellent for opening up arteries to provide more blood and oxygen to the heart, head, and extremities.

Vitamin B-6. As a natural diuretic, reduces water and water pressure from the cardiovascular system. Excellent in metabolizing fats, proteins, and carbohydrates.

Vitamin D. Essential for calcium assimilation. Most people with poor circulation are also calcium-starved, resulting in part from calcium becoming lodged in the cholesterol plaque in the arteries.

Vitamin F. This nutrient is also known as unsaturated fatty acids. These are essential for the dissolving of cholesterol and saturated fats in the bloodstream.

L-Methionine. An amino acid that acts as a "fat burner." Essential in the production of lecithin.

Apple Pectin. Helps to regulate cholesterol and also draws toxic metals out of the blood. It is said that apple pectin contains electromagnetic properties.

Capsicum, Garlic, and Ginger. Stimulate circulation and purify the bloodstream, increasing blood flow and regulating blood pressure.

Hawthorne Berry. Valuable for its heart-strengthening properties.

SYMBOLOGY OF POOR CIRCULATION

The variety of symptoms associated with poor circulation likewise means a variety of symbolic interpretations.

Cold Hands. Cold hands reflect doubt in your ability to handle situations with love, compassion, warmth, and feeling. Persons with cold hands deal with things in a matter-of-fact manner and without a working faith.

When we discuss circulation, we have to talk about the flow of blood, which is symbolic of spirit. Everything you do is infused with spirit, life, and faith. You either have a working faith and believe you can handle everything, or you have blind faith, where there is no true faith in your ability to cope.

A working faith says that your life's experiences have given you sufficient personal power to handle and master any situation with which you are faced, while blind faith is the religious type, which transfers the power of dealing with a situation to an external source. The belief here is that the person cannot handle it alone. When that proves true because of certain decisions made to validate subconscious expectations, the rational justification is, "God did not want me to do that." That is not the case.

Everything in life comes down to faith…belief in self. A person who lacks that fundamental belief is at the mercy of the material plane's energetic forces, situations, and circumstances. That could lead to feelings of being overwhelmed and unable to handle the event.

Cold Feet. Because the feet represent direction, cold feet take us along an uncertain path. You have questions about where you are going in life. Positive, true direction is a matter of faith in your decision-making process, and requires confidence, courage, and the ability to move forward in the manner you desire.

Heart Attacks and Stroke. We also know that poor circulation can lead to heart attacks, stroke, and even death. Remember that the heart is symbolic of emotions, and we can see how doubt, fear, and uncertainty, as well as the lack of a working faith, can lead to stagnation and poor circulation. Spirit cannot move forward in such an obstructed environment.

To validate a lack of faith in self, some people might be attracted to diets that provide emotional comfort, happiness, and security; such a diet is promoted through tradition and reinforced with advertising. In reality, many of these foods work against the individual.

Everybody with poor circulation should avoid hydrogenated fats and oils, and foods heavily laden with fat. Our emotional and cultural attachments to a particular food may make this difficult. Such attachments are a major reason why people cannot change their diets, making it difficult to attain and maintain a healthy weight, for example.

We can see how the diet, shaped by emotional choices, can ultimately create the physical reality needed to validate the expectations of self.

Hair Loss. Hair symbolizes strength, as recalled in the Biblical story of Samson. When understood symbolically, the *Bible* takes us from self-discovery to material mastery. All of the stories within the *Bible* are metaphors for presenting the Universal Teachings.

When you lose hair due to poor circulation, it is your mind's way of saying there is a lack of a working faith in self, and in your strength to deal with life.

Some would blame heredity (my father and grandfather were bald), and while that may be true, all it does is validate that the same concepts have been passed down from generation to generation. In fact, the *Bible* teaches us this in two different examples. In the New Testament, we read that the fruit does not fall far from the tree, while in the Old Testament, inequities of the father are said to be passed on to the children until the fourth generation.

It can be seen that in our individual growth, we end up emulating our parents—our living examples of how to be and act in the world. We develop the same concepts, and consequently over time we develop the same diseases and conditions as well. We claim these ailments and attributes as part of the family tree: our genetic inheritance. The reality is our concepts govern our attractions to foods, environments, and people, and all of these fulfill our subconscious expectations of what we are supposed to be in order to maintain the acceptance of our mothers.

We want acceptance from our mothers because at a deeply subconscious level, we know we entered the material plane, or world, through the birth canal. The truest part of your mind and self recognizes that we are spiritual beings encased in a body, which is a vehicle for operating in the material world. As spiritual beings we have a tremendous desire to return home to the peace and tranquility of the spiritual plane.

Consequently, we do not want to be rejected by mom, who holds the symbolic portal back to that plane. Mom's concept of what a woman or man should be is demonstrated by attitude and deed. Children observe this, and by the age of three have pretty much created their concepts. They begin to work toward fulfillment of the expectations of what they are supposed to be. In fact, we could spend the rest of our lives fulfilling those expectations.

While some of us seek mother's acceptance, others follow another path; they seek rejection as a form of acceptance. In the first example, the individual is more "like" mom or dad, based on gender. The person on a path of rejection chooses to be the opposite of the same-gender parent. Seeking approval or rejection are both valid forms of acceptance. (To read more on rejection as a form of acceptance, see Section I: From the Inside Out.)

Ringing in the Ears. Two symbologies are at work: one is the petty annoyance of listening to others, and the other is the inability to hear things clearly.

There is an old cliché that "you hear what you want to hear and see what you want to see." In this case, what you hear is distorted, and aspects of auditory communication are lost. A whistling noise is a constant annoyance. Consider this: what are you listening to that is a constant bother or that you do not want to hear? You need to uncover the underlying truths at work; otherwise, those issues may be the very things that lead you down the path to deafness.

Dizziness. Dizziness upon standing up quickly reveals the lack of a working faith. In this respect we are also looking at aspirations.

Rising quickly and moving to the next level is a matter of rising above "it," regardless of what or where that "it" may be, so without faith in self, how is it possible to rise above a situation? Without self-confidence to deal with a situation, you can be come disoriented, and lightheadedness stems from the disorientation. Both lightheadedness and memory issues are a result of lack in faith in self.

The head, blood, and air are all symbolic of spirit in different ways. The head is where thinking occurs, the blood carries oxygen, and air is where the spirit dwells in heaven.

If your circulation is too restricted to allow adequate blood flow to the blood-brain barrier, the brain will not get the vital oxygen it needs. In effect, the brain is starving to death. The brain is a bio-computer that the mind uses to operate the body, thus directing and working its way through material reality.

SYMBOLOGY OF THE NUTRIENTS

Calcium. Hardening of the arteries occurs when you have concepts that imply you lack the courage or confidence to deal with life from a position of strength, and this underlying feeling indicates a lack of working faith in self. In turn, this creates an inability to fully utilize your strength to deal with events and situations. Calcium, symbolic of that strength, is free flowing ions in meaningful amounts in the bloodstream that exist to protect the body on two levels. The first, and maybe the most important, is so the blood does not become too acidic. Acidity in the blood promotes development of disease. The second role of calcium is helping the blood to clot when there is a break, tear, or cut in the skin. This application of strength helps an individual avoid depletion, which leads to weakness.

Hardening of the arteries is interesting symbolically in that it validates a lack of a working faith in self. Physically, what is happening is that plaque is accumulating on the arterial walls. Cholesterol and calcium are the predominant components of plaque, both are vital building materials. Cholesterol is essential to the manufacturing of cells, hormones, and vitamin D.

When a person develops hardening of the arteries, blood flow through the circulatory system is restricted. Symbolically, this represents a lack of faith. Calcium symbolizes strength, so when this mineral is diverted from its proper duties in the body to contribute to hardening of the arteries and other conditions such as kidney or prostate stones, it is another example of how a lack of faith leads to a lack of strength.

Choline. Represents inner strength. When we talk about circulation, we are talking about clogged arteries. It takes strength to move forward in life and unclog blocked situations. Because choline, along with inositol, reduces fat and excess cholesterol by metabolizing them, they clear out the arteries and allow more blood to flow. It takes strength to allow spirit (symbolized by blood) to manifest in your life; not manmade concepts of spirit or the way that man approaches spirit, but truly a working faith in self as opposed to a blind faith. Blind faith is thinking that God is going to do it for you; however, that is not the case.

Inositol. Represents integrity. Inositol helps reduce fats and works hand in hand with choline. An aspect about circulatory issues and clogged arteries is that you are not allowing enough blood to get to the blood-brain barrier. This means that there is not enough oxygen (symbolic of spirit) getting to the brain. It takes integrity of self to pursue truth. It is much easier to follow manmade ways and manmade doctrines than it is to seek the truth of self.

Magnesium and Vitamin D. Symbolic of inspiration, magnesium combines with vitamin D (insights) to ensure your strength is well utilized. The B-vitamins, which represent different aspects of courage and confidence, also provide an open channel for faith and strength to flow freely, allowing spirit to nurture self on all levels.

Niacin/Niacinamide (the non-flushing form). Represents openness and receptivity. In circulatory issues we use it to dilate the arteries to allow more blood to flow to the extremities. What we are really talking about, from another point of view, is being open, being receptive to truth no matter how it comes at you, not having any preconceived ideas. Being open and having the courage and confidence to listen to something, to hear it, and not get caught up in the manmade ideals of what you think it should be because it does not necessarily teach us the truth of how life works or how to live within it requires openness and receptivity.

Pantothenic Acid. Represents inspiration, along with magnesium and vitamin D. These are three key nutrients that allow for inspiration, and life requires inspiration.

Vitamin B-6. Represents protection and regulation. In the circulatory sense, vitamin B-6, along with potassium, diminishes hypertension, because both work together to help regulate the fluid levels in the body. Vitamin B-6 also helps maintain the correct amount of white blood cells in the circulatory system, thus, it acts to protect.

Colds and Flu

Do you know anyone who has not had a cold, the flu, or some kind of respiratory infection?

A cold is a contagious viral or bacterial infection that affects only the upper respiratory tract, and has specific symptoms such as a stuffy nose, watery eyes, low fever, and an overall achy feeling, usually in the joints. While the flu also has specific symptoms, unlike a cold, the flu can attack either the respiratory or intestinal tracts, and either a viral or bacterial infection can spread, circulating in the bloodstream to any area in the body. Both colds and the flu generally spark mucus congestion in the lungs or sinus cavities.

In every infectious situation, whether it is a cold or influenza, there is usually a fever, which can also be spawned by nerve disease, or cancer. The basic metabolism of the body increases as antibodies are formed, and they create an army of fighters to combat the invading force of bacteria, viruses or other toxins. This is when the body creates a fever, also called hyperpyrexia. If a fever is left to run its course without being controlled, in extreme cases it can cause convulsions. Dangerously high fevers are seen in the most serious and contagious diseases, particularly in young children and older adults.

NUTRIENT AND HERBS TO ASSIST THE BODY IN FIGHTING COLDS AND FLU

The following will assist the body in expediting immune response for colds or infections:

Nutrients	Herbs
Beta-carotene (Vitamin A)	Comfrey Root
Vitamin C	Fenugreek
Zinc	Echinacea
	Garlic
	Goldenseal Root
	Slippery Elm Bark

Beta-carotene (Vitamin A). Preferred source of vitamin A because it is non-toxic and is converted to vitamin A only as the body needs it. Vitamin A is important in the maintenance of epithelial and mucosal surfaces and secretions as a form of primary defense.[23,24] It is also important for healthy function of the thymus gland as well as other body systems.

The thymus is active in the production of antibodies, which are proteins, or immunoglobulins, in the blood or saliva that stick to specific germs and neutralize them. Other immune system components that fight bacterias, viruses, fungi, and molds are lymphocytes, macrophages, and interferon.

Vitamin C. Stimulates immune response[25,26] and has a generally positive effect on the common cold.[27]

Zinc. Plays a fundamental role in normal tissue development, including cell division, protein synthesis, and collagen formation.[28] This is very important in the production of antibodies.

Echinacea, Garlic, and Goldenseal Root. All have natural antibiotic properties.

Comfrey Root, Fenugreek, and Slippery Elm Bark. These three herbs are highly effective in breaking up mucus and phlegm in the sinus cavities and lungs. They are the perfect herbal complement to infection-fighting nutrients. In addition to its efficacy against mucus, slippery elm bark also has astringent and anti-inflammatory properties.

SYMBOLOGY OF COLDS AND FLU

The key to mastery of any situation, in this case a cold or flu, rests in being able to read your inner-thoughts at work. Through understanding them, you begin to gain control over them and that leads to mastery and cure. Examining the symptoms of colds and the flu can help to provide the insight necessary to achieve understanding.

Stuffy Nose. Air—oxygen—is essential for everyone. Through the nose, the respiratory system feeds the blood with fresh, live oxygen and all of the "hidden" foods that are a part of the air.

As the Universal Teaching is recalled in John 4:32, Jesus once told his disciples that he had "partaken of food that they knew not of." The implication in this Teaching is that everything the body needs to exist can be found within the air, which is symbolic of the spirit.

As part of your defense system, the nose can tell you when something is offensive or unhealthy and should be avoided. Since everything is a symbolic reflection of thought, detrimental thoughts themselves often pass through this defense mechanism. This happens because of the use of artificial aromas, which are really man-made concepts that give off the appearance and smell of being wholesome and worthwhile.

The commercials seen on television constantly depict misconceptions as truth, most often involving the fare of fast-food restaurants. Eat this food, they tell us, and we will have a happy family life and enjoy great success. In reality, high-fat and salt content in these foods likely will work against your health. In this way, TV ads can circumvent the body's natural defense mechanism.

Symbolically, then, a stuffy nose indicates self-doubt in your ability to handle an upcoming event. Having a cold makes it easier to avoid the situation, so if you are plagued by nasal congestion, take note of when it happens relative to the activities and emotions of your life.

Watery Eyes. Why do the eyes water during a cold or flu? The standard perception is that it is because the eyes are irritated from the bacteria, etc. The more germane question here centers around the symbology of the eyes.

The eyes are your windows to the world. "For those who have eyes to see" is a Universal Teaching which explains that clear vision is the goal of true perception. How do you see yourself, your future? What is the belief system through which your world and life are filtered? If watery eyes plague you during a cold or at any time, reflect on what it is you do not want to see or may not be seeing clearly: do your concepts reflect or refract reality?

Low-grade Fever. What is the symbology of this common symptom of a cold and flu? Again the question becomes what fever represents symbolically. Very simply, it is anger. After all, a fever is synonymous with an elevated body temperature. What is it in life that "burns you up"?

As much as anger at other people, the fever may stem from a situation that first causes you fear and then anger at self because you feel fear.

Achy Body. Depending on the severity of your cold and often with the flu, you will develop body aches, usually in the joints. There are many reasons why the joints ache. The joints are areas of flexibility, and joints are indicative of having an unyielding or unbending attitude about what is occurring, either mentally or environmentally. If you have stiff joints during a cold or flu, take some time to examine the concepts within yourself that would promote stiffness. Remember that stiffness can also indicate unwillingness on your part to change, which might stem from a fear that change will put you at some disadvantage.

Congestion. Another aspect of a cold and flu is congestion. Regardless of the source, congestion is symbolic of an internal attack on your ability to cope with a situation that requires self-confidence at a spiritual level.

FLU-SPECIFIC SYMBOLOGY

Intestinal Tract. Although the flu can be very much like a cold, a key difference is that the flu can attack both the respiratory and intestinal tracts. Earlier in the text, we looked at the symbology of the respiratory tract.

The intestinal tract receives the liquid food that the stomach prepares. Once received, the liquid is further digested, and the nutrients are absorbed through the intestinal wall. Malfunctions occur when you choose not to accept and utilize the nutrients based on symbolic value, or when you choose to expel all material from the tract. A rapid expulsion of material usually occurs when certain thoughts are so unacceptable that the body seeks to reject them.

Each vitamin, mineral, enzyme, and co-enzyme has a symbolic interpretation, and each nutrient performs a specific function within the body. When a physical symbol is needed to get your undivided attention, the mind directs the brain to create the situation in the intestinal tract that will exclude a particular nutrient from being used, this, in turn, will create a shortage and set up the opportunity for a condition or disease to eventually manifest. This is in keeping with your self-image concepts, and is related to a current situation.

SYMBOLOGY OF THE NUTRIENTS

Beta-carotene (Vitamin A). Essential for healthy night vision. Symbolically, with proper vision, especially during periods of preparation (nighttime), you can avoid all of the doubt and frustration that accompanies aspects of preparing for a situation. Vitamin A strengthens vision, thus giving you greater insight.

When you can go into a situation totally prepared, courageously and confidently, the question of your image is not at risk. Without the doubt and fear, your reflection of your inner-confidence will show in an improved complexion.

Another aspect of vitamin A is that it is instrumental in protecting you from invasion from outside forces. This is because vitamin A feeds the thymus gland, which is the immune center. From here, T-cells rush out to do battle with invading forces. On a physical level, those forces can be allergens, germs, bacteria, viruses, fungus, or toxins from the environment, but these forces can also be thoughts from others that are projected onto you.

Vitamin C. Increases absorption of iron, which symbolically deals with faith and courage. Iron, as a major constituent of hemoglobin, helps carry oxygen to the cells, and removes carbon dioxide and carries it to the lungs for removal. Oxygen is symbolic of spirit because the Creator's home (heaven) is in the air (oxygen); therefore, it is symbolic of spirit, while iron, because it is an oxygen carrier, is symbolic of faith and courage.

Vitamin C plays a supportive role in the defenses of the body, and it ensures that the ability to maintain faith and courage are intact. When your courage and faith in self are compromised, doubt and fear set in, opening the door for frustration, anger, and resentment to take hold. All of this can lead to many different diseases, including cancer, as these emotions eat you up alive.

Zinc. Among zinc's roles are those involved in the sensory realms of taste and smell as well as its role in reproduction. Symbolically, zinc reflects those thoughts that contribute to courage, confidence, and expression.

Conditions That Restrict Breathing: Congestion, Asthma, and Emphysema

While congestion, asthma, and emphysema share some basic points, these conditions also have individual traits that necessitate separate discussion. Let us begin by defining some terms.

Congestion is an abnormal collection of fluid in the body, generally found in an organ. Blood usually comprises the congesting substance, although it can also contain bile or mucus. When we speak of congestion, we usually are referring to the type that makes breathing difficult, mainly because of mucus accumulation in the lungs. Sinus cavities can also become congested.

Asthma is a lung disorder marked by attacks of breathing difficulty, wheezing, and coughing, and causes thick mucus to be produced in the lungs. Asthma attacks can be triggered by stimuli such as allergies, infections, vigorous exercise, or emotional stress.

Emphysema is a lung disease categorized as a defect of the lung system. It causes over-inflation of the lungs and destructive changes of the air pouches, which make the lungs become too rigid. When emphysema occurs early in life, it is believed that it is the result of an inherited defect, or caused by damage of the air pouches.

Physical and mental symptoms associated with emphysema include anxiety, high levels of carbon dioxide in the blood, insomnia, confusion, weakness, appetite loss, congestive heart failure, fluid in the lungs, and lung failure.

Because the breathing difficulties experienced by persons with asthma can also cause undue stress on the lungs' air pouches, it seems logical that gaining control of asthma early in life not only is important for the immediate relief of symptoms, but there may also be long-term ramifications relevant to emphysema. Since compromised air pouches figure prominently in the development of emphysema, by controlling or eliminating asthma early on, it may be possible to avoid the full impact of emphysema as well.

NUTRIENTS AND HERBS TO SUPPORT IMMUNE FUNCTION AND BREATHING

To strengthen overall immune response and support the body in combating the symptoms associated with breathing congestion, include the following nutrients and herbs:

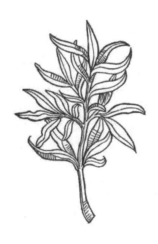

Nutrients	Herbs
Beta-carotene (Vitamin A)	Comfrey Root
Folic Acid	Fenugreek
Magnesium	Mullein
Niacin/Niacinamide	Slippery Elm Bark
Pantothenic acid	
Potassium	
Vitamin B-1	
Vitamin B-2	
Vitamin B-6	
Vitamin C	
Vitamin D	
Zinc	

Beta-carotene (Vitamin A). Due to its non-toxic nature, it is the preferred source of vitamin A, which is important in the maintenance of epithelial and mucosal surfaces and secretions as a form of primary defense. Beta-carotene is converted to vitamin A only as the body needs it.

Folic Acid. Has a direct nourishing and fortifying effect on the "front line" of the body's defense system.

Magnesium. Helps regulate the body's acid-alkaline balance. The body becomes more susceptible to disease when the blood is acidic.

Vitamin B-1, B-2, B-6, and Pantothenic Acid. Involved in nourishing the adrenal glands. These nutrients play a vital role because of the strain illness or stress places on the adrenals. When the adrenal glands are taxed and depleted, the result can be an under-performing immune system that can lead to prolonged recovery times for any illness or condition attacking the body.

Vitamin C. Stimulates immune response. It also has a generally positive effect on the common cold, fights bacterial infections, and reduces the effects of some allergy-producing substances.

Zinc. Plays a fundamental role in normal tissue development, including cell division, protein synthesis, and collagen formation. Zinc is very important in the production of antibodies, and plays an important role in nourishing the thymus gland, the "seat" of the immune system, and in liberating from the liver another source of thymus nourishment, vitamin A.

Fenugreek. A powerful herb used to support removal of mucus from the body.

Mullein. Highly effective in breaking up mucus and phlegm in the sinus cavities and lungs.

Slippery Elm Bark. Both an astringent and anti-inflammatory, which helps to reduce inflammation in the lungs. It also works at removing mucus from the body.

Symbology of Breathing Problems

In order to gain the clearest perception of asthma and emphysema, let us work from the youngest age up. The first thing that we find in looking at asthma in children is that infants can be afflicted with this condition based on hereditary factors.

Having said that, let us also consider the symbolic paradox that hereditary diseases do not exist. This position comes from a belief in reincarnation during which your soul returns to earth in a new body after the death of your previous physical body. This process allows you to continue to work on your soul and spirit until you master self, also called the great "I AM" within.

To that end, in each life cycle you choose your parents because they represent the concepts that you must overcome in order to become a master of the self. Since we chose our parents, we have to acknowledge the fact that we chose to be born with a particular disease, if it serves our growth. Because all disease is symbolic of particular thoughts, concepts, and actions, it holds the elements that you seek to understand as part of your path to mastery of these concepts.

An illness represents concepts in conflict with spiritual law, and that an illness appears to be hereditary is based on two things. First, there is a Biblical understanding that the concept needs to be worked out. This is demonstrated in Exodus 20:5 when the Creator said to the Israelites, "visiting the inequity of the fathers upon the children unto the third and fourth generation." Now what that means is that as each soul incarnates, it is thought that within four generations an understanding would be reached. When we go back to the metaphysical or the symbolic interpretation of the number 4, we find its meaning to be an advancement (moving forward in life) or a block (being stymied). Therefore, souls entering the fourth life cycle would have identified, understood, and controlled that particular conceptual difficulty, and hereditary disease would no longer exist.

The second factor in the heredity concept is that, as the Emotional Self gains understanding, it changes the diet of the Physical Self, and the diet determines the construction of the body. The diet changes the physical characteristics that will be passed on to offspring. The bodies of the fourth generation will be of a different cellular structure. Therefore, the result is a different level of health, and this is why there is no hereditary disease, only the concepts that remain to be mastered.

Asthmatic attacks have many causes, each dependent upon the concepts that the person is dealing with at the time. For some, a narrowing of the lungs' airways resulting from muscle spasms in the lungs causes the attacks. For others, it could be the swelling of the bronchial tubes or excess mucus in the lungs. Repeated asthma attacks can result in shortness of breath. Since air is symbolic of spirit, and spirit is symbolic of faith in self, the tie-in to shortness of breath can readily be seen.

Hereditary Disease. Asthma is often found in infants born into a family with a history of allergies. Heredity is in keeping with the understanding that each soul/person is here to work out/on a particular understandings that will facilitate mastery, and the need here is to understand/master sensitivity and fear.

Allergies. The allergies that induce asthma are often food-linked. Foods are a symbolic reflection of specific thoughts, feelings, and emotions, so each food that attracts or repels you has a deep emotional association attached to it. This is one reason most people do not abandon their cultural foods.

Understanding food allergies requires that you identify each food that causes you problems. Think back to your first memories associated with that food. An allergy to bananas, for example, might stem from a childhood incident in which your father threw a banana at your mother and hit her, she began to cry, a fight between your parents ensued, and the allergy was formed. In this case, bananas have become linked with aggression, violence, and profound sadness deep in your subconscious mind. You are sensitive about the situation, and that sensitivity carries over to the food.

Asthma attacks can be triggered by allergens other than foods. In these cases, understanding the reasons is a bit more complex on one level, but easier on another.

It is always easier to see things in others than it is to see things in yourself, and the same holds true for understanding the symbolic significance of something. If it is a part of you, then your vision is blocked by your defenses.

One of the most difficult things in life is to acknowledge that there is something wrong with your personality or emotional makeup. Even if the symbol you seek to understand exists outside of your emotional connections, it will still be distorted by your defenses but only to the degree that you are not willing to see the truth of the matter. In short: you will see what you want to see. Yet the reality is you need to see everything that you can and examine it symbolically to truly understand the forces or energies at work. You must learn to detach yourself as much as possible to get an objective view of what you are going through.

Children between three and eight years of age comprise the next age group that asthma seems to affect. The numerological symbology of these two numbers is significant. When a child reaches three years of age, he or she is starting a major life cycle. Three is the number of understanding. You must learn to understand that you and you alone are the cause of all of your situations, and you create all of your own problems. An unfortunate aspect of the Teaching "ask, and you shall receive" is that most people assume the requests are conscious, when actually it is the subconscious doing all of the asking in an attempt to fulfill expectations. So here you have a child that is trying to understand so many different roles, attitudes, positions, and feelings. This little person is in a true developmental state, so if doubt and fear are taught, interjected, or demonstrated, the child will doubtlessly feed on these emotions and make them his own.

After all, the child's role model has set the stage for what is expected, and when the child feels incapable of living up to those expectations, fear sets in—fear of failing and of being rejected—and it becomes easier to avoid the possibility of failure entirely by becoming incapacitated by illness.

The symbolic significance of the number eight represents material mastery. Man as master of self, being in balance and harmony, will master the material plane. When you add up any of the numbers that make up the number eight you will always come to the same conclusion, material mastery. Here is the math: seven (cycle) and one (unity), when a person is unified within self there is progression; six (man) and two (balance and harmony) create the same energy, advancement; five (senses) and three (understanding); and four (advancement) and four equals growth and forward movement.

Having examined the numbers from a symbolic perspective it is easier to understand why asthma would begin in the age span of three to eight years old.

Interestingly, asthma occurs before puberty twice as often in boys than in girls. Most boys are taught from the beginning the misconception that they must be leaders and providers, and be strong and independent throughout life. At the same time, they are not encouraged or taught that they are able; children in general are taught not to be powerful and not to have faith in their own ability to understand and master. So, they become infused both with the expectations placed on males and with doubt in their own ability to achieve, fearing even to try. Burdened with these misconceptions about life, boys develop asthma, or other conditions, as a means of coping with the paradox.

As time goes on, both girls and boys are affected equally during adolescence by asthma. While expectations for the two sexes are different at this point, they are equally stressful. This is a time when a person's personality and presence in the world begin to develop fully, and soon, these young adults will reach the time when they must go out into the world and make their mark, to be whom they think they are.

It is also during this particular timeframe that doubt and fear wreak havoc on an adolescent's courage and self-confidence. These emotions often manifest in breathing difficulties, a common, major symptom of asthma, emphysema, and congestion because the lungs are full of mucus. Symbolically, the breathing difficulty signifies that the person is dealing with thoughts, energies, forces, or situations so overwhelming that he or she begins to drown in their substance.

Congestion and difficulty, regardless of the source, always reflects strong self-doubt. It is through the action of your lungs that you receive the breath of life, and you inhale that which will nourish and sustain you. You exhale that which is used and no longer beneficial, that which would cause harm, damage, and possibly death if it were kept within the body.

The same can be said for man-made concepts, or misconceptions of truth. When you continue to rely upon these and do not exhale or purge them from your system through understanding their source, they can result in accidents, sickness, allergies, and sometimes death.

Other Asthma Triggers

Inhaling Foreign Substances. These substances can be minute physical particles, such as pollens, molds, or dust. In symbolic terms, a foreign substance represents an external thought that is being projected onto the individual. Remember, asthma can germinate out of allergies. This is in keeping with the basic understanding that allergies are a sensitivity problem, so the person with asthma is also highly sensitive to imposition, and on top of that, there is doubt and a fear factor.

Foreign thoughts, in the form of pollen, represent new ideas that could generate some type of change or growth. Molds, another source of asthmatic attacks, represent living, active, and invasive thoughts that pressure the individual into responses not necessarily in keeping with his or her attitudes and desires. There may not even be the capacity to carry out the actions that the thoughts may represent. Dust is symbolic of the everyday residue of life that seems to linger and annoy.

Airborne Pollutants. Another source of aggravation to the body can be gases such as chemical airborne pollutants.

A specific type of chemical may also have meaning, take cleaning fluid, for example. Suppose a child's father worked in a dry-cleaning plant. When the father came home from work each evening, he was always in a bad mood, so the child might develop an allergy to the cleaning fluid as a means of avoiding close contact with the father.

Other Triggers. Infections, exercise, and emotional stress can set off asthma attacks.

Symbology of the Nutrients

Beta-carotene (Vitamin A). Essential for healthy night vision. What is the symbolic significance of night vision? Night, itself, symbolizes a time of preparation. It is when, through your dreams, that you receive proper guidance on actions to take based on your personal patterns of behavior. If you cannot clearly see which path to take, then you will proceed with doubt, so it can be said that the night is symbolic of both preparation and doubt.

With proper vision, especially during periods of preparation (nighttime), you can avoid all of the doubt and frustration that can accompany dealing with a situation. Vitamin A helps you to see better, giving you greater insight into the situation. When you can go into a situation totally prepared and with clear vision, then the question of your ability is not an issue, and without the doubt and fear, your inner-confidence will show you the best path for accomplishing your goals.

Another aspect of vitamin A is that it is instrumental in protecting you from invasion from outside forces. This is because vitamin A feeds the thymus gland, which is the immune center. From here, T-cells rush out to do battle with invading forces. On a physical level those forces can be allergens, bacteria, viruses, fungus, or toxins from the environment. Symbolically, those external forces can also be the thoughts, deeds, and actions of others projected onto you.

Vitamin A is important for the outer cellular layer of many tissues and organs, such as the mucous membranes. The mucous membranes are the thin sheets of tissue cells that cover or line various parts of the body that open to the outside. Examples include linings of the mouth, digestive tube, breathing passages, and the genital and urinary tracts. The mucous membranes release mucus; mucus contains water, cast-off tissue cells, mucin, and white blood cells. Mucin is a carbohydrate that is the main part of mucus, and it is present in most glands that release mucus.

White blood cells, also called leukocytes, function in the destruction of bacteria, fungus, and viruses, and render harmless poisonous substances that may result from allergic reactions and cellular injury.

Folic Acid. A fortifier, this nutrient helps symbolically in building and defending your perceptions of the truth. Truth is always a relevant term, which is why you must know yourself so that you can see the truth of the Universal Teachings and look away from the teachings of man. The teachings of man instill doubt, fear, and other negative attributes that affect lives in a negative way.

Magnesium. As a facilitator, it assists in the assimilation of thoughts that lead to strength. From a position of strength, all actions taken, lead to a positive conclusion, but when you act out of fear, doubt, uncertainty, or with a lack of self-confidence, the seeds for failure are sown.

There is a Universal Teaching, from Matthew 25:29, appropriate to mention at this point, and it deals with strength: "For unto every one that hath shall be given, and he shall have abundance: but from him that hath not shall be taken away even that which he hath." In contemporary parlance, this means to use what you have been given in order to keep it and to receive more. The lesson is clear: if you have a faculty or a way of thinking, and you choose not to utilize it, you will no longer have access to it, and at that point, it can and will begin to work against you.

Niacin/Niacinamide. Represents openness and receptivity. The receptivity associated with niacinamide is due in part to the role it plays in growth, nerve function, metabolism, and how it affects the cardiovascular system, which is responsible for the delivery of the blood throughout the entire body. Blood, the lifeline of the body, represents spirit within the material realm. Blood carries all the nutrients to each cell within the body, it feeds and cleans the cells, and carries away the toxins that will destroy the body if left to collect.

In a similar fashion, poisonous thoughts left within the mind to operate freely will ultimately damage or even kill a person. All toxins, from both the thought and physical realms, must be eliminated from the system if there is to be true growth.

Pantothenic Acid. Symbolically, on one level this nutrient represents inspiration, due to pantothenic acid's nourishing of the adrenals. The adrenals produce hormones that help the body deal with taking quick actions based upon quick decisions, and this is reflected in the "flight or fight" concept.

When you face a daunting force, you might go into a state of fear, and your reaction to this fear is based upon your self-concept and self-confidence. The part of the body that reacts to the impulse of fear is the adrenal glands, which send out hormonal messages to signal body parts about how to react.

Pantothenic acid is the nutrient that represents your inspiration, courage, and confidence. This is because of the role it plays in growth, energy, and the health of the body. When you have tired or exhausted adrenals, you lack energy, and energy is directly related to enthusiasm, inspiration, and confidence.

Potassium. Represents balance and harmony, the keys to flexible thinking. When there is balance within, you can bend in any area or direction without fear of falling over or losing balance.

Vitamin B-6. Symbolically, on one level vitamin B-6 represents balance. In this instance balance is maintained through the correct amount of white blood cells necessary to keep the person in a good state of health, and vitamin B-6 acts to create balance within the system. This can be seen by how it works within the body by increasing the number of mature phagocytes.

It is interesting to realize how important balanced thinking is in regard to gaining strength, and without strength, you believe that you are helpless in dealing with the forces or energies of life. The truth of this perception is seen in the physical fact that a vitamin B-6 deficiency leads to impaired immune response and muscle weakness.

Vitamin C. Increases absorption of iron, which symbolically deals with faith and courage. Iron, as a major constituent of hemoglobin, helps carry oxygen to the cells, and removes carbon dioxide and carries it to the lungs for removal. Oxygen is symbolic of spirit because the Creator's home (heaven) is in the air (oxygen); therefore, it is symbolic of spirit, while iron, because it is an oxygen carrier, is symbolic of faith and courage.

Vitamin C plays a supportive role in the defenses of the body, and it ensures that the ability to maintain faith and courage are intact. When your courage and faith in self are compromised, doubt and fear set in, opening the door for frustration, anger, and resentment to take hold. All of this can lead to many different diseases, including cancer, as these emotions eat you up alive.

Vitamin D. Has a role in calcium absorption which tells us that vitamin D represents insight and, to a degree, understanding.

This interpretation is based on the fact that calcium represents strength; after all, it helps to build the bones of the body, and provides support. Without insight and understanding, it would be virtually impossible to achieve true strength. Look at how vitamin D is manufactured in the body, it requires sunlight, which is symbolic of insight and seeing clearly. Nothing is hidden in the light, especially if you have the eyes to see.

Zinc. Among zinc's functions are those involved in the sensory realms of taste and smell; it also plays a role in reproduction. Symbolically, zinc reflects those thoughts that contribute to courage, confidence and expression.

Through understanding the symbolic interpretations of the various nutrients, you can begin to see clearly how interconnected everything is. It is through the efforts made at "seeing and hearing" that one learns to see the truth in everything.

Constipation

Although constipation has many causes, the diet is the major contributing factor. Certain medications are also known to be a causative factor for constipation. It is interesting to look through the Physician's Desk Reference (PDR) and see how different drugs have side effects that can cause constipation.

One potential and often ignored cause is a compromised level of minerals, another would be an obstruction somewhere in the intestinal tract, a condition so serious it would require a medical procedure to remedy.

American eating habits and food manufacturing processes have combined to render ours a diet lacking in fiber, another major cause of constipation. People eat not only flesh food but also so much processed food, especially bread, pastries, white rice, and cereals. Most food products derived from grain do not incorporate the grain's protective fiber shell, which is often removed for better processing and quicker cooking.

Fiber has at least two important roles within the intestinal environment. Cellulose fiber breaks down and becomes foodstuff for some of the beneficial microbes that live within the intestinal tract. Fiber also acts as a gentle "broom" of sorts, sweeping against the intestinal villi, the fingerlike threads through which nutrients are absorbed into the bloodstream, and also moves matter along the digestive pathway to help ensure that nothing clogs the lining of the intestines.

Fiber in the intestinal tract acts as a triggering device. It absorbs water, swells, and pushes matter against the colon walls, which signals the brain to evacuate. Nerve endings within the intestinal wall sense the pressure and tell the brain to create the muscular motions that are necessary to move fecal matter through the colon. It is in this respect that a mineral deficiency can contribute to constipation. Minerals are essential for muscular contractions, so if minerals are low, the muscles will not efficiently move matter through the colon.

What some health professionals overlook is that almost all transactions within the body, outside of manufacturing and mitosis, are muscle-driven. Manufacturing refers to the glands' production of the enzymes and hormonal messengers that regulate and command the systems within the body, but even those substances are squeezed out of the glands by muscles.

Although we do not often think of it as such, constipation can be life threatening. As fecal matter sits in the colon, toxins from it are reabsorbed into the body.

Constipation can be eliminated by increasing fiber in the diet, eating more organically grown raw fruits and vegetables, increasing liquid consumption—particularly distilled water and organic fruit and vegetable juices—and avoiding milk and sodas. It is also best not to consume liquids at meals, which dilutes the digestive juices and could cause fermentation of foodstuffs, resulting in gas and bloating. Taking probiotics, such as acidophilus, helps digestion, assimilation, and elimination. Taking multi-minerals is also of primary importance because minerals participate in enzyme transactions as well as muscular transactions. Drinking aloe vera juice after each meal is another suggestion because this can act as a lubricant, as can oil and vinegar dressing on salads.

Finally, do not forget to exercise, which benefits circulation to the entire body, including the muscles involved in digestion and evacuation.

NUTRIENTS AND HERBS FOR CONSTIPATION

Nutrients	Herbs
Calcium	Apple Pectin
Magnesium	Butternut Root Bark
	Prunes
	Senna

Calcium and Magnesium. Both support contractibility and relaxation of muscle. This facilitates the muscular transactions necessary to move matter through the intestinal tract. They are also vital for proper elimination, as this too is controlled by muscles.

Apple Pectin. Along with other fibers is excellent for the intestinal tract. Fiber is beneficial for many different reasons such as: pushing matter along, absorbing toxins, and helping to absorb bile acids which prevent the breakdown of fats and the absorption of water to help matter flow easily.

Butternut Root Bark, Prunes, Senna. Are well known for aiding in bowel movements. They act like laxatives without the addictive nature of those types of products.

SYMBOLOGY OF CONSTIPATION

Constipation symbolically represents holding on to the past. This is indicative of an unwillingness to let go of past ideas, values, standards, and guides, all of which are based on the man-made concepts within the subconscious mind, and these concepts create your belief system.

When you hold on to the past ideas and concepts, and do not allow yourself to change, you limit yourself, and this, in turn, could create frustration, resentment, and anger. All of these energies are the beginnings of different diseases, and this is exactly what happens when a person is constipated, the toxic material is not purged from the system, so the poisons re-enter the body and corrupt it, and disease is born.

Concepts are something that must be purged and replaced with healthy ideas of how to live in keeping with the Universal Teachings that govern all life. It does not matter what causes the constipation, be it medication, lack of minerals, or a blockage, all these situations are also symbolic.

In the case of medications, the individual is seeking a man-made solution to an internal problem. Whatever the problem is that they are taking medication for will be tied into past concepts and the inability to move out of the past. Arthritis, symbolic of inflexible thinking, is similar to constipation. In both cases, the person can not let go of past concepts, ideas and standards as how to act/respond in every given situation. Constipation is simply holding tighter, and will kill you much quicker than arthritis.

One of the most common approaches to dealing with arthritis is taking pain medications and/or aspirins. The pain is alleviated but the disease and its destructive effects are still taking place. In time, the affected joints will wear out and need to be replaced. Again we see man-made thinking at work, without the true cause of the condition being dealt with. By changing the diet and understanding causes, true healing takes place.

Symbology of the Nutrients for Constipation

Calcium. Symbolic of strength, and it takes strength to deal with life. When you develop your personal power you can flow through with minimal angst because you know that you can handle whatever is placed in front of you. It also takes strength to let go of past concepts and ideas that you maintain about yourself. It is the holding on to the past that is the real detriment to health on all levels.

Magnesium. Represents inspiration and that is essential along with strength to enjoy/master the opportunities that life presents. When you are inspired you are willing and able to try new things, have new experiences and above all express in new ways. When you hold onto the past it stifles growth in expression.

In the end, without strength and inspiration the truth of constipation is experienced: death from toxicity.

Symbology of the Nutrients and Enzymes of Digestion

When we think of constipation, we do not normally think about nutrients being involved because on one level there is a lack of fiber in the diet, but on another level it is how the body functions.

In order for digestion to take place, enzymes are squeezed into the stomach, which is manipulated by muscles to mix the enzymes and food matter. The food matter is then broken down even further into chyme. The chyme enters into the intestinal tract, and these nutrients are absorbed along with toxins into the bloodstream while the fibers and undigested matter continue on. Muscular movement gently moves all of that material through the tract to a point in the colon, where it accumulates. Here it sits until the brain receives the signal to move it out of the body. At this point, the process of emptying the colon is accomplished through muscular transactions. Calcium and magnesium are required to facilitate the flow of electrical impulses from the brain to communicate with the muscles. Once the connection is made and the electricity flows, the muscles respond accordingly, and the toxic matter is released.

The person who is dealing with constipation needs only to identify and understand the concepts at work to have the strength and the ability to handle life's events. There is no need to hold on to the past (accumulated physical and mental toxins) as a form of security to deal with the present.

Remember that when fecal matter remains in the colon beyond the normal period of time for it to have been eliminated, the body will begin to re-absorb toxins in the colon, just as if we do not let go of our past, we will not have a healthy present and will not be able to achieve a healthy future.

Cramps

Cramps can occur in any muscle within the body. They are perhaps most often associated with menstruation in women or as a result of strenuous physical activity.

Cramps happen when a muscle contracts but does not relax. What causes it to contract, and what prevents in from relaxing? The quick answer: minerals. Cramping can be caused by a lack of them, particularly calcium, magnesium, potassium, or phosphorus.

Calcium and magnesium, especially, are vitally important in muscular function because they are catalysts, acting like light switches to facilitate the flow of electrical current, and this electricity stems from thought. Minerals allow the electricity of thought to make the leap from nerve ending to receptor sites on the cells of the muscles, and they transport the electrical impulses that tell the muscle what to do—thought energy, if you will—so that the muscle will contract or relax accordingly.

NUTRIENTS AND HERBS TO SUPPORT THE BODY IN DEALING WITH MUSCLE CRAMPS

Nutrients	*Herbs*
Calcium	Hops
Magnesium	Skullcap
Phosphorus	Valerian Root
Potassium	Wild Lettuce
Vitamin D	

Calcium. A mineral involved in neuromuscular excitability and transmission of nerve impulses. When calcium levels become low in the blood, increased neuromuscular irritability, seizures, and cardiac cramps are possible.

Magnesium. Deficiency symptoms include muscle fasciculation (involuntary twitching), tremors, and muscle spasms to name a few.

Phosphorus. Essential for calcium assimilation.

Potassium. Required to stimulate nerve endings for muscle contractions.

Vitamin D. Must be present for the assimilation and utilization of calcium. Vitamin D is so effective in helping the body to assimilate calcium that it has been used by itself to dissolve joint and spinal calcium deposits.

Hops, Skullcap, Valerian Root, and Wild Lettuce. All have calming, relaxing properties.

SYMBOLOGY OF CRAMPS

Cramps are symbolic of inflexibility to some degree. Because of the physical nature of cramping, wherein a muscle becomes somewhat rigid, cramps indicate a lack of flexibility in thinking.

To determine where doubt is at work in your life, look closely at the area where cramping occurs: legs, back, stomach, reproductive area, etc. Doubt in your ability to handle a situation causes a constriction in thinking, which is reflected in the cramping of the related muscle. To better understand the area of your life in which you may lack confidence, study the symbology of the body part or system afflicted by cramps. This exercise will give you insight.

Cramps also occur during particular parts of cycles. Life consists of cycles, and we are constantly going through them. This is why the cliché "history repeats itself" is so very true, especially when it comes to personal history.

SYMBOLOGY OF THE NUTRIENTS

It is interesting that there are four essential minerals for eliminating cramping in the body: calcium, magnesium, potassium, and phosphorus. The number 4 symbolically represents advancement on the positive side and a blockage on the negative side.

Remember that almost everything in the body is muscle-driven, so for movement to take place, muscles must act in harmony with each other. The realization of every task or journey undertaken by man is dependent on this harmonious movement.

Studying the symbology of the minerals involved in muscular transactions will allow you to see all of the essential ingredients and energies for getting a handle on life, and these energies allow for the mastering of life itself.

Daily life requires an enormous amount of strength to cope with the energetic forces from the emotional, social, material, and physical levels. Should you be confronted by something that challenges your personal belief system, you would require courage to stand your ground and stay committed to your convictions. When these situations occur, you must also look closely at your convictions—are they based on false, man-made concepts or on the insights and understandings that come from knowing Universal Truths? Do you have to defend your position and perceptions regarding how life is to be lived?

Calcium. Symbolic of strength. What is a cramping situation but something that stops you from moving forward, whether it is a belly cramp, a leg cramp or a back cramp. A cramp is when the muscle becomes so tight that it restricts use. What is it that stops you from utilizing what you have? Usually, it is doubt, fear and a lack of courage and confidence. Calcium, representing strength, works with magnesium (inspiration), to relax the muscles. Between strength and inspiration you have a regulatory mode of keeping the muscles agile and in perfect balance and harmony, ready to move forward in a moment's notice.

Magnesium. Magnesium symbolizes inspiration. Inspiration leads to flexibility of thinking because when you are inspired you seek more than one perspective. If you have and can manifest strength, courage, and inspiration in your every endeavor, you would be more open to seeing, you would be more flexible, and there would be no muscle cramping on any level.

Phosphorus. Symbolic of courage. Again, we can see how it, too, would work together with calcium (strength); both are essential in order to move forward in life. Movement requires an un-cramped ability, freedom of movement, freedom to go forward, and that takes courage.

Potassium. Potassium symbolizes balance and harmony. It is essential for the physical functioning of the body, and it reflects the need for balance between material and spiritual considerations.

This illustrates the point that a fine balance must be maintained in all aspects. Life, like health, has to be maintained in proper balance, or it can become distorted, and these distortions can lead a person to become so engrossed in the material plane that they become unbalanced. Were you to become potassium-depleted, you would begin to experience cramping and a tendency toward water retention. With water being symbolic of the material plane, we can see where the dependency or co-dependency on the material becomes dominant and overwhelming.

Vitamin D. Represents inspiration. If you have inspiration, it is easy to move forward when your muscles are working properly.

Diabetes

Diabetes is a metabolic disease affecting how the body uses glucose, or blood sugar.

One indication of diabetes is that the person suffers from the constant need to drink fluids, often with no other symptoms. An unconscious person with diabetes insipidus or Type I during surgery or accidental injury will still produce great amounts of urine, so if enough fluids are not given, the patient becomes severely dehydrated and develop electrolyte and mineral imbalance.

Another type of diabetes is Type II diabetes mellitus. Here the main cause is a defect in the parts of receptor cells that accept the insulin. The disease tends to run in families but may be triggered by outside factors such as physical stress, obesity and ingestion of too many refined carbohydrates.

The pancreas releases insulin when it detects sugar in the blood stream. Insulin also promotes the transport and entry of sugar into the muscle cells and other tissues while lowering the amount of sugar in the blood stream.

When the pancreas does not produce enough insulin, the symptoms of diabetes mellitus develop, including weight loss, tiredness and lethargy. As with diabetes insipidus, the symptoms in diabetes mellitus also include frequent urination and increased thirst, but these are often accompanied by weight loss and increased appetite. Sugar levels in the blood and urine will be high, in addition, the eyes, kidneys, nervous system, and skin may be affected. Infections are common and hardening of the arteries often develops.

There are several diabetes-linked complications, many involving the eyes or vision. For instance, diabetic amaurosis is a form of blindness that can be caused by bleeding into the retina. Cataracts are another vision problem that seems to be common in both Type I and Type II diabetes. Problems arising from poor circulation and infections are also a concern for those with diabetes. A related skin disorder, xanthoma, which produces yellow bumps on the skin in uncontrolled diabetes mellitus, disappears when the disease is brought under control.

When diabetes is present, the body cannot process all of the starches and refined sugars coming into the system from our diets. The pancreas, which has the sole responsibility of producing insulin for the body, becomes overloaded. The emotional/mental aspects need to be changed, and this change is equal or even greater than the need to change the diet.

Nutrients, Amino Acids and Herbs to Support Circulation and Insulin Production

The following will assist your body in increasing metabolism, insulin production, circulation to the extremities, and beta cells in the pancreas; in opening arteries; and in neutralizing acidity in the blood.

Nutrients	Amino Acids	Herbs
Chromium	L-Glutamine	Blueberry Leaf
Iodine		Cedar Berries
Niacin/Niacinamide		Goldenseal Root
Vitamin B-1		Kelp
Zinc		

Chromium. The primary role of chromium is to maintain normal levels of blood sugar (glucose) that act as fuel for the body. If glucose levels are high, supplementation lowers them; if levels are low, supplementation raises them.[29]

Iodine. A component of the thyroid hormone helps regulate the body's production of energy, promotes growth and development, and stimulates metabolism. Metabolism is a strong factor in the body's ability to burn fuel (glucose, fat).

Niacin/Niacinamide. Aids in the metabolism of fats, carbohydrates, and proteins.

Vitamin B-1. Needed for carbohydrate metabolism.

Zinc. Needed for the synthesis of insulin. Zinc binds to insulin and enhances its activity.

L-Glutamine. An amino acid that lessens the craving for sweets.

Cedar Berries. Used to stimulate the pancreas. If there are beta-cells left in the pancreas, where insulin is produced, the combination of herbs will stimulate them.

Goldenseal Root. Supports lowering blood sugar levels.

Kelp. Provides iodine, which is essential for thyroid hormone production. The hormones regulate metabolism helping to burn off some of the stored fat (energy). That is what fat is, stored energy, and too much of it becomes a problem.

SYMBOLOGY OF DIABETES

Diabetes is a disease that affects how the body deals with sugar. Sugar in this context refers to glucose.

Glucose is a simple sugar found in certain foods, especially fruits, and is a major source of energy in both animals and humans. Glucose, when eaten or produced through the process of digestion of carbohydrates, enters into the bloodstream from the intestines. The excess glucose that is not immediately used as fuel for the body is converted into glycogen, which is usually stored in the muscles and liver. When the body requires additional fuel it converts glycogen back into glucose.

It is here in the conversion process that problems arise, and diabetes is able to manifest. Immediately there are two insights as to the cause of diabetes on an emotional level. The first deals with the concept of sugar itself, the second deals with the inability to convert thought into action. In other words, it relates to having the power or fuel (glucose) but not the ability to use (metabolize) it properly.

Sugar, by common understanding, is a substance that is sweet, and is also a substance that can make other things taste sweet. Questions arise here about what the person dealing with diabetes thinks is sweet, and why he or she cannot deal with it.

Sugar, particularly processed sugar, is an empty food—by that I mean it has no nutritional value, and does nothing good for the body. In truth, sugar is totally unnecessary and may actually be more detrimental than is realized. For instance, if food is foul, rotten, spoiled, or vile tasting, it can be doctored with sugar to make it taste good. In that disguise, it bypasses the taste buds and enters into the system. This very technique, in fact, is used to sneak medicine into children. It may also be a way that the major food peddlers pawn off less than healthy food onto American consumers.

Sugar is symbolic of the desire to have and enjoy the sweets of life, while each person has very personal sweets, there are certain ones that everyone shares. For example, everybody wants to have a great job and make lots of money.

In the material world, money has been portrayed as the key to happiness. So everyone pursues money for the purpose of being happy, content, and fulfilled. Yet, when you look at all the people who have money and who still appear unhappy, what does that say? For many of these individuals, the solution they seek is to acquire even more money and things. Money is used to buy the sweets in life: gold, diamonds, bigger homes, fancier cars, and expensive designer clothing. Unfulfilled, some people use their money to purchase sex, drugs, and other diversions that they hope will help them to feel good about themselves.

Sugar, much like the money-bartered sweets that it reflects, is an empty substance that cannot truly satisfy any hunger on any level in a nourishing way. I use the term "nourishing" because when anything does not contribute to your growth and welfare, be it a situation, person or substance, then by that virtue alone it works against you. This is recalled in Matthew 12:30, the Universal Teaching: "He that is not with me is against me." Much like the sugar that a diabetic craves, money, and the sweet things it can buy, cannot fill the craving within.

The second problem with this condition is the inability to convert stored or circulating glucose into action. Action creates the need for more fuel, so as you burn it your body must convert glucose, and even glycogen, into fuel. It is the same with your thoughts, and there are many reasons why a person would have trouble converting thoughts into actions: feelings of unworthiness, a lack of ability, or fear might block these actions.

Thoughts are precursors to action, and every thought that you have requires an action on one level or another. If you have the thought that you are hungry, then you may go to the kitchen to satisfy that thought, but once there and having eaten something, you may still be hungry for the feeling of being satiated. This requires yet another action because the feeling of being satiated is still not accomplished, so you eat more to reach that point of being fulfilled or satisfied. Now you have all this food/energy stored—some call that stored energy fat—and you continue to eat, storing more because the right action that would lead to fulfillment and being satiated has not yet been experienced because you have not yet found the proper food that will nourish you.

Obviously the food that will nourish you is not outside of you but is within your own mind and it is your mind that directs your life. Guided and motivated by your ego, your mind is always seeking to fulfill self-expectations. If you believe, as many diabetics do sub-consciously, that you are unworthy of having the sweets of life, then you will not be able to properly metabolize glucose, or sugar, in your body. Hence, diabetes may occur.

Going back to diabetes insipidus, we note that this form of the disorder is marked by extreme thirst and heavy urination. It is fascinating to realize that water, the object of thirst, is symbolic of life in the material plane. This is in keeping with the understanding that air is symbolic of the spiritual plane, and without water or air (oxygen), life would cease. Another aspect of this is the understanding that humanity is a spiritual entity within a material vehicle. I use the term vehicle because the body serves the same purpose as a car: you use it to go from place to place, and it carries your consciousness around within the material plane.

Without air, you will die, and without water, you will die. The secret is in finding balance. An extreme thirst indicates that the individual has not found the truth that will quench their thirst for the self-acceptance that leads to fulfillment, and the heavy urination symbolizes the need of both body and mind to cleanse themselves of those toxins that can destroy them.

With diabetes, there are high levels of acid in the blood. This symbolizes the mind's efforts to eliminate those concepts that are eating at the person with poisonous, acidic thoughts about how life should be. I say "acidic" here in the sense that these thoughts that are based on man-made teachings are empty and hollow, just like the sugar that causes diabetes.

In diabetes, the heavy urination problem stems from a deficiency of a hormone that regulates the amount of urine made by the body. This transaction, as well as all other hormonal or enzymatic exchange within the body, is the result of thought. Every transaction in the body results from a stimulus, and the brain is a part of each of these actions. The brain receives its directives from the mind, which tells it what functions must be carried out and when, but the body also is a vehicle with its own Divine Intelligence. It seeks to care for itself by carrying out certain transactions without the appearance of conscious thought; however, the mind has controlling influence over the brain and, consequently, over the body. If there is a need for diabetes to manifest as a way to help the individual soul to understand some of the concepts that it must work out and bring into harmony, then the mind will tell the brain to slow down the production of a particular hormone, for example, insulin because the mind is the controlling factor in all matters of life and health.

Another cause of diabetes insipidus is the kidneys' failure to respond to the hormone that regulates urine production. The kidneys remove the wastes that are in liquid form from your bloodstream, and if this system failed, your body would be poisoned to death. The kidneys act to balance the blood's liquid content, they balance the water levels in the body as well as the acidity and alkalinity of the blood. Kidney problems can also mean an imbalance in your life, and you may need to consider physical and spiritual cleansing.

Spiritual cleansing is the process of eliminating man-made ideas, values, and standards that are based on misconceptions and wrongful interpretations of the truth. Man is always striving to enslave his fellow man by creating artificial roles or circumstances that appear to give more power to some and less to others. For example, roles of the sexes make one more dominant, or having more money makes some more powerful than others. In truth, from the perspective of the Universal Teachings, everyone is equal.

Kidney disorders are indicative of a spiritual cleansing problem. When the kidneys malfunction, the place to look is in the inability to cleanse the misconceptions of truth from the belief system. The mind is holding on to some concept or idea about material life, and this means you are maintaining potentially lethal concepts and ideas in your body and in your life.

With the other type of diabetes, diabetes mellitus, the main cause is the failure of the pancreas to release enough insulin into the body. The pancreas works in conjunction with the liver to convert stored sugars into usable sugar for fuel and energy, and also produces enzymes for digestion. The pancreas is symbolic of your ability to take certain thoughts and ideas and make them work; it can provide you with the fuel (courage and strength) to carry on.

The pancreas releases insulin when it detects sugar in the blood stream and the more sugar, the more insulin required. Based on this awareness, insulin is symbolic of the extra effort, coupled with courage and confidence, an individual must have and use to take a thought through the controlled process required to convert it into physical action.

Insulin also acts as an agent to regulate metabolism. This validates the symbolic interpretation that insulin is tied into courage and confidence, and it is with these two attributes in hand that the speed, or metabolism, of moving through a project or the digestive process, is determined because the more courage and confidence a person has, the easier it is for them to move through most endeavors.

It is also believed that diabetes mellitus may be a defect in the parts of cells that accept the insulin. Here again, we have a situation in which thoughts are influencing the cells in order to achieve a certain condition within the body, and this holds true for both good and bad health. In this case the cells are being prevented from accepting thoughts that will help them convert thought energy into action energy.

It is documented that this disease tends to run in families, but this is true only from the perspective that children are taught by example about how to live and eat. In other words, genetics can load the gun but lifestyle pulls the trigger. Some of the foods comprising staple diets are rooted in cultural tradition, so that the individual's lifestyle is a reflection of that culture. Here is found the tendency for diseases to run in families. This was understood in the past, as written in Luke 6:44, and is reflected upon in the Universal Teaching, "every tree is known by his own fruit."

When the pancreas does not produce enough insulin, the symptoms of diabetes mellitus emerge, including weight loss, fatigue, and lethargy. Looking at the symbology of insulin it is easier to understand how weight loss, lethargy, and fatigue evolve. Keep in mind that fatigue and lethargy are viewed as two separate energies.

Weight loss is symbolically tied into the opposite of confidence, doubt. Doubt does many different things to an individual, but in this case it is working to prove to the person that they do not have the strength (muscles and weight) to carry on and move forward from where they are. The fatigue goes hand in hand with this perspective. Symbolically, fatigue is more often than not borne out of doubt in your ability to deal with the upcoming, or even daily, situations. Lethargy, on the other hand, is symbolic of a lack of inspiration. Here the individual has no motivation, and there is nothing on the horizon that can be seen to inspire forward movement. Fatigue may incorporate seeing what is ahead, but when the doubt kicks in forward movement stops.

Medically, diabetes mellitus is broken down into four main types. From a numerology standpoint, the level of diabetes should also provide great insights as to the concepts involved. The symbolic meaning of 4 is advancement. Another way to look at the number 4 is in the components 3 and 1, or 2 and 2, which make 4. Looking quickly at the other numbers involved: 3 equals understanding; 1 equals unity, and 2 represents balance and harmony. If there is balance and harmony between the male and female, and the spiritual and material, then it could be said that you are in true unity within your self, and in unity there is understanding, and understanding and unity lead to advancement on all levels.

Each aspect of the four types of diabetes is reflective of the level of doubt and fear at work. For instance, in Type I diabetes, also called insulin dependent diabetes, the person is symbolically dependent upon an external source for motivation, inspiration, courage, and confidence, and without this external source, death will occur.

Type II, non-insulin dependent diabetes, most often develops in overweight adults because of the weight aspect, this type of diabetes has more than one symbolic interpretation. There are many different reasons for being overweight, so for the purpose of staying on track with the metabolism perspective, let us say overweight people also have the same trouble as diabetics. They cannot act at certain levels of thought, and usually these are thoughts that would enhance the person's situation. Do not overlook the reality that many people who are overweight are also rich, with their wealth acquired through all manner of circumstance.

Regardless of the reasons a person is in that situation, the basic cause remains the same: it is one's inability to convert certain thoughts into specific actions. Although let us not forget that persons with Type II diabetes do have the ability to acquire material things, so there is enough courage and confidence to go after goals, but not necessarily the ability to utilize the courage and confidence to attain those goals. While Type II diabetics are not totally dependent upon an external source, they usually need a drug to control the disease.

Type III, or gestational, diabetes occurs in some women during pregnancy. This happens because some women believe that they are not capable of being a mother, that they are too young for the role, or they do not have the strength to care for a child. However, as time goes on after the delivery, the mother gains more courage and confidence in her abilities to care for the child. At this point the diabetes disappears, but it seems to set the stage for Type II diabetes to occur later in life.

The changes people go through after their children move out merit mention here because "empty-nesters" are again faced with dealing with the future. There are no longer children to take up the time, so these parents must again, or for the first time, express themselves as individuals. The transition is difficult for some, and many diseases are created at this juncture.

Type IV diabetes includes the other types of diabetes linked to disease of the pancreas. As mentioned previously, the pancreas is symbolic of your ability to take certain thoughts and ideas and make them work. They can provide you with the fuel (courage and strength) to carry on. Once again, it is obvious that courage is a vital ingredient to the mastery of life and health. Health is a symbolic reflection of the state of consciousness the individual is experiencing at any given time.

Type IV diabetes is sometimes linked to hormonal changes and even the side effects of some drugs. Here again you can see how thoughts, influencing hormones, can have far reaching effects. Each hormone within the body plays a specific role in the overall health of the person, so each hormone can be influenced by the particular thoughts that relate to the function that it has.

The fact that drugs can cause diabetes and other poor health conditions is symbolic of the imbalance in life when one relies on man-made approaches to handling a situation. Instead of following a natural approach to living and health, industrial society chooses to follow a path that leads to disharmony, and this dis-harmony is reflected in our dis-eases.

Another factor that can cause Type IV diabetes is genetic defects. In this scenario, the body is corrupted from the beginning. Some would then say that the emotional causes that drive food and sweets consumption are not valid in this instance. Although that statement seems true, the fact is the soul has chosen to occupy that particular body to work out those concepts that relate to that particular disease. Herein lays the whole question of hereditary diseases.

We have examined symbolically all the symptoms in diabetes mellitus except increased appetite, which is in keeping with the need to continually consume the sweets of life, even though there is no way to utilize it. This is one of the circumstances that leads to hoarding behavior. Hoarders think that what they have is not enough to deal with life, so they constantly require more. The greater the doubt, the more is required to fulfill the hole in the confidence.

There are different types of physical complications associated with diabetes, for instance, diabetic amaurosis, the blindness linked to diabetes.

Blindness is very interesting symbolically, it deals with a fear of looking into the future or of looking at self. In either direction, the fear is such that it shuts down the outside world as much as possible. Deafness, although it is not a direct consequence of diabetes, is another attempt to disconnect from the external sounds (voices) coming in, and close off unwanted input.

Cataracts are a vision problem that seems common in people with either Type I or Type II diabetes, and this is yet another form of shutting out the picture of reality.

Poor circulation in the feet and legs is another common affliction among those with diabetes. Think a moment about the purpose of the feet: you choose a direction or goal, and the mind directs the feet to take you there. Difficulties here signal doubt at work with regard to your direction in life.

SYMBOLOGY OF THE NUTRIENTS

Chromium. A trace-mineral essential for good health. The primary role of chromium is to maintain normal levels of blood sugar (glucose), which acts as fuel for the body.

It is noteworthy that chromium can both raise and lower blood sugar levels. This indicates the ability to exercise control over the emotions. When emotions get out of hand in one direction, you burn more energy in rage and anger, but when your emotions shut you down, your energy levels likewise shut down because there is apathy and indifference. Symbolically, chromium reflects an ability to control the emotions.

Iodine. The primary micronutrient that nourishes the thyroid gland and is a component of the thyroid hormone, which regulates mentality and speech, and aids in the condition of the hair, nails, skin, and teeth. Symbolically, the thyroid gland is affected by attitudes stemming from image and expression. It is situated in the neck in front of and on each side of the trachea, and close to the larynx. Therefore, it plays a part in the balance between your material and spiritual considerations.

Interestingly, people with sluggish thyroids are generally overweight. Symbolically, this would indicate that a person is imbalanced in how they deal with life, based on doubt or fear. On the other hand are those with a hyperactive thyroid. This group has a hard time maintaining a balance that will give them the strength to deal with life, and this imbalance of strength also comes from doubt or fear. In both instances, understanding the root concept is necessary to understand the forces at work in creating the imbalances. Iodine regulates the body's production of energy, promotes growth and development, and stimulates the rate of metabolism.

Iodine symbolizes inspiration because without inspiration there would be no motivation for growth and development. Without inspiration to generate enthusiasm, there would be no energy or desire to do anything.

Niacin. A B-complex nutrient that promotes growth and proper nervous system functioning. That is why niacin is symbolically a facilitator and expediter.

One of the ways niacin works in the body is to dilate blood vessels, which allows blood freer access to the extremities. This additional blood is analogous to giving a hand to handle a situation, and the feet to carry you in the proper direction. Because blood symbolizes spirit, niacin symbolically gives you more courage and strength.

Vitamin B-1. Necessary for healthy mouth, skin, eyes, and hair. It is needed for carbohydrate metabolism and is essential for nerve tissues, muscles, digestion, and normal heart function. Vitamin B-1 symbolizes courage, and courage is important for all tasks and accomplishments in life.

Zinc. Involved in the production of insulin, it is also a component of male reproductive fluid. By virtue of these and its many other roles, it is symbolic of expression. Courage and confidence, the symbolic significance of insulin, grow and develop with and because of expression. Without expression there would be stifled and very limited growth, just as zinc deficiency could cause diarrhea, lethargy, dermatitis, mental disorders, skin lesions, anorexia, a loss of taste, growth retardation, and sexual immaturity. By examining each deficiency symptom through the perspective of expression, the connection can be seen.

L-Glutamine. Lessens the craving for sweets. Because of its symbolic function as insight, it can easily cross the blood-brain barrier, and insights lessen the craving for sweets because with insights comes self-knowledge. Self-knowledge, the key to excellent health and personal mastery, is the goal of humanity. It is when we can accept and love ourselves that we will be able to "love thy neighbor as thyself" (Mark 12:31), and even more powerfully, to "love one another; as I have loved you, that ye also love one another" (John 13:34).

Diarrhea

Diarrhea is a problem for both young and old. Regardless of the cause, when diarrhea is present any food that has been ingested is rapidly expelled from the system. If it continues to the point of dehydrating the body, more than nutrients will be lost; the condition can become life threatening.

Stopping the diarrhea as quickly as possible is of paramount importance. The best way to accomplish this task is by tackling the problem head-on. Since diarrhea is more of a symptom than a disease, we need to attack it symptomatically. The first step is to eliminate the parasite or germ causing the condition. Next, increase the amount of fiber foods. You could also use carob powder because it will gel the bowels; mix it in food or drinks, and this will cause the stool to become firmer.

By stopping the diarrhea process, all food that is consumed will remain in the body longer, affording the system an opportunity to extract the nutrients it needs for replenishing.

In Mexico, where this condition is more common, the people do two interesting things. They squeeze fresh lemon juice over all salads before they eat them, and when diarrhea does strike, they eat plenty of cheese, which gels the bowels.

Generally, what creates diarrhea is a bacteria or fungus within the intestinal tract that the body is trying to expel as rapidly as it can because the body's own intelligence has identified it as a threat to the body. With diarrhea there is such a rapid expulsion of the liquid portion of the waste in the intestines that electrolytes are lost and nutrients are not absorbed into the bloodstream. It is also possible that the lack of nutrient uptake could be created by faulty digestion.

When you lose electrolytes and minerals, you set the body up for other problems because minerals are involved in enzymatic processes. Minerals are co-factors that allow biochemical processes and exchanges to take place, and are also catalysts that facilitate other transactions. When there is a mineral deficiency, the body will utilize what is available for the most essential functions. This can be problematic because the secondary and tertiary issues are not well cared for because there are not enough nutrients available to meet all of the nutritional requirements of the body.

Here is a chain of events that demonstrate what a lack of nutrients due to diarrhea can cause. Due to rapid expulsion, calcium uptake is diminished. Of course this could also come as a result of poor nutrition, where the pancreas and stomach lining did not produce enough digestive enzymes, then digestion would be impeded and nutrient availability is therefore limited. The first signs of a calcium deficiency are muscle aches, spasms and palpitations, and this could manifest in many different ways including a fatal heart attack. Calcium is a conductor of electricity and chemical processes essential for life. When the electrical flow of the body is affected health is compromised, and compromised health could be fatal. Another telltale sign is the slow process of clotting when you cut yourself.

When there is a lack of sufficient calcium ions in the bloodstream the body intelligence will pull calcium from the bones. This is done to try and keep the body in an alkaline state, and germs cannot live in an alkaline environment.

In addition, the process of supplying the bloodstream with calcium can cause osteoporosis. This is especially true if calcium supplementation is not used.

In dealing with diarrhea, two of the best things to do immediately are to consume carob powder and cheese. Carob gels the bowels, and cheese will literally gum up the system, slowing the loss of fluids and electrolytes.

HERBS TO SUPPORT THE BODY IN COMBATING DIARRHEA

The following act as congealers and liquid-absorbing agents, helpful in solidifying the stool and regulating bowel movements following diarrhea.

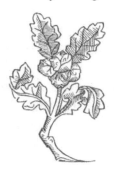

Herbs	
Acacia	Garlic
Bayberry	Pau D'Arco
Blackberry	Rhubarb
Carob	White Oak
Charcoal	

Acacia and Carob. Absorbs discharges and soothes irritated linings of the intestines.

Bayberry, Blackberry, Rhubarb, and White Oak. All are known as powerful astringent herbs traditionally used by healers in combating diarrhea.

Charcoal. Absorbs liquid and excess gas.

Garlic and Pau D'Arco. Used to kill bacteria.

Symbology of Diarrhea

Diarrhea symbolizes thoughts that are so alien, uncomfortable or threatening that you seek to get them out of the mind and system as quickly as possible. It is also important to look at the symbology of the lost minerals: calcium for strength, magnesium for inspiration, potassium for proper balance and harmony in material considerations; and phosphorous for courage.

You must also look at the events surrounding you at the time diarrhea strikes from the perspective that it is a reflection of any thoughts at work at the time. The presence of diarrhea indicates you are involved in something that is uncomfortable, unfriendly, or potentially life threatening, owing to dehydration and the accompanying loss of nutrients and minerals. When I say life threatening, I do not mean that death is imminent, but rather that there is a great loss of vitality and vigor.

It is said that diarrhea is a form of constipation. When we look at constipation symbolically we see that it represents holding onto the past. Thoughts move a person forward, out of the accustomed comfort zone, which affects the ego in a negative way because it threatens the life of the ego.

One of the primary purposes of the ego is to maintain its own identity. This takes us back to living our lives by seeking to fulfill our subconscious expectations of whom we think we are supposed to be, and this guarantees the continued existence of the ego.

To come to a place of enlightenment, a place of continual awareness, or a place of mastery, one must let go of the ego, and the only way one can achieve that is through understanding. The ego operates on an emotional plane more than in any other realm of thought. The emotions, which are extensions of concepts, are triggered by stimuli, which then trigger emotional responses.

When you do not feel equal to this new opportunity, primarily because it conflicts with old ideas of self, then the new idea has to be quickly eliminated to maintain status quo, and diarrhea may very well be the way it is eliminated.

Digestion, Assimilation, Utilization, and Elimination Issues

Good health is the result of many factors—the way we think, the air we breathe, the water we drink and the food we eat.

Two of these factors are summed up in the expressions: "you are what you eat," and "you are what you think." The types of food that you eat determine the nutritional health of your body. If the food is predominantly cooked, then its nutritional value would be much lower than that provided by raw vegetables. If the diet lacks the fiber found in living foods and is heavy in dairy products or fats, such as hydrogenated oils or saturated fatty acids, you can bet that there will be difficulties on many levels, but especially in regard to the food digestion, assimilation, and utilization process. These difficulties will be experienced across the entire channel of digestion, which is most like a canal or long tube with an opening at either end. It includes the mouth, the esophagus, stomach, intestinal tract, and colon.

DIGESTION

Digestion begins in the mouth. When you see, smell, or taste something, messages are transmitted to the brain, which signals the first step in the process: production and release of enzymes to aid in the digestive process by the salivary glands. As masticated, or chewed food continues down the esophagus into the stomach, the second and most major enzymatic process takes place: the pancreas and stomach lining both secrete enzymes that ensure further digestion. The pancreatic gland produces enzymes that digest proteins, fats, and carbohydrates. The hormone insulin for the facilitation of sugar into the cells is also manufactured here.

When problems arise in the pancreas, digestion is disrupted, and constipation can result. If the sugar in the blood that is used as fuel is not metabolized properly, there is an accumulation of that sugar. When the blood sugar levels stay high, it could mean the disease diabetes is at work. (For more information on this process, see also Diabetes.)

Once the enzymatic contributions of the stomach lining and the pancreas have been added, the resulting liquid, called chyme, moves into the duodenum for further digestion. When the chyme enters into the intestinal tract, the process of assimilation begins. At this point, the nutrients in chyme are molecular in size.

ASSIMILATION

Complete assimilation depends on the small intestine being clean and having a thriving colony of friendly bacterial flora. Complete, effective assimilation depends on two factors. First is the quality of the food ingested: was it fresh, organically grown raw food, or did it come out of the freezer or a can? The second factor is the quality, or thoroughness, of the digestive process itself: to what degree has the food been broken down, and is the quality of the chyme such that the nutrients will be able to pass through the intestinal wall?

The amount of nutrients coming into the system and the amount assimilated determines your level of health because everything you have assimilated into your bloodstream through the villi will now feed your individual cells. This underscores the need both for consuming good food and having efficient cleansing processes. Often, it is necessary to reinforce and supplement the natural cleansing process because of all the toxins entering the body. It creates a load over and above the normal wastes that the body produces in the feeding of the cells and removing the waste that they generate.

When the diet is not of organic quality or is overly processed, the body is being fed a chemical mixture of "food products" that is heavy in artificial colors, flavors, flavor enhancers, preservatives, modifiers, and other chemical ingredients added for various purposes. These chemicals end up in the raw materials that cells use to repair themselves and regenerate, and many are toxins with the potential to damage the body. The body is programmed to render them harmless, eliminate them, or store them in fat cells.

Toxins may first be broken down into harmless substances. What cannot be broken down and eliminated will be stored in the fat cells. What cannot be eliminated or stored will end up being incorporated into building material as the cells divide and create offspring, and this sets the stage for possible disease or illness.

UTILIZATION

When we talk about utilization, we are talking about the availability of the nutrients in the bloodstream. Once nutrients are in the blood stream, other issues and questions come into play, such as: are there other nutrients that complement each other and that are vital and necessary for the utilization of other nutrients? Much like nature, nothing stands alone. This is one of the reasons why "magic bullets" do not work. They block the symptom and never deal with the root cause of the problem. Utilization is being able to utilize the nutrients within the body, not just assimilate them into the bloodstream. They can only be utilized by finding their counterparts, their allies and comrades, if you will, that work in conjunction with them.

ELIMINATION

The body's overall elimination process involves four systems. The respiratory system is used for eliminating carbon dioxide, spent air, and other detrimental gaseous substances. The urination process is used because the kidneys eliminate liquid wastes. The skin uses perspiration to vent steam and liquids. Lastly, the intestinal tract passes all used and unused solid material from the body through defecation, completing the elimination process.

The solids, water, and gases are taken from the bloodstream, converted in the liver and then dispersed, the water and gases are placed back into the bloodstream for elimination, and the solids are passed through with bile into the intestinal tract for elimination.

The need for keeping the intestinal tract clean and healthy cannot be emphasized strongly enough. Fiber plays an essential role in cleaning the intestinal tract, and this is why a diet rich in fiber is important. It can be supplemented with fiber tablets and powder.

Fiber acts as an intestinal broom, pushing matter through to the colon for elimination. Along the way, it absorbs liquid and swells, pushing matter against the colon walls where nerve endings receive and send signals. When enough bulk matter is assembled, the mass pushes against those cells, which tell the brain that tells the muscles to eliminate the matter.

Another vital aspect of cleansing is to eliminate any unnecessary mucus in the system. Mucus is created from dairy-based products as well as some whole grains, and mucus can accumulate in the intestinal tract, blocking assimilation pathways.

Taking probiotics is one step you can take to ensure better assimilation. Probiotics are beneficial microbes that protect the host from foreign entities entering the bloodstream. Additionally, they provide the body with B-complex vitamins, which helps to prevent disease. The best-known probiotic is lactobacillus acidophilus, which is found in yogurt, acidophilus milk, and supplements. While probiotics could and should be consumed periodically to ensure a healthy flora colony, it is particularly important to take them after a course of antibiotics, which destroy friendly flora in the intestinal tract, allowing other forms to flourish. (See also Candida Albicans.)

A clean colon aids proper elimination and helps to ensure there is no retention of toxic materials.

Nutrients, Enzymes, Herbs and Flora to Support Digestion, Assimilation, Utilization and Elimination

The following supports the body in eliminating indigestion and heartburn, improving digestion, bettering intestinal health, eliminating mucus, and normalizing eliminations.

For the Pancreas	
Nutrients	*Herbs*
Manganese	Dandelion Root
Selenium	
Zinc	

Manganese. Supports detoxification pathways. Stores of it are found chiefly in the human liver, kidney, pancreas, lungs, prostate gland, adrenals, and brain.

Selenium. Good for the liver and pancreas. It is a natural antioxidant and appears to preserve elasticity of tissue by delaying oxidation of polyunsaturated fatty acids.

Zinc. Plays a part in the manufacturing of insulin in the pancreas.

Dandelion Root. Stimulates bile production, benefits the spleen, and improves the health of the pancreas.

For the Intestinal Tract	
Herbs	
Cedar Berries	Licorice Root
Gentian Root	Wheat Bran
Goldenseal Root	

Cedar berries. Stimulate the pancreas.

Gentian Root. Its focus of activity is on those glands and organs involved in digestion, such as the liver and pancreas. It also works on the gallbladder.

Goldenseal Root. Lowers blood sugar; stimulates the pancreas.

Licorice Root. Strengthens the pancreas and spleen.

Wheat Bran. Lowers blood-glucose levels and stimulates the pancreas to produce insulin.

For Cleansing the Intestinal Tract	
Flora	*Herbs*
Probiotics	Apple Pectin
	Butternut Root Bark
	Clay
	Dandelion Root
	Flax Seeds
	Marshmallow Root
	Psyllium Husks
	Slippery Elm Bark

Probiotics. Friendly microbes that assist the body in maintaining good health. Are essential in all digestive functions.

Apple Pectin. Helps to regulate bowels and elimination. It also draws toxic metals out of the blood. It is said that apple pectin contains electromagnetic properties.

Butternut Root Bark. Has a mild laxative property.

Clay. Has the ability to absorb toxins. We want to prevent toxins from getting into the bloodstream, because once in the bloodstream, damage will occur. This is especially true if the immune system and liver are not operating at absolute top efficiency.

Dandelion Root. Improves liver function. Bile and certain enzymes produced in the liver aid in maintaining proper intestinal flora.

Flax Seed. Provides "pushing and sweeping" benefits.

Marshmallow Root. Soothes mucous membranes. Used internally to treat inflammation and mucosal afflictions.

Psylium husks. Act as brooms. They provide no nutrient value, but they are used as scrapers that push through bulk and provide fiber that helps the body eliminate waste.

Slippery Elm Bark. Effective, both internally and externally, against sore and inflamed mucous membranes.

SYMBOLOGY OF DIGESTION

When we see food, the brain tells the salivary glands to produce enzymes that will begin to break down the food. The minute you begin eating, the digestive process is under way, and through the digestive process, the body seeks to break food down into its component parts. Eventually, the food is turned into a useable liquid, and is broken down to molecule size so that the cells can use the material. The body can then bring building material into its interior system through the intestinal tract, and from there the material is drawn into the bloodstream through assimilation and is ultimately distributed throughout the body for utilization by the cells.

The digestive process is symbolic of how we deal with thoughts that are presented to us on a daily basis. Every time a thought is presented to you, it is subjected to certain subconscious processes. In one of them, the thought is compared to your conceptual database. In your subconscious mind, the thoughts and things that are accepted as true are obviously easy to digest and assimilate into the self. There are other aspects of the thoughts that are examined from a conceptual point of view as well. Thoughts that match your concepts and belief system are then brought into the mental system, and each thought triggers a response or a reaction of some sort. Some ideas or thoughts presented are so uncomfortable that you may regurgitate them, just as you would quickly expel the food that does not settle well in your system.

There are different levels of disagreements leading to indigestion. These include nausea, acid indigestion, heartburn, and upset stomach. Nausea indicates an unsettling thought that can cause a person to lose balance, momentum, and centeredness. Some thoughts initially sound fine and are in keeping with the belief system; they pass through the body's defenses because they appear innocuous and agreeable. As the digestive process continues all the way to the concept level, something changes. When the subconscious mind has an opportunity to look at the thought, the mind realized something about this thought would be in conflict with the belief system, and there we have the beginnings of indigestion. Indigestion indicates that the thought being presented is not something the person can easily stomach, digest, or accept. This is based on subconscious concepts.

Acid indigestion and heartburn are more common than one might think. While they are a chronic problem for some, those who suffer from these symptoms occasionally are dealing with something uncomfortable that has been presented. When we speak about something being presented, it is an acknowledgement of the ways in which the mind/body "sees" a presentation. One type of presentation is sound; sound conveys many different things, and stimulates concepts and patterns. Hearing a horn or siren produces a physical change within the body.

The first sign that there may be a digestive problem will be an upset stomach. This is because the idea or thought presented was so unacceptable that an upset stomach ensued.

Presentations can also be visual, aromatic, or energetic (something you can sense). For example, you can meet someone and become nauseated because the energy the person emits is not in accord with your own energy. Each of these types of presentations can trigger a past association that was positive or negative. When this occurs, it means you have a PEA (personal emotional association) with that particular trigger.

There are many different ways in which we are confronted with thoughts (food) that will be digested and dealt with accordingly. Sometimes thoughts are presented and everything is wonderful, with no indigestion. At another time, those same thoughts could end up creating a disease or condition. This occurs because the time, place, and events you are involved in have a different energy, one that may not be in keeping with where you are at, where you are headed, or where you desire to be.

Thoughts that are presented are going to be broken down into component parts on a molecular, or fundamental, level, just as food would be. At that point the mind will initiate a couple of things. First, it will seek out that which will provide strength and growth, in much the same way as the body uses nutrients. The information that is central for the health of the body is first to be utilized. The mind also seeks to identify threats to its status quo, which is analogous to the way the body tries to render harmless or eliminate toxins from consumed foods. What cannot be eliminated is stored in fat cells, and what cannot be either eliminated or stored ends up being incorporated in the body. Thoughts are handled in the very same way. Consequently, there are thoughts that will add strength and those that will debilitate.

The body will occasionally hang on to certain toxic thoughts, which set in motion those processes necessary to manifest a disease or condition that symbolically reflects your overall concepts, and your personality that has been created based on those concepts. Very simply, you will be attracted to those foods and thoughts that will affirm your self-expectations and in doing so, you will end up creating the disease or symbolic manifestations of that personality type. For instance, if you have a tendency to be inflexible in your thinking, you might be attracted to foods that will create physical conditions that will create inflexibility in the joints. One tendency might be to consume an excessive amount of dairy products to provide calcium that cannot or might not be assimilated, and then calcium deposits could form. A protein-heavy diet would generate large amounts of uric acid in the blood, which would work against the joints. The synovial membranes would be damaged, causing synovial fluid to leak out, thus creating the disease of arthritis. Everything that is consumed, whether it is a solid, liquid, gas, or emotional thought, has a direct effect upon the body through the multiple processes undertaken by the mind and body.

When you find yourself in a specific situation and want to examine your thoughts, determine what aspects are disagreeable and the intensity of those feelings. Once you have awareness, you have the opportunity to change it by making a strong move or a subtle alteration of attitude. This alone would be enough to change the energy of a situation; through awareness you can make a choice to reject a particular thought or presentation so that it does not create any acid indigestion.

If you experience occasional heartburn or indigestion, look around to see what is going on. Make note of what you are doing, and whom you are with. Yes, a meal may be involved, but the meal is not the issue. Rather, it is the energy surrounding the meal, the conversation, the emotions, and the music—whatever has triggered your mind to tell your pancreas not to secrete the necessary enzymes to completely digest the food and break it down into a usable form.

Interestingly, though it is not part of the digestive process, sore throats from colds or the flu are also indicative of something that is hard to swallow. The prevailing situation, concept, or presence is so difficult to take, in fact, that the person becomes angry, in addition to having a sore throat. Anger will soon manifest in fever, and the person may even throw up, if the issue is sufficiently disagreeable.

Symbology of Assimilation

We touched on this during our discussion of digestion. The body responds to thoughts, and some thoughts are agreeable or usable, providing something worthwhile, but other thoughts can be harmful. When there is assimilation of harmful thoughts, it is in keeping with the mind's desire. The mind may need to provide the body with material that will adversely affect the body, and this will create a symbolic reflection of a particular type of condition or disease.

Symbology of Utilization

When we speak about utilization, the same symbology applies. The body has its own Divine Consciousness, and it knows on some levels what to do with what it gets. The mind is just the same. Anything that is presented to the mind through any of the senses will be utilized by the mind in its attempt to fulfill self-expectations, and this is why it is vital to have as much clarity and self-understanding as possible and to make sure clarity and self-understanding is an ongoing process.

People are like onions. The more layers we can peel back, the better we are able to get to the incredible core of consciousness that is connected to the All. This aspect of you has power beyond belief. This is the True Self of the Creative Continuum; the self that will manifest the power of being Divine, and it seeks that which is helpful and beneficial.

Symbology of Elimination

The symbology of elimination is different from the standpoint that it is an ongoing process, and it is tied into the internal detoxification process. Digestion, by contrast, is a short process: you consume a food (or thought), you analyze it, digest it, break it down, assimilate what you can, utilize what you can, and then reject the rest. The body is in a constant state of being, dying, and rejuvenating. If we are constantly rejuvenating, it raises this question: if the body renews itself, what is it that causes us to age, becoming decrepit and diseased?

The answer is twofold. On one hand, it is a matter of the physical diet. Are you eating a chemical-laden, overly processed diet full of bad fats, or do you consume mostly fresh, raw organically grown fruits and vegetables? If you do eat meat or fowl, were they organically fed, free-ranging stock? The body processes everything that comes into it, and at the same time, it is detoxifying itself and sloughing off toxic material such as sick, mutated, and dead cells. Toxins enter the body from the air we breathe, the water we drink, and the food we eat. If our bodies were not in constant detoxification mode, we would become so intoxicated that we would die very young. The same thing can be said for toxic thought.

Aging also results from the thoughts you accept as true. Examine yours well and thoroughly to determine if there is truth or nourishment in what is being presented. Are you buying into thoughts or concepts that appear pleasing or sweet, but in reality are detrimental to your well-being? The quality and quantity of the building material that you provide to your body and mind will determine your level of health. If you do not employ the process of seeking, knowing, and understanding self, you expedite the dying process.

The dying process happens because the individual is not attracted to foods and thoughts that will promote health. His or her conscious choices are based on emotional needs, which override the inherent desire to be healthy. The subconscious concepts and patterns of behavior divert the person's attention away from healthy living and toward detrimental living in order to fulfill subconscious expectations and manifest symbolic representation of the concepts at work, and the end result can be a medical condition or disease.

When you do not eliminate the toxins and waste—in this case the invalid, man-made concepts that no longer serve you—you can become constipated. Another form of not letting go of the past is kidney problems. If the kidneys fail, death is not far behind. When you can eliminate toxic thoughts from your life and nourish yourself with truth, harmony and balance, you will have excellent health on all levels.

In as much as death is the beginning of a new cycle in one respect, premature death reflects a type of rejection from the current life. The rejection may not always be contemporaneous but rather could be the result of accumulation.

A person can be constipated for a day, three days, or five days, but after a certain period of time the level of toxicity builds to the point that death becomes imminent. The same is true in cases of kidney malfunction. When there are difficulties with elimination, it simply indicates an unwillingness to let go of the past. To some degree, we can understand this because so many of us have been trained to stay within a particular framework of reality because it is understood, safe, and secure. By the same token, if you hold onto that which is detrimental even though it appears to be safe and secure, you can end up expediting your own demise.

Symbology of the Pancreas

The pancreas is interesting symbolically owing to its roles in manufacturing insulin, helping us to utilize the sweets of life, and because it is a digestive enzyme. It is symbolic of your ability to break down thoughts presented to you, allowing you to more effectively utilize them.

Problems with the pancreas indicate a difficulty in breaking down for digestion what is coming into your life. If you are coping only with great difficulty and feeling overwhelmed, you do not believe you have the wherewithal to break down and utilize what is coming into your life. Have you ever felt trapped by a certain situation? This may manifest as chronic indigestion until the situation passes or you determine its meaning.

The reality here is it is only your belief system that is caught in the situation. Reality itself is only a reflection of what dwells within, based on concepts. When the external is not flowing and working, it is a reflection of the internal conflict.

Symbology of the Nutrients

Digestive Enzymes. The digestive process has many different symbolic lessons for the seeker. Digestive enzymes and the raw materials needed by the body to manufacture them give a degree of insight into the processes of thought analysis.

There are three major types of enzymes: proteases to break down proteins, amylases to break down carbohydrates, and lipases to break down fats. These different enzymes indicate there are also different ways to deal with thoughts presented to you. Each new thought, event, situation, or person requires an individualistic look. There may be commonalities between situations, but each will have unique aspects that require a separate perspective and approach.

We must also think about the thought processes and what types of insights and understandings are needed to get the maximum out of what is being presented to us. With the body it is simple, all we need do is examine the physical attributes: vitamins, minerals, proteins (amino acids), fats, and carbohydrates. These are the components of digestive enzymes.

What is it that gives us the ability to best break down thoughts, to digest them and extract truth from them for the best possible utilization? The most nourishing of thought and perception systems are the Universal Teachings. These are the laws and principles that govern everything in the universe. They provide an understanding of how the human mind functions as well as insight and truth about why we do what we do. Learning to incorporate these Teachings into your life will open the door to mastery.

Universal Teachings are the fundamental tenets of every religion, regardless of how they are presented. Fundamentally speaking, the truth is the truth; eon after eon, every spiritual master and teacher has presented the same insights and understandings. To gain the most sustenance from thoughts, you must be able to digest them properly, and this can be accomplished by incorporating the Universal Teachings into your daily life.

The Teachings do not have a nutritional counterpart. Whereas vitamins are co-enzymes and minerals are co-factors that both undergo changes and combine with other factors to create something new, the Universal Teachings are concepts or guides that are whole and complete, they do not change; they are the immutable laws of life.

Manganese, Selenium, and Zinc. Digestive enzymes, on the other hand, have components to help make them whole and complete so that they can function properly. This is why selenium, zinc, and manganese are essential for their roles in the production of digestive enzymes. Let us look symbolically at those productive efforts.

Selenium represents protection and cleansing. How appropriate it is that that we must protect ourselves from some thoughts that are presented to us. Some thoughts are negative in nature; they undermine and make you feel bad about yourself. Other thoughts are designed to instill certain specific responses, one being guilt. Selenium is essential in the processes of providing protection and cleansing. Cleansing is another aspect of the digestion process, and it must be carried out to its conclusion to eliminate those entities, in any form, that no longer serve us well.

Zinc is important in the digestive enzyme construction process and also facilitates actions within the body. Zinc plays a fundamental role in expression and a supporting role in our defensive capabilities. Symbolically, it represents a working faith. A working faith is required to get the most out of digesting thoughts, examining and extracting from them the kernels of insights and understandings that will support true expression and the ability to complete a cycle or process. A great example is undertaking an endeavor because you must have faith in self to realize you know the things to do in order to get a project or task accomplished.

Finally, manganese symbolizes will and intent. Having the intent to accomplish something is one thing, but having the will, the courage, and the faith to manifest it is another. This is why these nutrients work together to facilitate the digestive process. In this situation selenium to protect, zinc to have faith and express, and manganese to manifest the nourishment that has been extracted from the thought.

Emphysema

(See Conditions That Restrict Breathing: Congestion, Asthma, and Emphysema.)

Energy Problems (See also Hypoglycemia, Low Blood Sugar.)

A significant number of people deal with energy issues; chronic low-energy levels has been one of the most common concerns voiced to me by clients during all my years as a body/mind nutritional counselor.

Low energy can stem from several causes, including anemia, a condition in which the body is not producing enough oxygen-carrying red blood cells to support all of the body's cellular activities, and oxygen is an essential nutrient for energy transactions.

Another essential nutrient for energy production is pantothenic acid, also known as vitamin B-5. Pantothenic acid has a major role because it becomes a part of co-enzyme A in the Krebs cycle. The Krebs cycle is a biochemical transaction within that takes place in the mitochondria. The mitochondria are found in every cell in the body, they are the fundamental producer of energy for the cells/body. Fats are the primary food source for the mitochondria, which uses fat to produce ATP (adenosine triphosphate). This is present in all living cells. It serves as an energy source, and is the main energy molecule the body utilizes.

Additionally, pantothenic acid, along with vitamin C, plays a major role in supporting the health of the adrenal glands, which are the body's stress centers, and when they become overtaxed, there are consequences.

One consequence is the adrenals can no longer maintain a sufficient level of protective power, and as the adrenals' effectiveness diminishes, the immune system also becomes compromised, losing some of its ability to protect the body.

There will be stress-induced flare-ups of conditions such as the various forms of herpes, including fever blisters and shingles; while the viruses that would cause them are normally held in check, a taxed immune system can no longer hold them at bay.

Other conditions may also appear or become exacerbated in times of stress, including canker sores; menopause symptoms, both the early onset of menopause and symptoms in menopausal women; allergies; acne; chronic fatigue syndrome; fibromyalgia; and hypoglycemia (low blood sugar).

Energy problems develop because the adrenal glands fail in their role related to maintaining proper blood sugar levels in the bloodstream. If they are exhausted due to stress they cannot communicate with the liver effectively, and this means that the liver cannot release glycogen into the bloodstream. Without glycogen converting to glucose, the cells have virtually no fuel, and energy levels plummet.

To understand the process, consider this scenario. You are driving your car and the gas gauge moves to "empty." You pull into a gas station and begin to fill the tank, leaving the pump nozzle set on automatic. When the tank fills to a certain level, the nozzle automatically clicks off, and no more gas goes into the tank.

Now let us say your body is a car and the adrenals, its driver. The adrenals monitor sugar in the bloodstream, so when sugar levels get too high, the adrenals communicate to the pancreas to secrete insulin, which brings the sugar levels back down into normal range. When sugar levels return to normal range, the adrenals once again communicate to the pancreas and tell it to stop insulin production. A problem arises when food or sweets are coming into the body every couple of hours. The body is constantly being fed, so food is continually being converted into glycogen, which will become fuel for the body.

In order to maintain homeostasis in the body, the adrenal glands are constantly communicating to the pancreas regarding needed insulin production. After several hours of this back-and-forth effort, the adrenals are exhausted, and the pancreas also becomes exhausted with all of the insulin production. Once that happens, the pancreas can no longer continue to produce adequate amounts of insulin on an as-needed basis, and the body begins to experience hyperglycemia, or high blood-sugar levels, and eventually, diabetes.

NUTRIENTS TO HELP ENERGY PROBLEMS

(See Hypoglycemia, Low Blood Sugar.)

SYMBOLOGY OF ENERGY ISSUES

Remember that oxygen is spirit, so again we are back to an issue of faith and confidence. Consider for a moment that fire cannot take place in the absence of oxygen and that fire is, in fact, a form of rapid oxidation in which energy and heat are released. It also takes the presence of spirit to release the power, heat, energy, and love that is encased in all things. Without spirit, virtually nothing will transpire or be transformed.

When we talk about low energy, we also need to think symbolically along the lines of inspiration. When you are inspired in life, you have all the energy you need to go out and do battle with the forces of the material plane. These forces are both within you (your thoughts and belief system) and without (your family, your work, living environment, hobbies, etc). When you are truly inspired, then you can find things you desire and want to do, and you will be motivated. The doubt and fear that dwells within all of us is contained so that we can pursue our desires.

Persons who suffer from chronic fatigue and fibromyalgia may also be lacking in inspiration; they are also quite affected by their own doubt and fear, which makes them unsure of what they would like to do, so their energy remains low until they refocus.

Symbology of the Nutrients

(See Hypoglycemia, Low Blood Sugar.)

Fertility Problems (Male and Female)

It is astounding to read reports that imply there are over 2 million couples who cannot have children because of infertility problems. There are many causes for infertility in each sex, and some of the problems lie in psychological areas such as not wanting to remain in the relationship, not wanting the responsibilities or stress of parenthood, or even fearing the rigors of parenthood. Still others are conflicted by their career goals or a reluctance to take on the financial burdens of having and raising a child.

All of these psychological factors cause internal stress, and stress depletes the body's nutritional reserves. Poor nutritional reserves coupled with an inadequate diet causes even greater depletion of the essential nutrients necessary for the proper functioning of the reproductive system. With these factors in mind, one ideal approach to resolving these issues would be to replace as efficiently as possible all of the nutrients that the body would require. I will say from experience that through using specially designed nutritional programs that are available in the marketplace, fertilization can take place. Even women with endometriosis have had success in becoming pregnant.

Like every other condition within the human body, the inability to conceive has multiple causes. In women, two common physical causes are blocked fallopian tubes and endometriosis. Another cause may be an allergy that the body develops toward the egg. I have seen this in gay women who are trying to conceive; usually this develops in the partner that becomes the "dominant male" of the relationship and seeks to become pregnant.

Within each human body are both female and male hormones, so people are, in essence, both female and male. In some gay women who are trying to conceive, the mind/body has difficulty because childbearing is contradictory to concepts a gay woman maintains about herself, her identity, and her sexual role. You can begin to understand why the body would attack the eggs as an alien invader. In order to protect itself, the egg would create an impenetrable shell—because all living things have an innate desire to survive and live—thus, fertilization would be impossible in this scenario.

Irregular menstrual periods in the woman may also make it difficult or impossible to predict ovulation, while male infertility factors can include a low sperm count, weak motility factors, or both.

In many cases of infertility, the odds for a successful conception and pregnancy can be greatly strengthened through improved nutrition.

Nutrients, Amino Acids and Herbs for Male Reproductive System Support

Nutrients	Amino Acids	Herbs
Beta-carotene (Vitamin A)	L-Arginine	Damiana
Calcium	L-Cysteine	Ginseng Root
Folic Acid	L-Glutamine	Sarsaparilla
Inositol	L-Methionine	Saw Palmetto
Magnesium		
Manganese		
Pantothenic Acid		
Niacin/Niacinamide		
Selenium		
Vitamin B-12		
Vitamin C		
Vitamin E		
Zinc		

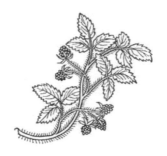

NUTRIENTS AND HERBS FOR FEMALE REPRODUCTIVE SYSTEM SUPPORT

The following should be included in the diet to support a woman's overall health during the reproductive cycle, as well as during pregnancy and lactation:

Nutrients	Herbs
Beta-carotene (Vitamin A)	Capsicum
Folic Acid	False Unicorn Root
Iron	Gotu Kola
Niacin/Niacinamide	Red Raspberry
Pantothenic Acid	Wild Yam Root
Unsaturated Fatty Acids	
Vitamin C	
Vitamin D	
Vitamin E	
Vitamin B-1	
Zinc	

Beta-carotene (Vitamin A). The preferred source for vitamin A. It is non-toxic because the body converts beta-carotene into vitamin A only as it is needed. Vitamin A is a fat-soluble nutrient that plays an important role in the formation of bones, teeth, and skin. It is necessary during pregnancy and lactation since fetal requirements for vitamin A increase the maternal need it. Many experts advise a 25 percent increase over pre-pregnancy intake.

Calcium. A mineral necessary for metabolism and the building of bones and teeth.

Folic Acid. Necessary for growth, cell division, and red blood cell formation. It helps with reproduction, and is necessary for the health of the glands and liver. There is evidence that adequate intake of folic acid during childbearing years may reduce the risk of neural tube defect pregnancy. About 25 percent of normal pregnant women in the United States have marginal to low serum levels of folic acid.

Inositol. Necessary for hair growth, fat and cholesterol metabolism, and lecithin formation.

Iron. Supplementation is essential for almost all pregnancies, especially for women with low serum ferritin levels. Studies indicate that 20 percent of pregnant women in the United

States enter pregnancy with low iron stores and may have difficulty meeting the increased iron demands of pregnancy by diet alone. The recommended daily dietary intake is 30 mg of supplemental iron throughout pregnancy.

Magnesium. Essential for the metabolism of potassium and calcium. It also plays a role in neuromuscular activity and impulse transmission.

Manganese. Plays a role in enzyme activation. High levels of this nutrient can be found in the bones, liver, and pituitary gland.

Niacin/Niacinamide. A B-complex nutrient that plays a role in growth and the proper functioning of the nervous system.

Pantothenic Acid. Essential for growth, contributes to energy functions, and is necessary for the skin.

Selenium. Preserves tissue elasticity and works with vitamin E.

Unsaturated Fatty Acids. In regard to fertility, unsaturated fatty acids are essential building material for making hormones, as well as helping the body to build tissue.

B-complex Vitamins. Should be considered during pregnancy for two reasons: (1) B-vitamin blood levels generally decline during pregnancy, hormonal changes, and (2) fetal levels exceed those in the mother, reflecting active transport across the placenta.

Studies indicate that B-6 needs tend to increase in pregnant women whose diets are rich in protein. Vitamin B-6 is necessary for the proper functioning of both nerves and muscles, including pressure-sensitive nerve cells and cardiac muscles. Vitamin B-1 is important for carbohydrate metabolism, digestion, and heart function. Vitamin B-12 helps form normal red blood cells and a healthy nervous system, and is important for its role in DNA synthesis.

Vitamin C. Essential for the absorption of inorganic iron and strong immune system function. Plays a role in collagen production. Pregnancy increases the need for vitamin C.

Vitamin D. Facilitates calcium absorption and participates in bone metabolism. Important in the reproductive cycle; studies have shown that vitamin D plays a role in promoting positive calcium balance in pregnant women, and one of its metabolites (25-hydroxy vitamin D) freely crosses the placenta.

Vitamin E. Essential for the hair, skin, and mucous membranes. It also participates in the synthesis of hemoglobin. The motility and fertility of sperm are in proportion to the amount of vitamin E in a man's semen. Studies using both laboratory and farm animals show that testicles degenerate with inadequate amounts of vitamin E.

Zinc. Aids in the metabolism of phosphorus and protein. It is a component of male reproductive fluid. Zinc also participates in the metabolism of RNA.

L-Arginine, L-Cysteine, L-Glutamine and L-Methionine. Amino acids are vital to the production of sperm as well as having a healthy uterus. The majority of seminal fluid is composed of arginine, which helps with male sterility, especially sperm motility. Methionine, a methyl donor and detoxifying agent, is needed anywhere that rapid growth or development is taking place, such as sperm production.

All herbs listed are taken to tone the male and female reproductive systems.

PSYCHOLOGICAL CONSIDERATIONS

Shaky finances, ambivalence about your partner or relationship, conflicting career aspirations, and a fear of the lifestyle changes and responsibilities associated with parenthood can all play a part in sabotaging fertility at the subconscious level. These are all legitimate reasons that one or both partners may have for not wanting to have a child at a particular time, yet without honest discussion between the partners, these feelings may never be consciously expressed; they may only serve to block conception.

When a couple consciously wants to have a child but cannot conceive or carry a pregnancy to term, then along with any health or nutrition issues involved, it is important to look at the subconscious energies and concepts at work. Both parties must equally share in the desire to have a child.

SYMBOLOGY OF INFERTILITY

Speaking in a general sense as well as in symbolic terms, everybody starts out being fertile with the capacity to reproduce. What changes? Much of the answer can be found in assessing the nourishment of the body. Without proper physical nourishment, it is difficult for the body to create an internal environment that will support life, let alone reproduce it.

Looking symbolically at those statements, if your mental environment (at the psychological, emotional, and conceptual levels) and the concepts within your subconscious mind tell you that you do not have the ability to express yourself, then it will be very difficult to reproduce.

Children represent an aspect of self. After all, children do contain the DNA of the parents and create personalities that reflect the parents, either from a position of acceptance or rejection. (For more on rejection as a form of acceptance, see Section I: From the Inside Out.)

Looking at some of the physical causes for infertility, we can see symbolically that blocked fallopian tubes indicate the woman has the ability to express self in terms of eggs being produced; however, there is a blockage. Something is impeding the woman's ability to express herself. Maybe it is a lack of authority or fear of expression, but some subconscious concept along those lines is preventing her from being able to express her innermost thoughts and bring forth creative expression. Her ability to change her reality and to grow and mature is hampered on some levels.

Endometriosis, on the other hand, indicates that the concepts relating to being a woman are misconstrued. From all outward appearances, we are looking at and working with a female (and female energy), yet subconsciously, the woman's ability to truly express herself and to bring forth or nurture life is impeded in some way. There are concepts at work telling her that she cannot or is somehow unworthy of reproducing.

The same thing holds true for the male. Symbolically, infertility in men can be identified as a lack of expression or the man's doubt in his ability to express himself, bring forth new life, or attain personal power. If the man's sperm count is beyond the functionally sterile level, he probably has the ability to impregnate, but another issue is at work, and it may be that the motility of the sperm is weak.

In this scenario, the man feels no power or strength to project thoughts forward and create a new reality, and he may feel he does not have the ability to project personal power into situations to elevate himself. Man-made concepts tell him he cannot push forward in life.

In each of these cases, what we are really talking about are concepts that may say to the person that he or she does not have the right, the authority, and certainly not the power to be able to accomplish the goal of bringing forth another aspect of expression and personal power. After all, if they cannot conceive a child, how will they propagate their lineage and pass on all that they are?

SYMBOLOGY OF THE NUTRIENTS

Virtually all nutrients vital to good health are involved in reproduction, so we will not go through their individual symbology at this point. Let it suffice to say that when you have a healthy body, the physical environment is conducive to producing a child. It also takes courage, stamina, insight, understanding, a working faith, emotional control, and much more to achieve reproduction. In the same vein, when the energies of a man or woman are together in a way that does not allow doubt or fear to hinder creativity or creative expression, then fertilization can take place.

Fertilization is a unique concept because it requires that many different, yet specific aspects, be in place for it to take place. One is an environment that is conducive to growth, another is energy to stimulate that growth. We may think of someone who is constantly creating something new—ideas, concepts, thoughts, or inventions—as having a fertile mind.

For a couple trying to conceive, it is a matter of creating a symbolic representation of their unity, and having a child is a symbolic manifestation of their ability to create, communicate, bring forth life, express themselves, and validate their male or female roles.

Some couples can get pregnant easily but cannot seem to carry the child to full term. This indicates some type of doubt at work, either in the relationship, finances, or perhaps parenting skills. Other considerations like career, living environment, and future plans are also part of the mix that influences thought and, consequently, the energy of the pregnancy.

Every woman who cannot conceive and every woman whose pregnancy ends in miscarriage is dealing with issues at a deep subconscious, psychological level; these are concepts that prevent certain energies from manifesting in their life.

Assuming that there is not any blockage of the fallopian tubes or the presence of endometriosis or other conditions, there really is no reason why a well-nourished woman cannot conceive. The infertility exists in the subconscious concepts that would block that conception.

Some women produce eggs that cannot be fertilized for various reasons. In those instances it may very well be because of certain concepts within the subconscious mind that the body attacks the eggs. The immune system identifies the eggs as alien invaders, so the eggs themselves fortify their protective casing so that nothing can penetrate, including sperm; thus, there is no chance of fertilization, and pregnancy is avoided altogether. Autoimmune issues require deep examination and a willingness to change in order to express the self differently.

All herbs listed are taken to tone the male and/or female reproductive systems.

Gallstones

Gallstones are a misnomer; they should be called gall clumps because the "stones" are really globs of cholesterol that become clumped together in the sac-like gall bladder. Gallstones are primarily the result of too much fried food and a diet high in saturated fats, and this is why the stones have a cholesterol-type base. There is a process often recommended within the health food industry that can be used to dissolve them.

Here is the procedure: Take three tablespoons of cold-pressed olive oil and one teaspoon of freshly squeezed lemon juice, and wait for fifteen minutes. Repeat the process until you have consumed six to nine ounces of olive oil. Then eat a large salad. This entire process should be started on an empty stomach first thing in the morning. If you should happen to throw up, simply rinse out your mouth with water. Do not swallow the water, and then continue the process.

The very first bowel movement that you have will contain gallstones. In all the years that I have been suggesting this approach, I have never heard of one problem other than the taste of the olive oil, and it has been effective time and time again.

SYMBOLOGY OF GALLSTONES

Gallstones represent several things: the inability to utilize sustenance effectively, the inability to break down sources of energy and power to provide the proper material for the individual to move forward in life, and a fear of expanding the mind that can result in failure to accept new thoughts and insights—it is a sad fact that most of us are more comfortable with maintaining the status quo than we are with change. There is an inability to digest, break down, and utilize new thoughts that are being presented.

When there are gallbladder problems, look at your diet symbolically. Do you maintain an affinity for certain foods because they are in keeping with cultural and family traditions? These particular foods may represent security, happiness, acceptance, or even approval. It is hard to give up these emotional connections, and this is one of the reasons it is so difficult for people to change their diets. The change must come from within and must involve not only knowing that certain foods are harmful to health, but also understanding the emotional connections and concepts behind them. One example is men who eat meat because they think it makes them strong and virile. Realize that the food is not the source of true power and virility. This message is just a man-made concept, promoted and reinforced through marketing. The reality is that power is a conceptual thing; you already have the strength, it is just a matter of manifesting it. If there are beliefs within the family lineage that you do not have the power to manifest that strength to be or do whatever you set your mind to, then, regardless of what the diet is, you are not going to.

People are attracted to those foods that will create a physical condition to manifest the subconscious expectation of how the self should be. This extends to any conditions or diseases the person might have, whether it is arthritis, diabetes, poor circulation, or heart attack. These ideas come from family history. We are what we eat and what we think. The path to self-mastery is a matter of discovering what it is you think about who you are and then getting a handle on that. By understanding them, the concepts that motivate your thoughts and actions and the patterns of behavior that work through you, you begin to change your responses to stimuli that trigger behavioral responses. You begin to literally change your mind.

In changing your mind, you change your likes and dislikes, and you also change the emotional needs that you have because as you grow and understand, you gain control over the emotions. They no longer have the power that they do when you stand in the realm of the unknowing self.

Glaucoma

Glaucoma is a disease of the eyes marked by increased pressure within the eyeball, which soon damages the optic nerve. Over two million Americans alone are estimated to suffer from this disease, with those numbers increasing daily. An interesting aspect of this condition is that people with glaucoma have a tendency to be thiamine deficient. [30]

With everything that is currently known about glaucoma, at least one aspect remains in question: what causes the drainage canal behind the eye to become inflamed and, therefore, blocked? The purpose of this channel, called the Schlemm's canal, is to allow the fluid within the eye, called aqueous humor, to drain. Fluid constantly enters the eye, so when a blockage occurs, drainage is prevented. Pressure builds up behind the eye because none of the fluid is able to exit.

The most common type of glaucoma is open-angle. It is without symptoms in the earliest stages, producing an entirely painless increase in eyeball pressure. Side, or peripheral, vision can be affected, but only slowly. Those at greatest risk are anyone with a family history of this disease, African Americans, the severely nearsighted, diabetics, persons over sixty-five years of age, and anyone taking hypertension drugs or cortisone.

"Glaucoma can't be cured, but can be controlled," states author John Kirschmann in his best-seller, Nutrition Almanac. [31] He recommends a diet rich in vitamin A as well as the B-complex vitamins, especially inositol, for those afflicted with the condition.

According to an article in The Journal of Holistic Medicine, [32] vitamin C can help glaucoma by increasing osmotic pressure in the blood, which, in turn, pulls fluid out of the eyeball. Doctors in Rome found a dramatic drop in the eye pressure of all their glaucoma patients within two hours after a single dose of vitamin C was used. An Ohio optometrist found substantial drops in eye pressure and improved vision in his glaucoma patients when they took 500 mg of vitamin C morning and evening for up to four months.[33]

NUTRIENTS AND HERBS TO SUPPORT EYE HEALTH

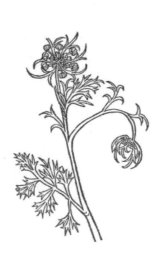

Nutrients	Herbs
Biotin	Eyebright
Choline	Ginger
Folic Acid	
Inositol	
Niacin	
Pantothenic Acid	
Vitamin A	
Vitamin B-1	
Vitamin B-2	
Vitamin B-6	
Vitamin B-12	
Vitamin C	

Biotin. Necessary for the manufacture of fats, the metabolism of carbohydrates, and the breakdown of proteins into urea. It also affects proteins in converting amino acids into sugar for fuel/energy.

Choline. Part of the neurotransmitter acetylcholine, which is essential for the transmission of impulses (electrical energy) through the nervous system. It is released at some neuromuscular junctions, at some neuroglandular junctions, and at synapses between certain brain and spinal cord cells. In most parts of the body, acetylcholine leads to excitation.

Folic Acid. Another vitamin that has a direct nourishing and fortifying effect on the "front line" of the body's defense system.

Inositol. Closely associated with choline and biotin; also needed for the growth and survival of cells in bone marrow, eye membranes, and intestines. This nutrient is vital for hair growth and can prevent thinning hair and baldness.

Niacin. A B-complex nutrient that promotes growth and proper nervous system function.

One of the ways that niacin works in the body is to dilate the blood vessels. This allows blood freer access to the all the cells and tissues of the extremities, such as hands and feet.

Pantothenic Acid. Also known as vitamin B-5, pantothenic acid helps in the utilization of other vitamins, especially vitamin B-2.

Vitamin A. Essential for all vision, especially healthy night vision. Vitamin A deficiency is a major public health problem.

Beta-carotene is the preferred source of vitamin A, which also serves as an antioxidant. It is a potent quencher of singlet oxygen, a highly reactive molecule form or configuration believed to be responsible for aging. It breaks down DNA so that reproduced cells are flawed and weak. This leads to aging and disease. Because it is converted to vitamin A only as needed, beta-carotene does not cause hyper-vitaminosis A, the way high amounts of fish liver oil can.

Vitamin B-1. Necessary for healthy mouth, skin, eyes, and hair. It is essential for nerve tissues, muscles, digestion, and normal heart function.

Vitamin B-2. Functions as part of a group of enzymes involved in the breakdown and utilization of carbohydrates, fats, and proteins. B-2 is also good for cell respiration and the maintenance of good vision, skin, nails, and hair.

Vitamin B-6. Required for the proper absorption of vitamin B-12, the production of hydrochloric acid, and magnesium assimilation.

Vitamin B-12. Helps form normal red blood cells and a healthy nervous system. It is very important in the production of myelin, a sheath that covers and protects the nerves. It also plays a role in making folate available to the cells and helps the body metabolize fats, carbohydrates, and proteins more effectively.

Vitamin C. Needed for healthy teeth, gums, and bones. It strengthens the blood vessels and also helps to detoxify the effects of heavy metals often found in drinking water, for example, lead.

Eyebright. A traditional herb for eyes.

Ginger. A circulatory stimulant. Considered a "packager" because it carries nutrients throughout the system.

SYMBOLOGY OF GLAUCOMA

There is a constant replacement of fluid in the eye. When the drainage canal becomes blocked, this creates one of the conditions for the disease of glaucoma to arise. This is a symbolic reminder that there should constantly be a fresh look at our material considerations and perceptions of life.

When we hold onto the past and continue to look at things according to the same perspectives and through the same conceptual filters, problems can arise. Life has its own innate, ongoing cleansing process. Part of that cleansing process is learning to look at things anew, which affords fresh insights; through them, greater understandings are realized. This ultimately allows for growth on all levels. When this does not happen, and people continue to relate to the events and situations in life from old perspectives, that may very well be when pressure builds up within an individual. The pressure stems from a belief that what the person is seeing at this point in life cannot be handled. Each person has personal concepts that will create conflict within the body. Where disease strikes in the body is indicative of that person's particular conflict.

It is interesting that medical science has determined that the number 23 should represent a significant threshold of pressure within the eye. In accord with the symbolic interpretation of numerology, these two numbers add up to 5—coincidentally the number of the physical senses that a person uses to navigate through life. Of course, there are the intuitive senses that can also help us to navigate clearly. I use the term "navigate" because the senses keep us informed of where we are at any given moment in time. Additionally, they protect us from outside forces that could have a negative effect upon us if we lose our way. For example, consider toxins that we are able to avoid through the sense of smell or taste, and the dangers we skirt around because we may see or feel something that could cause harm. The five senses are a key to mastery in life when they are developed to their highest potential.

Uncontrolled glaucoma causes blindness by pressing against the optic nerve over time. What is the symbolism here? The optic nerve has three important regions: the margin, the nerve fibers, and the cup. What I find most interesting in this is that the number 3 symbolically represents understanding. Understanding is required throughout life, as the *Bible* reminds us we "have eyes to see" and to "know what is before thine eyes, and all the mysteries will be revealed." These are key Universal Teachings.

Symbology of the Nutrients

Biotin. Symbolizes liberation through cleansing. In glaucoma, the fluid that is supposed to be replaced on a daily basis, symbolic of having a fresh look at life, is blocked from draining; therefore, cleansing is blocked and must be restored for clarity.

Choline. Symbolically represents inner-strength and life requires a true inner-strength to move forward. When strength and personal power are lacking, doubt and fear have an opportunity to manifest in your life. One result may be glaucoma, which can hinder your ability to see clearly. Doubt and fear have created a number of problems for people, and these problems manifest in different ways, but blindness, one of these problems, is the ultimate result of those who no longer wish to see.

Folic Acid. Symbolically speaking is a fortifier. It helps to fortify and strengthen every aspect of being. In this application we are seeking to fortify and improve the ability to perceive self and life from a different point of view.

In order to truly move forward you must be able to see yourself clearly. Introspection is something that should be done on a daily basis, if not moment by moment. This is especially true when symbols arise that require questioning. It is through questioning the self that answers lead to insights and understandings as to why we do what we do. This, in turn, gives us strength to eliminate destructive habits.

Inositol. Represents integrity, which is closely associated with choline (inner-strength) and biotin (liberation through cleansing). When you think about integrity's role in life, you can see how essential it is to have true inner-strength. Integrity has different definitions. Here we want the benefits of integrity to be able to have the courage to move forward on what we clearly perceive and understand what needs to be changed. Creating blindness is not the way to eliminate unwanted situations from your life.

Niacin. Represents openness and receptivity. In this formula it is absolutely essential that the canal that drains the fluid from behind the eye remains open. When it becomes inflamed it stops the cleansing and fresh fluid cannot enter. This, in time, will cause blindness. This is also true of concepts that create the ideals, values and standards that you use to live your life. If they are not examined and that which is useless is not removed or eliminated then you lose perception of the truth of life and the true role of self.

Vitamin A. Significantly, this nutrient represents the ability to see into the doubt that exists within the self. You could even say that vitamin A aids in self-examination by its role in improving (internal) vision.

If you have glaucoma, it may well be that there are things going on in your life that you are no longer willing to "look at" and deal with. We arrive at this perception because of glaucoma's potential to cause blindness.

When you doubt your own ability to handle things, forces are set in motion that will create a way out of the conflict. In this case it appears that taking a fresh look at things is not in keeping with the inherent belief system. I would not be surprised if these individuals also suffered from arthritis, which also represents a form of inflexibility. Through self-examination, you can begin to see the truth of who you really are as opposed to who you think you are supposed to be. This insight will lead to new vision, and a fresh perspective on life.

Interestingly, vitamin A also supports immune function, and glaucoma is frequently the result of inflammation constricting the flow of fluid from the eyes. With proper vision, you can avoid the doubt and frustration that accompany your preparation for any situation in life. Vitamin A helps you to see well, thus, giving you greater insight into the situation, and going into a situation totally prepared gives you courage and confidence. When you have those energies at work and in hand, you need not doubt your ability to master a situation.

Another aspect of vitamin A's symbology is that it is instrumental in protecting you from invasion by outside forces. Vitamin A is needed for the health of all mucous membranes, and it feeds the thymus gland, which is an immune center. It is from the thymus gland that T-cells rush out to do battle with invading forces. On a physical level those forces can be allergens, germs, bacteria, viruses, fungus, or toxins from the environment, the very elements that could cause the inflammation. Forces can also be thoughts, attitudes, and energies from others that you willingly accept into your conscious realm of reality, done to help you fulfill subconscious expectations of self.

Vitamin B-1. Acts as a facilitator. Among this nutrient's many roles is that of protector of your eyes, and your eyes allow you to see the world. By constantly assessing and adjusting your concept-based perceptions, you are able to see things in a new light. This gives you an opportunity to change existing situations and create new ways of handling events and interacting with people.

Vitamin B-1 facilitates the ability to control emotions. This also plays a major role in glaucoma because adverse physical reactions, in this case an inflammatory response, are always the result of conflict between subconscious ego expectations and spiritual directives.

Vitamin B-2. Represents courage. It works with vitamin B-1 (confidence) in supporting eye, skin, and hair health. Confidence and courage are required in every endeavor, and if one was lost, it would impact the way you see yourself as well as the way in which others see you.

Both traits are required to constantly examine, or re-examine, thoughts and situations from fresh perspectives. Doubt and fear are always present in some arena of our lives to some degree, which is why fresh looks are so important; they can help us identify where those two energies are at work affecting our perceptions.

Should you be confronted by something that challenges your personal belief system, you would require courage and confidence to look at and understand these new thoughts in order to get any potential benefit they have to offer. Without the benefit of taking a fresh look, you would miss entirely the opportunity to digest, assimilate, and gain sustenance from new or re-evaluated thoughts.

Vitamin B-6. Symbolically represents regulation as well as protection. In order to view things clearly, it is imperative to have regulation when you examine something, whether it is an object or a concept. If the optic nerve is damaged then sight becomes distorted, and that alone will create many uncomfortable situations in which you may very well require protection to survive.

You must always be aware to a decent degree in order to protect yourself from the manmade ideas that are constantly projected on you and society as a whole. Without protection you are vulnerable to outside influences that will create damage within your life on many levels, including the physical.

Some ideas require regulation by emotional response, and others, a protective mode so as not to destroy a current position or stand on issues/concepts. These regulating, protective thoughts are necessary to keep the body in a state of good health because thoughts actually change its biochemistry in response to external stimuli or emotional responses to a given event.

Vitamin B-12. Symbolically represents a working faith. Without faith and fortification (folate), new life (red blood cells) and expression (cells as a reflection of self) would not take root and produce viable results.

It takes an internal working faith, which stems from past successes, to truly accomplish the difficult things in life.

Vitamin C. Symbolic of material/physical protection. On both levels, physical and metaphysical, insightful awareness is essential to remaining healthy and free of danger.

Vitamin C increases absorption of iron, symbolic of faith and courage. Iron is contained in hemoglobin, which caries oxygen to the cells. It also removes carbon dioxide and carries it to the lungs. Oxygen is symbolic of spirit because air symbolically represents heaven. Tying together these symbolic interpretations, we can see that vitamin C (protection) is essential for faith and courage/strength to grow.

High Blood Pressure (Hypertension)

High blood pressure, or hypertension as the medical community calls it, has many different causes from faulty internal processes, such as a breakdown in the communication between the nerves and the cells that comprise the heart as well as the muscles surrounding the arterial system leading to improper muscular tension and conditions that ultimately will be called a disease.

Hypertension is also the result of today's fast-paced, anxiety-filled lifestyles, which are conducive to the creation of stress and tension—two underlying causes of hypertension. Stress, tension, and anxiety are not entirely physical diseases, although they do cause them. Instead, they are the result of emotional and mental attitudes about and reactions to situations.

Internal reactions at emotional levels cause slight chemical reactions within the body. An excellent example of this is when the phone rings in the middle of the night. This event will trigger a biochemical reaction within the individual. One such change will be a diminishing amount of calcium in the body, and when calcium is compromised it creates an imbalance between sodium and potassium. This, in turn, will cause the body to retain fluid, putting pressure on the cardiovascular system, and as a result could elevate blood pressure. Another affect of this chemical stimulation is that the body may begin to tighten up as the muscles contract. This contraction places excessive pressure on the cardiovascular system as well, leading to elevated blood pressure.

NUTRIENTS, AMINO ACIDS AND HERBS TO SUPPORT NORMAL BLOOD PRESSURE

There are many dangers to uncontrolled high blood pressure; stroke and death are but two. Include the following in your diet to help reduce high blood pressure through the elimination of excess water, muscular tension and vasodilatation.

Nutrients	Amino Acids	Herbs
Calcium	L-Taurine	Apple Pectin
Magnesium		Cayenne
Potassium		Garlic
Vitamin B-6		Hawthorne Berries
Vitamin D		Hops
		Valerian Root

Calcium. Acts as a calmative on the muscles.

Magnesium. Helps to nourish the nerves and the brain, it is also used in the utilization of choline, a fat-dissolving vitamin. Fats/cholesterol and triglycerides in the blood create circulation problems.

Potassium. Works along with vitamin B-6 in maintaining proper water balance. Often times, an imbalance in osmosis creates pressure on the arterial system.

Vitamin B-6. Aids in maintaining correct water balance in the blood and tissues.

Vitamin D. Ensures the effectiveness of calcium.

L-Taurine. An amino acid is found in high amounts in the heart and central nervous system. Taurine aids in the metabolism of cholesterol and triglycerides.

Apple Pectin, Cayenne, and Garlic. All have the ability to equalize blood pressure.

Hawthorne Berries. Tone and strengthen the heart muscle.

Hops and Valerian Root. Calming herbs to the nervous system.

Symbology of High Blood Pressure

Symbolically, hypertension provides us with a great deal of insight and knowledge. It shows, from the physical perspective alone, that the individual is lacking faith in self on some level, that there is a belief that what they are confronting is more than they can handle, and that there is a lack of faith, confidence or courage. The truth is you do possess all of the abilities to deal with any situations that confront you.

When you think about what causes hypertension you can see the validity of the symbolic perspective. Hypertension has three fundamental causes as we discussed earlier. The first that we will examine is the imbalance in the osmosis in the body, meaning that there is too much fluid being retained in the system. The way to maintain proper fluid balance is by keeping the potassium/sodium relationship in harmony.

When you look at the symbology of both potassium and sodium you can begin to see how those two must maintain a particular balance within the self in order to maintain the courage and confidence necessary to go out into the world and deal with life and the issues and forces an individual is confronted with.

Another causative factor in hypertension is stress, which refers to emotional stress and corresponding muscular tension. These are really a reaction to what is seen and heard, and how the individual responds to those stimuli. All of that is tied into the concepts within the subconscious mind. This is reflected in the belief system that an individual maintains about how life is supposed to be lived, how they are supposed to deal with things, and how they should and should not act in regards to certain stimuli, events and situations.

By making judgments (man does even though he is religiously taught or instructed not to) a person will end up getting upset about what they may see and/or hear. This can make a person angry or tense, and that reaction creates pressure on their cardiovascular system which, in turn, can set the body up for hypertension.

Along those same lines, hypertension can lead to strokes and heart attacks. When that is examined it can be seen that the energy of anger can get somebody so worked up and out of emotional control that they really can "blow their lid." It can easily be seen where a stroke or heart attack would occur.

Heart attacks are the result of accumulated emotional responses and attacks. Again, these emotional responses are based on the value judgments, subconscious concepts, and patternistic expectations of the individual. After a period of time the person can no longer handle the attacks, regardless of how subtle they may be. People respond to everything that they see and hear, especially when it is directed towards them.

The individual that is hypertensive is working with the belief system that instills doubt and fear that they cannot handle the situation that they find themselves in. These individuals require understanding and when we look at the nutrients that are involved in helping the body to eliminate hypertension it gives us a greater clarity as to what concepts and the emotional stances within the individual need bolstering.

SYMBOLOGY OF THE NUTRIENTS AND VARIOUS HERBS

Looking at the nutrients that are symbolically involved in alleviating hypertension reinforces the truth of what is necessary for a person to possess to deal with life from a position of strength. Because when looking at hypertension symbolically, we see that the fundamental causes are the reactions to what we see and hear, and this is based on the subconscious concepts that we maintain. The other cause is an imbalance of the osmosis within the body, and this, too, is based on concepts centering on the person's material considerations.

The nutrients that are required to allow the body to come back in to balance and harmony are calcium and magnesium.

Calcium. Represents strength, and what could be truer than having the strength to be able to see and hear the things that go on and not allow it to affect you in a negative way. To see and hear, and yet not make value judgments is strength. Judgments have the potential to make you angry, resentful, or uptight.

When a person begins to get uptight that is when they begin to constrict the arteries through muscular tension, and reduce the amount of bloodflow through the arteries creating hypertension. It takes a lot of strength to deal with life and to look within the self to understand what is creating the reactions that one has. Some people believe on some levels that they do not have the strength to handle what they are confronting, yet the truth of life is no one is ever placed in a situation they cannot master.

Magnesium. Represents inspiration, and is yet another key to eliminating hypertension. When we look at life we know it also requires a bit of inspiration. You need to have some degree of inspiration to even want to handle all the things that you are confronted with.

Knowing that you have the strength, you can become inspired. You can see how the role of calcium and magnesium is so vitally important to well-being. It is interesting symbolically how magnesium is involved in so many different functions within the body, demonstrating how vitally important inspiration is in living a vibrant life.

Potassium. When a person understands the concepts that motivate them, they have more of a moderate, balanced, and regulated approach for handling the material plane. This is why potassium is also very important in regulating blood pressure within the system, because, symbolically, potassium represents balance and harmony.

When these energies exist within the individual, and when the body has adequate amounts of these nutrients, it creates an environment that prevents high blood pressure from taking hold. Hypertension cannot take root and manifest in a person's life because things are seen from a balanced perspective, and things are understood because one has the internal strength and the insights necessary to move forward without getting uptight about the situation.

Vitamin B-6. Represents protection and regulation. This nutrient is also integral to eliminating hypertension, especially when it is caused by an imbalance of fluids in the body. The fluid retention that creates this imbalance is symbolic of the imbalanced approach to dealing with life in the material plane.

It can be seen that the imbalance in the material plane is vitally important to understand. Many individuals are unbalanced because they are using material objects, such as foods, money, drugs, and sex as a way of trying to fulfill emptiness within.

Our society teaches us to look outside of the self to satisfy all of its internal needs, but the truth of the matter is that whatever it is that a person thinks they require is just that, thoughts. These thoughts are based on concepts within the subconscious that may not be understood.

Vitamin D. Represents insight, and life requires insights to some degree. One of the aspects of insights is that they are necessary in order to be able to utilize your strength.

Strength, to some degree, is always present—even if sometimes you do not see it. Sometimes you may feel you cannot handle a situation, and yet there it is in front of you. Again, remember that we are always co-creating our reality. Therefore, we are never placed in a situation that we cannot handle or master.

Apple Pectin. Included in this recommendation for eliminating hypertension. Apples are symbolic of knowledge, and knowledge is the key to everything. Knowledge of self is the ultimate key to mastery, and it is essential to have self-knowledge, in fact, it is taught in the *Bible*: "Know thyself and the truth will set you free."

Hypoglycemia (Low Blood Sugar)

Hypoglycemia is the medical term for low blood sugar, and is generally caused by poor dietary habits or an excess of stress. It is surprising how many people constantly feel tired and run down, even after a full night's sleep. Are you in this group, or do you know someone who is? Chronic tiredness—even after sleeping up to 12 hours a night—is perhaps the most identifiable of hypoglycemia's symptoms, which also include irritability and headaches.

Hypoglycemics are the people you do not talk to until you give them something sweet to eat or drink in the morning to raise their blood sugar level, but nourishing the adrenals might be a better solution. Pantothenic acid, vitamin C, and a little dash of licorice root strengthen the adrenals so that there is good communication between them and the liver.

Many people try to deal with this problem by taking B-12 injections or stimulant herbs high in caffeine such as Guarana, Ephedra (Ma Huang), or other types of herbs that are high in caffeine. This approach is not the answer, and is only a form of relief without addressing the true cause. These herbs work by stimulating the central nervous system, which is an unhealthy approach to the problem. One approach that will work and will help the person feel like a human being again lies within good nutrition and dietary changes.

Knowing how difficult it is to change eating habits, I have researched and found the nutritional elements that will help the body to correct hypoglycemia. First, let us examine how low blood sugar is created. As we stated, one cause of low blood sugar is brought about by stress, and when the body is subjected to stressful conditions, it depletes the fuel supply, so more fuel must then be added to the system.

The adrenal glands are involved with blood sugar regulation. They tell the pancreas when to start and stop insulin production. Insulin (a hormone produced by the pancreas to regulate the blood glucose level) is used to shuttle blood sugar into the cells. When too many refined carbohydrates are eaten requiring constant communication from the adrenals to the pancreas, exhaustion can begin to set in.

The adrenal glands communicate with the pancreas throughout the day. By 3:00 p.m. it is exhausted from telling the pancreas to start and stop insulin production, and the last message that the pancreas received was to start insulin production. As insulin production continues, blood sugar levels decrease. When blood sugar levels are too low it is the responsibility of the adrenal glands to tell the liver to release more glycogen (blood sugar) into the bloodstream, but because the adrenals have been talking to the pancreas all day it cannot talk to the liver and sugar levels continue to plunge.

NUTRIENTS AND HERBS TO SUPPORT THE ADRENALS IN ENERGY PRODUCTION

Nutrients	Amino Acid	Herbs
Folic Acid	Aspartic Acid	Eleuthero Root
Pantothenic Acid		Gotu Kola
Vitamin B-12		Licorice Root
Vitamin C		

Folic Acid. Works in conjunction with B12 to ensure that anemia is corrected and/or prevented.

Pantothenic Acid. Provides nourishment to the adrenal glands. The adrenal glands work with the pancreas in maintaining proper blood sugar levels; this helps in keeping the energy levels up.

Vitamin B-12. Has been used by the medical profession for years to provide energy to tired and run down individuals.

Vitamin C. Helps support the adrenal glands, which are responsible for regulating sugar in the bloodstream. They work in conjunction with the pancreas and the liver. By supporting the adrenal glands you end up having better control over hypoglycemia.

Aspartic Acid. Helps in increasing stamina and endurance as well as resistance to fatigue.

Eleuthero Root. Has been used for centuries as a tonic and is highly invigorating.

Gotu Kola. Feeds and stimulates the brain as well as the body, and creates alertness.

Licorice Root. Also nourishes the adrenal glands.

SYMBOLOGY OF HYPOGLYCEMIA

In examining hypoglycemia symbolically we find that it represents a lack of inspiration, enthusiasm, and motivation. The hypoglycemic person never seems to have the energy to do what needs to be done, or even what they say they want to do.

When a person lacks inspiration and enthusiasm it generally can be traced back to a bout of doubt or fear. These feelings and attitudes about self reside within the subconscious concepts that the person operates with, and these concepts are reinforced through repetitive actions, patterns of behavior that the individual performs.

In almost every case there is a lack of completion, which can be tied into a success-failure concept and its corresponding pattern of behavior. The person has the ability to be a success, but failure is often the route that is chosen. This is in keeping with the subconscious expectations of the person.

Another area to examine in hypoglycemia is the blood. The blood represents spirit and sugar represents the sweetness of life and the material plane. If an individual does not have the wherewithal in their own mind, and the faith in self to utilize their energy and spirit effectively and take control of their destiny, then hypoglycemia sets in. With hypoglycemia there is an amount of doubt and a lack of confidence manifesting in that person's life. Of course this can be said for almost everyone, but each person deals with their issues according to the way that the concepts were presented to them as a child and by whom they were presented. Low blood sugar can also represent low self-esteem because it all revolves around a lack of faith in one's ability to do things. An individual with hypoglycemia is often overwhelmed to a point where they are operating out of doubt and fear, and may be totally uninspired to the point that nothing motivates them and nothing interests them.

SYMBOLOGY OF THE NUTRIENTS

Hypoglycemia, low blood sugar, is symbolic of different subconscious concepts at work, and often, in conflict. It becomes abundantly clear what is energetically lacking within the person when examining the nutrients symbolically. The nutrients that are essential for restoring the body's balance, harmony, and energy are pantothenic acid, folic acid, vitamin B-12 and vitamin C.

Low blood sugar symbolically translates into a lack of inspiration. Its fundamental cause, as with most diseases, is conflict within the subconscious. This conflict exists because subconsciously the person does not believe that they have the right, authority, ability or the wherewithal to do what they desire to do on a conscious level. The conflict is between desire and limiting subconscious concepts, and is supported by doubt and fear.

Pantothenic acid. Symbolic of inspiration, is vital to energy production within the body, and is part of the Krebs cycle. This cycle produces energy within each cell. Pantothenic acid also helps to nourish the adrenal glands, which are symbolic of courage and confidence. They communicate with the liver, symbolic of protection and transformation, to release glycogen, the sugar that the body runs on. The glycogen is in the bloodstream so that fuel is available for the cells to perform their functions.

Folic Acid and Vitamin B-12. Symbolic of facilitation and a working faith, respectively. Without inspiration in life (pantothenic acid), a working faith (vitamin B-12) and something to facilitate the desire to succeed (folic acid), nothing would be accomplished.

Vitamin C. Symbolic of protection, and without the feeling of protection as a form of strength, it can be understood how hypoglycemia would be symbolic of a lack of inspiration. Through subconscious concepts that one maintains and the experiences that reinforce those concepts, the individual looses faith in their ability to do things. Additionally, they are not inspired about what is going on in their life.

It can be shown consistently how the symbology of the nutrients validates the nutritional approach necessary in order to bring the body back into balance and harmony. Life itself is a matter of seeking balance and harmony, having the inspiration, feeling protected, and having a working faith, knowing that you can deal with anything that comes along.

Another aspect to hypoglycemia is the feeling of being overwhelmed. Again, this would end up making an individual feel emotionally down, robbing them of their strength and faith within themselves. When you feel overwhelmed it is a statement of not being able to handle everything that you are confronted with. The truth of the matter is, if you are faced with a certain situation it is your co-creation and, therefore, you can handle it. You have just created an opportunity for self to master a particular situation, concept, and pattern of behavior. Another way of looking at patterns of behavior is to see them as patternistic responses and outcomes of certain stimuli.

Whenever a person is affected by hypoglycemia, they will also have, to some degree, allergies and Candida Albicans. It would be worth the time to read the symbology and nutritional approaches to both of these situations.

Immune Health Concerns

In today's world of AIDS and other degenerative diseases, we are faced with the fact that our bodies—especially our immune systems—are no longer able to defend us. There seems to have been a weakening of that system. Why is that so? There are always two sides to every story. For the purpose of our discussion we will touch on two aspects that are instrumental in weakening the immune system.

First, we need to recall the latest research that is taking place in regard to stress. It is being demonstrated and proven that stress adversely affects the immune system. Stress taxes the adrenal glands that secrete hormones that carry messages to the other glands on how and/or what to perform or manufacture. All the glands of the body are tied together in a complicated system, and each and every aspect of life within the body is dependent on each other. This is why it is so important to maintain a proper nutritional balance within. In this way you are providing the system with the needed ingredients to function correctly and, thus, provide optimum health and eliminate the opportunity for disease to take hold.

It appears that stress depletes nutrients that are vital to the health of the immune system. When this happens the immune system does not perform at efficient levels and illness becomes more prevalent. The inability of the immune system to destroy invaders sets up a condition in the body that allows invaders to take hold, it is then that we are infected with some sort of germ.

At the same time another situation can take place which may be the cause for all of the autoimmune diseases. Here is what happens: The bacteria that surrounds us all the time—on our skin, in the air and on the food we eat—enters into our bodies. Since the immune system is not strong enough to attack and destroy all of the invaders, some of them have the time and the ability to adapt to the new environment, our bloodstream.

While in the bloodstream, they are able to enter into healthy cells and become a part of those cells. This creates a condition where the antibodies do not know what to attack because the invaders are now a part of the cells that the body has always recognized as its own, so now these mutated cells have an opportunity to multiply. The result is sick cells that have the ability to destroy the body. Arthritis is thought to be one such condition, an autoimmune disease. AIDS may very well be another one of these types of diseases, which brings us back to the true cause, a much-weakened immune system.

Now that we have dealt with stress as one of the causes of this condition, we must look at the other cause, nutritional deficiencies, which is more difficult to correct.

Poor nutrition has been the cause of countless diseases throughout time. Scurvy, rickets, and pellagra are just a few examples. Nutrition, or more correctly, nutrients are the building materials of the human body. They are the building blocks, cement, wood and nails of life— nothing is created within the human body without an adequate supply of nutrients. Neither is any system able to maintain itself without the proper nutrients in the correct amounts.

When you try to maintain good health but do not have all the right nutrients or proper amounts, you will not have a sound and healthy immune system.

To reiterate, the two causes of a weak and ineffective immune system are stress and poor nutrition. Stress is a perception and attitude problem that requires a particular form of adjustment, whereas nutrition is a dietary and supplementation adjustment.

In regards to the dietary changes the most obvious would be to include more fresh fruits and raw vegetables. More specifically, increasing garlic, onions, celery, watercress and carrots would be especially helpful, and decreasing all fried and fatty foods along with curtailing the amount of meat, fish and fowl that you eat would also be wise.

NUTRIENTS AND HERBS TO IMPROVE RESISTANCE TO STRESS AND INFECTION

Nutrients	Herbs
Beta-carotene (Vitamin A)	Astragalus
Choline	Codonopsis
Folic Acid	Echinacea
Inositol	Ligustrum Berries
Magnesium	Reishi Mushroom
Pantothenic Acid	Shiitake Mushroom
Selenium	White Atractylodes
Vitamin B-1	
Vitamin B-2	
Vitamin B-6	
Vitamin B-12	
Vitamin C	
Vitamin E	
Zinc	

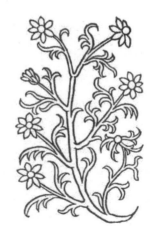

Beta-carotene (Vitamin A). Your vegetarian source of vitamin A. The beauty of vitamin A is that it helps mature antibodies in the thymus gland and protects all mucus membranes exposed to the environment.

Choline. Essential for the health of the liver and kidneys. Essential for the health of the myelin sheaths of the nerves; the myelin sheaths are the principal component of the nerve fibers. It is also important in the transmission of the nerve impulses.

Folic Acid. Is involved in the formation of white blood cells and lymphocytes, the front line soldiers of the immune system.

Inositol and Vitamin B-1. Wonderful for nerves.

Magnesium. Activates more enzymes in the body than any other mineral. Lack of magnesium may be involved as one of the causes of one kind of leukemia, or cancer of the blood.

Pantothenic Acid. Stimulates the adrenal glands and increases production of cortisone and other adrenal hormones; can improve the body's ability to withstand stressful conditions. Pantothenic acid has been demonstrated to enhance the activity of macrophage and natural killer cells in the body. It is necessary for antibody production, part of the humoral branch of the immune system.

Selenium. Appears to prevent certain kinds of cancer.

Vitamin B-2. Protection of cellular respiration.

Vitamin B-6. Must be present for the production of antibodies and red blood cells. Improves T-cell levels and mitogen stimulation.

Vitamin B-12. Helps the placement of vitamin A into body tissues by aiding carotene absorption or vitamin A conversion.

Vitamin C. Fights bacterial infections and reduces the effects on the body of some allergy-producing substances.

Vitamin E. Prevents saturated fatty acids and vitamin A from breaking down and combining with other substances that may become harmful to the body. The B vitamins and ascorbic acid are also protected against oxidation when vitamin E is present in the digestive tract.

Zinc. Is essential, it seems, to "mobilize" vitamin A from the liver, so that it can perform its usual bodily functions. Protects the immune system and supports the T-cells. When zinc intake is decreased, the thymus atrophies.

Astragalus. Increases in phagocytosis, interferon, and cancer survival.

Codonopsis. Increases phagocytosis, red blood cells, and T-cell transformation.

Echinacea. Induces living cells to excrete more interferon, which the cells already manufacture. Bolsters the body's defenses by magnifying the white blood cell count. Echinacin, the active constituent of Echinacea, stimulates interferon-like activity. It protects cells against virus related diseases, such as herpes influenza, canker sores, etc., and has the ability to stimulate T-cell activity.

Ligustrum Berries. Increases the number of white blood cells in cancer patients.

Reishi Mushroom. Increases phagocytosis, macrophage, and cell-mediated immunity; suppresses tumor growth in mice.

Shiitake Mushroom. For the immune system.

White Atractylodes. Increases white blood cells and phagocytosis.

SYMBOLOGY OF THE IMMUNE SYSTEM

The symbology of the immune system is really very simple; it is designed to protect the ego and the self from negative attacks, which are presented, inferred, and demonstrated on a daily basis. It is also designed to protect one from the sarcastic and cutting remarks, as well as those said in jest, which often times have a put-down effect.

When examining the immune system, it can be seen as a conglomeration of different energies at work, for example, when looking at the components such as T-cells, T-helper cells, killer cells, phagocytes and white blood cells (to mention a few), it indicates that a high degree of awareness is necessary to protect the self. By converting the different components into symbolic terms we can then see that it indicates that there are many different ways in which the self seeks to protect itself from attack. The attack can originate outside of the person or from concepts within that generate forces that must be dealt with and nullified.

Internal concepts that you operate with can seek to hinder the self from growing into the living light that it can be. Each aspect of the immune system serves different functions, and overall it works to protect the self. It is the same with our consciousness in the sense that there are suggestions, attitudes and verbal aggressions that are projected onto us and toward us from others. These come in many forms and yet the end result is the same. These attacks are designed to hinder, limit, debilitate, put down, insult and embarrass. All of these are attacks that are designed to undermine the individual.

To be healthy on all levels, which will manifest as good health externally, you must have awareness about yourself at all times, and this can be accomplished in different ways. One absolutely necessary aspect is to develop the skill of listening to others. This is done in order to identify when a negative thought or concept is being presented.

By seeking to understand the concept that has been presented and heard, not that the put down has been experienced, but how it will affect the individual in terms of responding. There will be a response because there is always a response. It may be at that moment and it may be that the response will take place later, against somebody else, or in another arena altogether. The scenario could be where an individual gets upset at their computer, at the mouse, and picks it up and throws it against the wall and breaks something. Obviously there is anger and frustration in that transaction. Where did it come from? Often reactions are something that may have been brewing from a previous encounter, or it could have been a different situation altogether, or a person that may have said something.

By having a healthy immune system, symbolically, your awareness is about you at all times. By being in such an alert and conscious state of mind a person will be able to sense auditorially and/or vibratorially, how it is that someone is communicating with them or seeking to attack them in subtle ways. It is the subtle attacks that are the hardest to see and defend against, and this is especially true when a person faces life unaware of the reality of how it works.

Often when a person is under attack and they subconsciously allow the attack to have an effect on them, it is fundamentally because they are in doubt about a situation. From a different point of view, all of us experience doubt and fear in one arena or another within our lives. There are some transactions, events, people, situations, and feelings that literally trigger doubt and fear within an individual, this, in turn, gets past the immune system, so to speak, the defenses, and can be debilitating.

One of the best things that someone can do for their immune system on an energetic level is to really work at maintaining awareness. Listening to what other people say and seeking to understand self is one of the primary keys to mastery in life and control over the emotions.

In as much as the immune system protects an individual from attack from others, the defenses that are used to protect self from others can also symbolically suppress the true Inner Self. When the immune system falters and the individual becomes sick, whatever is affected in the body is a symbolic indication of where the conflict resides. It goes back to what we said earlier about how sometimes the attacks are from within. It is because of an individual's doubt within self and their abilities to handle a particular situation that they will end up creating stress within their life and that will lower the immune system. This then provides an opportunity for an invasion to take hold and root.

The truth is that a condition, disease, or accident is, in reality, doubt manifesting very strongly. This is usually in regards to a particular upcoming event or situation that the individual is about to confront or is seeking to avoid.

SYMBOLOGY OF THE NUTRIENTS

The immune system is one of the most vital systems within the body. Fundamentally, it protects the self from external forces that can cause damage. When we examine the nutrients that are involved in the proper functioning of the immune system, and look at them symbolically, we see what it really takes to withstand the forces of life. Additionally, it can be understood from another point of view why some people do not and cannot deal with those forces.

One reason is because they are malnourished as a result of not only the diet but also the spirit and personal power. This is the consequence of having been taught to look externally and not internally.

Choline. Represents inner-strength. Repeatedly we come across the same concepts, the same energies that are essential for well-being, for defending the self against external forces.

Folic Acid. Being a facilitator or a fortifier, helps to fortify and strengthen the individual.

Magnesium, Pantothenic Acid, Vitamin B-2. Pantothenic acid and magnesium represent inspiration. Both of these nutrients are essential for the immune system. Interestingly, vitamin B-2, which works to protect cellular respiration and defending the cells, represents courage symbolically. Keep in mind the importance of all the nutrients because they each have a contributing effect upon the whole. Here we see that courage and inspiration go hand in hand in combating invading negative thoughts. You have to be strong in your understandings so that regardless of the presentation of thoughts to you, you are clear enough not to accept them and allow them to debilitate your inspiration or courage. Once again we see the same premise that it takes some degree of courage to deal with the onslaught of forces that one is confronted with on a daily basis.

Selenium and Zinc. Also essential to the function of the immune system. Zinc symbolically represents expression and a working faith. Once again we see the need to express one's self especially if one is being attacked. Attacks can come in the form of subtle put-downs, jokes at a person's expense, and out and out negative statements. A person must also know that they have the confidence to deal with events and situations, including certain people in their lives in a positive way, and they can handle everything from a position of strength.

Selenium provides protection and cleansing. The cleansing is an important aspect of the immune system because as the immune system is destroying pathogens, mutated cells, invading entities—if you will, negative thoughts—and devouring them, rendering them harmless, the mind/body must also eliminate them.

Vitamin B-6. Also tied into protection, represents regulation. In the immune system it helps in regulating the white blood cells, and white is symbolic of spirit. In this case, white blood cells are phagocytes which patrol the body and destroy invading pathogens or invading forces. It is within our abilities to identify negative thoughts, a negative input from an external source, and to be able to nullify it so that it does not cause any damage or harm.

Vitamin B-12. Represents a working faith and is tied in with courage.

Vitamin C. Like vitamin B-6, is also symbolic of protection. The need of the body and the functioning of the immune system demonstrate how there are certain fundamental energies that are essential for the immune system/mind to protect the self: courage, working faith, and the ability to discern invading forces and thoughts and nullify them before they can act in a negative way upon the self.

Vitamin E. If you recall in the beginning of this Work we talked about vitamin E being symbolic of self confidence and a reduced need of external support in matters of dealing with a working faith. Look at this interpretation from the point of view that when a person has self-confidence, they have a working faith and fundamentally they feel that they can deal with anything that comes their way. They can protect self because they know they have the confidence to be able to handle it. It is when people get caught up in doubt that the systems within the body become vulnerable to attack from others, from bacteria, which is only symbolic of negative thoughts coming in from external sources.

You can see that the immune system and your ability to defend yourself and be in a position of strength at all times is what the symbology of the immune system is in its totality. Know that when you nurture yourself with the proper thoughts as well as the proper nutrition, and maintain a positive outlook you have the beginnings of a healthy immune system. When you seek to understand and discern what is being presented to you, you will know how it is going to affect you. Having that knowledge you can make the necessary changes and attitude adjustments so that what is presented does not have a negative effect upon the self.

We know that so much of this information, in terms of the immune system, seems to be redundant and at the same time we know that we cannot stress enough the issues at hand in terms of what is essential for defending yourself and working from a position of strength in dealing with everything that an individual must deal with in life.

Impotence

In today's high-stress world, we often find ourselves unable to perform in life as we once did. This applies to all aspects of life, but one of the most frustrating areas is sexual expression, with the result being an inability to perform.

The causes go beyond simple stress, for example, in some instances a person may have poor circulation. Others deal with diabetes, some with side effects from medication, and some suffer from psychological causes.

There is an herb that has been in use for centuries to assist man in maintaining his "nature." This herb, often taken in tablet or capsule form or as a tea, is called yohimbe.

The inner bark of the tropical West African tree Corynanthe Yohimbe contains several indole-based alkaloids, of which yohimbine is the most prominent. It causes increased vasodilation and peripheral bloodflow in combination with stimulation of the spinal ganglia that controls the corpus spongiosum (erectile tissue). This action produces an erection in the male. Other pleasurable effects are warm spinal shivers—which are especially enjoyable during coitus and orgasm (bodies feel like they are melting into one another)—psychic stimulations, mild perceptual changes without hallucination and heightening of emotional and sexual feeling. Effects last about two hours.

Yohimbine is also a mild serotonin inhibitor. It has been found that when larger than normal amounts of serotonin are produced in the body, blood pressure, nervousness, depression and exhaustion are increased. There is a possibility that some forms of impotence are not psychologically based or due to any waning of one's glandular manhood, but may simply be the result of increased serotonin levels in the brain. Conversely, substances that inhibit serotonin are likely to have an apparent aphrodisiacal influence. This response, however, is the natural sex chemistry of the body being liberated pharmaceutically from the blockage of the serotonin.

Normally, there are no undesirable after-effects. Individuals with sensitive stomachs may experience some queasiness or mild nausea for a few minutes shortly after drinking the tea, so it is best to sip it slowly. Persons suffering from blood pressure disorders, diabetes, hypoglycemia, active ailments, or injury of kidneys, liver, or heart should not use yohimbe. It is a brief-acting monoamine oxidase inhibitor and should not be used by persons under the influence of alcohol, amphetamines (even diet pills), antihistamines, narcotics and certain tranquilizers.

Yohimbe works directly on the sex center of the brain as well as other organs. In the brain, it inhibits serotonin, which we stated earlier increases blood pressure, exhaustion and feelings of depression. Also with high serotonin levels there is generally a loss of interest in sex.

Yohimbe has been found to be very effective in reestablishing a sexual relationship, and is safe for both men and women to take.

NOTE: Psychological counseling is highly recommended as most impotence problems arise from feeling of inadequacy and often reinforced through assertive/successful mates.

NUTRIENTS AND HERBS TO HELP IMPOTENCE

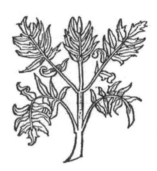

Nutrients	Herbs
Zinc	Damiana
	Dong Quai
	Siberian Ginseng
	Yohimbe Bark

Zinc. Nourishes the prostate gland as well as being important in sperm production.

Siberian Ginseng, Dong Quai, and Damiana. Are all famous for their aphrodisiac-type properties.

Yohimbe Bark. Contains yohimbine, a strong sexual stimulant. Also used as a general tonic. Can be used by women.

SYMBOLOGY OF IMPOTENCE

Impotence is very close, symbolically, to the inability to fertilize an egg. When we talked about reproduction we talked about doubt and fear of expression. Here the point is driven home even more because of the inability to perform as a man should perform under certain circumstances. The concept that would create this kind of a situation is a feeling of inherent weakness, a lack of maleness, a lack of strength, a doubt in one's ability to express oneself, or a lack of ability to satisfy or please another human being.

What is really interesting about impotence, symbolically, is that an erection is created when blood is directed into the penis. When you recall that the symbology of blood is spirit flowing through the body, faith in self, or faith in one's ability to do things, you can see where a working faith can achieve an erection. When seen through that understanding, it is easy to see how a strong doubt in one's expression, and ability to perform in life would manifest symbolically as impotence.

Obviously there are always rational logical reasons why one is impotent. It may very well be because of a medication, or an injury. If it is because of medication then you have to take a look at the disease that is being treated. Looking at it symbolically you will see that it too would fall into the particular realm of thoughts that would be conducive to the occurrence of impotence.

Symbology of the Nutrients

As discussed earlier there are many causes for impotence. Symbolically it boils down to the lack of the ability to express oneself. Obviously there are underlying feelings of inadequacy, questions about one's manhood, virility, or ability to perform, and in essence the individual believes that they cannot.

Zinc. There are many roles for zinc within the body. Zinc is essential to the workings of the prostate and sperm production, and symbolizes a working faith, fundamental support, and expression.

In this instance it fundamentally supports a working faith that is lacking as well as supporting the ability to express. There may be a fear of expressing one's thoughts and opinions. Go back to the old adage: children should be seen and not heard. Well, that can have ramifications into adulthood where one has a tendency to be quiet, to be withdrawn, to avoid confrontation and in time this may affect one's performance.

Poor circulation and taking medications are other causes. Whatever the medication is being used for is also symbolic. Like with poor circulation it is a lack of faith, a lack of spirit, or a lack of confidence. It all comes back to self-expression.

The beauty of nutritional symbology and body functions and diseases is that every which way that you look at it, it proves itself to be true.

Intestinal Cleansing

The need for fitness of the intestinal tract cannot be emphasized enough. Like the importance of the other cleansing organs, it is imperative to excellent health that this particular system be free of mucus and other factors that would have a tendency to clog the villi.

The villi, which look like little fingers, have openings between them from where they hang in the intestines. This opening is where the nutrients are absorbed into the bloodstream for distribution to all parts of the body. If the villi are clogged for any reason, then the amount of nutrients that should be entering into the blood and providing food for the cells, is diminished. In addition to decreased nourishment, there is the fact that the body makes the effort to absorb what it can through the villi openings.

The body does not know what it is bringing into the bloodstream; it only knows that it should be absorbing anything that is available to it. With this in mind it becomes important to remove all the harmful pollutants that are in the intestines as quick as possible. The sooner that this is done, the quicker the body can respond to the nutrients that are available to it.

HERBS AND FLORA TO ASSIST THE BODY IN INTESTINAL CLEANSING

Herbs		Flora
Apple Pectin	Garlic	Probiotics
Butternut Root Bark	Marshmallow Root	
Cascara Sagrada	Psyllium Husks	
Clay	Pumpkin Seeds	
Comfrey Root	Rice Bran	
Dandelion Root	Slippery Elm Bark	
Flax Seeds		

Apple Pectin. Used for its electromagnetic properties to draw metals to it so that they can be excreted from the body.

Butternut Root Bark. For its mild laxative property.

Cascara Sagrada. An aid in restoring the natural tone of the colon. Used in smaller amounts in folk medicine to treat liver disorders and gallstones. Herb to treat jaundice and other hepatic conditions.

Clay. Great for pulling toxins to it so that they can be eliminated from the body.

Comfrey Root, Marshmallow Root and Slippery Elm Bark. All mucilaginous in quality. Because of their slick adhesiveness, they coat the lower bowels with a nutritious substance that strengthens as well as heals.

Dandelion Root. Works on stimulating the liver, which is your chemical factory and helps protect the body by encasing toxins in fat.

Flax Seeds, Psyllium Husks and Rice Bran. Offer fiber to push bulk through and to help absorb toxins.

Garlic. One milligram of its major constituent, allicin, is estimated to equal fifteen standard units of penicillin.

Marshmallow Root. Soothes mucous membranes; internally, treats inflammation and mucosal afflictions.

Pumpkin Seeds. An anthelmintic (parasitic killer).

Slippery Elm Bark. Effective, both internally and externally, against sore and inflamed mucous membranes.

Probiotics. Your friendly intestinal flora that need to be replaced, and by having an abundance of probiotics within the intestinal tract you create a hostile environment for Candida. Candida flourishes in the absence of healthy intestinal flora. (See the Candida Albicans section for more information.)

Symbology of Intestinal Cleansing

The intestinal tract is another aspect of your self-defense system, and 70 percent of the immune system is active in this environment because it is protecting the body from pathogens, toxins, viruses and anything that would seek to enter the body that would be detrimental. So, when you think about cleansing the goal is to first minimize the intake of toxic-forming material, which is obviously symbolic of toxic thoughts. By avoiding negative associations, people and thoughts, you end up protecting yourself. Cleansing or keeping this environment clean is vitally important. From the symbolic perspective, it is being aware of what is being presented to you at all times, because sometimes negative thoughts and suggestions are hidden in something sweet, something flavorful that has the appearance of being desirable and yet, in reality, will end up containing a toxin, a poisonous thought that could undermine your courage and confidence. The toxin can then feed upon a doubt or fear and, by doing so, undermine the health of your spirit. As Francis Bacon said, "A healthy body is a guest chamber for the soul; a sick body is a prison."

Another aspect to cleansing is the colon, which is a part of the intestinal tract. When fecal matter sits in the colon, the toxins are reabsorbed. Constipation represents the inability to let go of past thoughts and ideas, and when that happens, if a person remains constipated for too long they will become poisoned once again. Holding on to the past can have the same effect. It limits your growth, stifles your health and will ultimately cause your demise.

SYMBOLOGY OF HERBS AND FLORA

We will only discuss symbolically apple pectin and probiotics.

Apple Pectin. Chosen for the simple reason that there already exists a universal symbology for it; the apple represents knowledge. This is derived from the biblical story of Adam and Eve. It is the act of Eve eating the apple and the knowledge that followed that gives apples its symbology. Eve, after consuming the apple made the determination of what was good and what was bad. In reality, we are not supposed to judge anyone or their actions. We are, however, supposed to have knowledge. We are supposed to be able to see, evaluate, and choose what is beneficial for self and avoid that which is detrimental and could be harmful to us.

The apple pectin in this cleansing program represents the ability to make proper choices by avoiding acceptance of negative and toxic suggestions and thoughts. Apple pectin helps in the cleansing of man-made concepts from the self by regulating the bowels. It also helps to regulate cholesterol, blood pressure and it acts as a magnet to draw arsenic and lead to it so that they can be eliminated from the system.

A quick symbolic examination shows the importance of having self-knowledge. Holding on to the past makes a person toxic, and toxins kill. High cholesterol leads to poor circulation, a lack of faith in self, and is extremely damaging to the spirit. High blood pressure is another lack of faith in dealing with things. This, too, can cause death via stroke or heart attack.

Probiotics. The friendly flora; bacteria that live in the intestinal tract that assist the body in maintaining good health. The way that they help is a byproduct of their metabolism of the B vitamins. The B vitamins are co-enzymes, and what this means is that within the body they combine with other nutrients and substances to become enzymes.

Symbolically, we could say that probiotics are the insights, thoughts, little things in life, pearls of wisdom, Universal Teachings, those fundamental principles that yield so much when applied and worked with. In regards to the cleansing aspect, nothing would be more wholesome and beneficial than building a cleansing program based on the Universal Teachings. The Teachings provide those insights and understandings that allow the individual to create the energies, courage, and confidence necessary to live a healthy and vibrant life free from the toxic concepts of man; a healthy life based on the spiritual laws that govern the All.

Probiotic strains produce the B vitamins that facilitate the cleansing process. This, in turn, allows the person to move through life with courage and confidence, and be in harmony with the Creative Continuum.

From a different point of view, we are constantly co-creating our reality based on our subconscious expectations. If you do not understand your expectations of self, who you think you are supposed to be and how to act in given situations, then your creations are not in your true control. They are just manifesting the subconscious expectations to validate what it is you believe about yourself, which has nothing to do with who you really are. We are so much more than we appear to be.

Kidney Cleansing

The kidneys filter the bloodstream and extract the toxins for elimination. There is the possibility that calcium and certain forms of pollution may accumulate in the kidneys, and they may have to work overtime to keep the bloodstream free from reabsorbing the toxins made water soluble by the liver.

Herbs to Assist Your Body in Regaining Nutritional Balance

As you feed your body organic foods and natural supplements you will see the following results. The supplements will assist the body in dissolving calcium deposits and neutralizing the acidity of the blood.

Herbs	
Buchu Leaf	Juniper Berries
Celery Seeds	Parsley
Hydrangea	Uva Ursi

Buchu Leaf. Urinary disinfectant; mildly diuretic. It is used mainly for diseases of the kidney, urinary tract and prostate.

Celery Seeds. Aids and stimulates diuretic activity.

Hydrangea. Used for bladder and kidney disorders, including kidney stones, inflammation, and backache from kidney trouble.

Juniper Berries. Acts directly on the kidneys. Highly volatile oil content (especially terpinol). Its primary application is as a diuretic.

Parsley. A wonderful diuretic.

Uva Ursi. Have disinfectant and other properties, and acts as an antiseptic in the urinary tract. It is also used for bladder inflammation, kidney inflammation, and kidney stones.

SYMBOLOGY OF KIDNEY CLEANSING

(See symbology of Kidney Infections and Stones.)

Kidney Infections and Stones

When we talk about the kidneys, the most obvious conditions to examine are kidney infections and kidney stones. Your kidneys are a filtering device that help you maintain proper ratios of nutrients. From one point of view they protect the body because they are not going to give up anything that the body requires, such as a vitamin, mineral, or amino acid if it knows that particular nutrient is still required for proper functioning of the system.

Kidney infections can have many different causes, but the treatment for the infections is rather simple. Many people take cranberry as a way of dealing with them. Cranberry is good from the perspective that it prevents the bacteria from adhering to the urethra walls, and kills the infection.

To eliminate a kidney infection, or any type of infection in the body, the following nutrients are essential.

Nutrients	Herbs
Vitamin A	Echinacea
Vitamin C	Garlic
Zinc	Goldenseal Root

To dissolve kidney stones the following nutrients and herbs are highly effective.

Nutrients	Herbs
Magnesium	Gravel Root
Vitamin D	

Magnesium. Lack of magnesium can lead to calcium deposits in muscles, skeleton, heart and kidneys, and can cause alterations in heartbeat.

Vitamin A. A fat-soluble nutrient that is important for the healthy function of the thymus gland, in addition to other systems in the body.

   The thymus is very active in the production of antibodies. Antibodies stick to specific germs and neutralize them. Other aspects of the immune system that fight bacterias, viruses, fungi, and molds are lymphocytes, macrophages, and interferon.

Vitamin C. Stimulates immune response. It also has a generally positive effect on the common cold.

Vitamin D. Needs to be present for the assimilation and utilization of calcium. In fact, vitamin D is so effective in helping the body to assimilate calcium that it has been used by itself to dissolve kidney stones, joint and spinal calcium deposits.

Zinc. Is essential, it seems, to "mobilize" vitamin A from the liver, so that it can perform its usual bodily functions. Protects the immune system and supports the T-cells. This is very important in the production of antibodies.

Echinacea. Induces living cells to excrete more of the interferon, which the cells already manufacture. Destroys the germs of infection directly, and bolsters the body's defenses by magnifying the white blood cell count. It protects cells against virus-related diseases, such as herpes, influenza, canker sores, etc. Has the ability to stimulate T-cell activity.

Garlic. Has been proven to increase resistance against bacterial infection.

Goldenseal Root. Known to contain natural properties that kill bacteria.

Gravel Root. Works with vitamin D to help break up calcium deposits in the body.

SYMBOLOGY OF KIDNEY INFECTIONS

Whenever we think about kidney infections from a symbolic point of view there are a couple of different things to consider. First is that there is a breakdown in the cleansing, an unwillingness to let go of some past thoughts and retain them, thus, poisoning the system. When a person cannot let go of the past it becomes toxic and destroys the body. Another important point is that kidney infections make physical intercourse uncomfortable; therefore, it can act as a deterrent to that form of communication.

Eliminating toxins and bringing in new material is vital to a healthy body. This is why we have nine openings in the human body for cleansing and for our emotional and spiritual evolution: two eyes, two ears, two nostrils, mouth, anus, and urethra. Women have ten openings in the body, but the vagina is for expression, not cleansing per se. Even though there is an elimination of the uterus lining, it is not an ongoing process. It starts after menses and ends after menopause, and is directly tied into the ability to bring forth children, which is a form of self-expression.

Through the eyes and ears we bring in fresh ideas. Through the nostrils we are breathing in spirit, faith in self. Through the mouth we are consuming sustenance of the material plane, and gaining sustenance from that which we consume. When we look at the anus and urethra we can see that it is the elimination of the wastes of our consumption. The things that are no longer of value to us, we eliminate. What we are also supposed to be eliminating are those concepts, ideas, values, and standards that do not serve us and are no longer of value. That is why kidney infections represent the inability or unwillingness to let go.

SYMBOLOGY OF KIDNEY STONES

Kidney stones symbolically indicate that the individual is not only unwilling to let go of the past, but their sense of personal power is not being utilized to its fullest extent. We know this because kidney stones are made of calcium in most instances, and calcium is symbolic of strength.

Because of certain ideas an individual maintains in the subconscious mind they are unable to fully utilize the strength that they have, and these ideas prevent the body from building on that strength. In the filtering process, the person tries to keep the calcium (strength) from manifesting but they cannot stop it. It comes down to a matter of using it, and again we return to another Universal Teaching that says, "use what you have and more will be given." If you use the strength you have you can build upon it, and as you do you become stronger because you have a working faith in your ability to handle things.

The ability to prevail over obstacles lies within a working faith. When you lack a working faith in self then there is doubt in your ability to have the strength to overcome or even do whatever it is that you are confronted with. The cause of doubt is that you are relying on past concepts, and in this case, kidney stones will form and cause a problem.

What is interesting from a symbolic point of view is the way kidney stones are dealt with. You need magnesium and vitamin D to dissolve them since they are made of calcium. Symbolically, magnesium represents inspiration and vitamin D represents insight, and inspiration and insight help you understand and move forward in life allowing you to utilize your inner-strength.

There is a new medical technique for getting rid of kidney stones using sonic vibrations. All sounds, including the spoken word, are carried as sonic vibrations. From that perspective, it may be that the person needs to speak out and manifest their strength as a way of utilizing their abilities within.

Symbology of the Nutrients

When examining kidney issues there are fundamentally several problems a person can have, and all are incredibly serious, life threatening, and painful. Since we will not discuss herbs symbolically, we will look at the nutrients necessary to eliminate kidney stones.

Calcium. Symbolically represents strength. Kidney stones bring us back to the fundamental principles of calcium assimilation because they are calcium ions aggregating in the filters within the kidney. Since calcium represents strength, it is apparent that the person that has kidney stones has a tendency not to utilize their strength to their fullest abilities, and has some subconscious issues within their own concepts regarding their strength.

Magnesium and Vitamin D. Symbolically represent inspiration and insight. These two nutrients are necessary in order for the body to utilize calcium effectively. When a person has insight, and if it can be related to looking within the self, we can see the truth of things, including the truth of who we are. This is not what we believe we are, not who we have been programmed to think we are, but who we truly are. We are spiritual beings entrapped in a material body. Because we are spiritual in nature we are endowed with all the gifts of the Creator, and this means that we truly have the insights necessary to be able to do whatever we set out to do, and we can begin to see that we can do things well.

When people draw on the Universal Teachings for knowledge and insights they perform even better. One Teaching tells us to "draw on our past successes." In that way the strength, knowledge and energy of a past accomplishment is brought into the now of whatever the person is confronting. Another Teaching tells us to "look back in order to see ahead." This Teaching informs us of the nature of cycles and patterns of behavior, and in this case is in regards to the current endeavor that a person is undertaking. The Teachings allow a person to use their inspiration and insights to develop their strength, knowing that it truly exists.

Life is more a matter of utilizing your strength and power than allowing it to lie dormant out of self-doubt, and in this case, create malfunctions. The other ways that symbolically tell the individual that their strength is not being utilized and is dormant within the body are calcium spurs, kidney stones and prostate stones. These are all indications that a person is not using their inner-strength to the best of their own abilities.

Leg Aches

Leg aches indicate different things, and can have multiple causes. A person could have suffered an injury, but more often than not, leg aches are the result of a lack of minerals within the system.

The role of minerals within the body is very similar to the function of light switches within the home. Minerals are catalysts, and as such they allow biological transactions to take place. In our analogy of the light switches they allow the energy of thought, which is converted into electricity, to travel through the nervous system and make the leap from nerve ending to receptor site on a muscle. When there is not an adequate amount of certain minerals within the body then the energy cannot make that jump. Therefore, the muscles will either be flaccid/relaxed or they will cramp. The cramping is the muscle contracting without the message to relax, and this is the beginning of the leg aches.

The minerals that are required for proper operation and communication are calcium, magnesium, phosphorus and potassium. These are instrumental in the body's ability to contract and relax muscles. Leg aches, "charley horses," restless leg syndrome, tossing and turning in bed, having a hard time falling asleep, PMS cramps and growing pains are an indication that the body is compromised in the areas of calcium, magnesium, and potassium.

NUTRIENTS TO HELP ALLEVIATE LEG ACHES

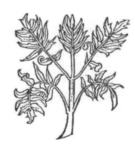

Nutrients
Calcium
Magnesium
Potassium
Vitamin D

Calcium. A mineral involved in neuromuscular excitability and transmission of nerve impulses. When calcium levels in the blood are low, symptoms of increased neuromuscular irritability, seizures and cardiac cramps are possible.

Magnesium. Deficiency symptoms include muscle fasciculation, tremors, and spasms.

Potassium. Necessary to stimulate nerve endings for muscle contractions.

Vitamin D. Needs to be present for the assimilation and utilization of calcium. In fact, vitamin D is so effective in helping the body to assimilate calcium that it has been used by itself to dissolve joint and spinal calcium deposits.

SYMBOLOGY OF LEG ACHES

Symbolically speaking, leg aches relate to the feelings and thoughts that an individual has about their ability to support his or herself in the current situation. It could also indicate an upcoming situation that is already in the making but has not yet shown itself in the immediate present. We arrive at the inability to support oneself symbolically because the legs support the trunk of the body, and the trunk is symbolic of the material plane.

Sometimes leg aches occur only in one leg, and when that happens it is necessary to examine the particular leg affected. If the right leg is affected, then the issues relate to your concepts that deal with your faith in self in regards to the situation. It calls into question your ability to support yourself and your faith in self. If the left leg is affected, the issues relate to your ability to support yourself in the material plane. In this case, there is a financial issue that is brewing, or currently taking place. When faith in self is required to deal with things on a non-material level your right side would be affected, if it is a matter of faith in self dealing with things in a material way such as finances or business, your left side would be affected.

Some events are so taxing and questionable that they could affect both legs at the same time, and could possibly involve the back as well.

SYMBOLOGY OF THE NUTRIENTS

Looking at the symbology of the nutrients involved in maintaining proper muscular function we see how the symbology of aches play out. It can easily be seen how each mineral involved validates the other, and how their symbolic energies are necessary to confidently handle the many situations and events in life that we may find ourselves in on a daily basis.

Calcium. Represents strength. It can be seen how in dealing with life it takes strength and fortitude to withstand some of the obligations that are placed on an individual. It is especially difficult when a person is making changes in their life. In some family environments the traditional and cultural obligations and responsibilities prevent or work against an individual changing, and to do so would bring rejection from parents. Even friends might be upset when a person seeks to grow beyond their current level of life.

Magnesium. Represents inspiration. One has to be inspired to be able to continue to do battle with opposing energies, and these energies are both external and internal. The internal forces are those that seek to keep a person within their traditions and expectations of self. All of this relates to the concept of the desire to return to the Spiritual Plane. (For more on this topic, see Section I: From the Inside Out.)

There are many different things that can inspire an individual. Materially, it may not matter how much money they may, or may not, be earning. For some, just having a family is enough of an inspiration to keep them going. Regardless, there is always something that inspires us to move forward.

Potassium. Represents balance and harmony. When an individual lacks strength (calcium) and inspiration (magnesium), balance and harmony diminishes and they begin to loose their confidence on all levels. They doubt that they have the internal fortitude or strength, and to some degree become imbalanced in their approach to situations. This in turn starts a cascade of events that will ultimately lead to a physical condition or disease. (See also Osteoporosis.)

Liver Concerns

Like the kidneys, the liver is a live-or-die organ for the body. The liver performs vital functions, the most important being the creation of glycogen. The liver stores energy in the form of glycogen, and when the body is not being fed, glycogen is broken down and converted into glucose, the sugar (fuel) the cells use. This conversion of glycogen into glucose is important in maintaining the blood glucose level. Glycogen becomes glucose, the sugar that the cells use as food, and the entire human structure requires sugar as fuel.

The next vital function is to render harmless any chemical that is not natural to the body. It is identified as an alien invader, the immune system attacks immediately, and the liver becomes involved as the blood passes through. The detoxification process kicks in and the liver stores the toxins in fat cells as a "prisoner." In this way it cannot harm the rest of the population of cells.

The liver is adversely affected and placed in a stressful situation by fried foods, heavy consumption of fatty foods (including meats), alcohol, smoking, and living and/or working in a polluted environment.

When the liver is being cleansed it functions better, which helps the digestive system to perform more efficiently. This helps in the elimination of toxic material from the body. The liver is also tied into the kidneys by processing the toxins into water-disposable products. That way the kidneys can work with the material to get it out of the body.

NUTRIENTS TO ASSIST THE BODY IN DETOXIFYING

Nutrients	Herbs
Choline	Beet Root
Inositol	Chicory Root
Lecithin	Dandelion Root

Choline and Inositol. These two nutrients are often found together and are considered lipotopic vitamins, translated simply: fat burners. In this program they are used to break up and dissolve fatty deposits in the liver.

Lecithin. Keeps cholesterol more soluble, detoxifies the liver, and increases resistance to disease by helping the thymus gland carry out its functions.

Chicory. Has properties very similar to dandelion. Often used for jaundice and spleen problems. Promotes the production of bile, release of gallstones, and elimination of excessive internal mucus.

Dandelion Root. Stimulates liver activity, encouraging the elimination of toxins from the blood. It stimulates the flow of bile and excretion of urea. Successfully used with hepatitis, swelling of the liver, jaundice, and dyspepsia with deficient bile secretion.

SYMBOLOGY OF THE LIVER

The liver is a manufacturing organ and converter of substances; it must be free from excess fat, otherwise its functions become hindered, just as one must be free from pent up energy and pent up emotions. As they sit and continue to generate more energy in the form of anger, resentment or frustration they are increasing the heat/energy within a particular gland, organ, or system. This will invariably cause an illness within the body, and will cause cells within that particular environment to mutate or become corrupted. It takes inner-strength to combat some of the internal as well as external forces in life. Forces such as anger, frustration, resentment and guilt must be dealt with from a position of strength. In the same regard, it takes inner-strength to transport energy (the movement of fats into the cells) into action (the use of fats by cells to build and nourish themselves) to create a material reality. The human body and all of its transactions are lessons on how to master life. It takes insights, understandings and control over responses to ensure mastery.

It is easy to see how inner-strength is essential to the cleansing of past ideas and concepts from the subconscious mind. If we do not cleanse our minds of man-made teachings, then we are doomed to follow in our parents' footsteps because history repeats itself. As we learn in Ecclesiastes 3:15, everything in the universe flows in cycles.

The liver has many functions. It's a sugar for the blood manufacturer, a cleanser, a detoxifier, a chemical manufacturing plant and converter. It takes the sustenance that spirit provides and converts it into material manifestation. You use inner-strength everyday to co-create your reality, and reality is the physical manifestation of your subconscious expectations in action.

Here is the quick and easy explanation of how we co-create our reality. Everything in the universe is composed of atoms, and atoms have a positive or negative electrical magnetic charge. The human brain generates electrical magnetic energy waves which are either positive or negative, attracting or repelling whatever it needs to fulfill expectations. The reality of a person's life, immediate surroundings and personal situations are a reflection of expectations.

Through the generating power of the brain people draw to them exactly what they need. This is true both positively as well as negatively.

SYMBOLOGY OF THE NUTRIENTS

Choline. Symbolically, it represents inner-strength. Choline's biochemical transactions reflect this concept. When the substance combines with phosphoric acid (a form of courage) it produces lecithin (protection) to nourish and protect the myelin sheath covering of the nerves (communication). This allows for clean, strong signals to be sent.

Choline prevents fats (stored energy) from accumulating in the liver, which performs cleansing tasks for the body among other important functions. Looking at this symbolically, it is when energy is not being used in the pursuit of mastery that there is a doubt or fear at work. Otherwise, the action would move toward the attainment of mastery. People can appear to be busy, but they do not move forward on a personal level. They are engaged in busy work, which acts as a distraction from real progress.

Inositol. Represents integrity and is closely associated with choline (inner-strength) and biotin (liberation in a cleansing way). When you think about integrity's role in life, you can see how essential it is to have true inner-strength. It also takes a degree of integrity to examine the self honestly. When a person can look at self it allows for the detoxification process to work without impediments, and this facilitates growth and development.

Low Blood Sugar

See Hypoglycemia.

Memory Problems

Have you ever started to introduce a friend or colleague to one another and you could not recall their names? How about looking at a phone number and by the time you looked back at the dial or push buttons you do not recall the last two or three digits? These are everyday occurrences that make you feel very uncomfortable, but you can take heart, for these are "normal" situations according to the experts. Even though the experts tell us that a little bit of forgetfulness is common it does not help to alleviate the fear that something is wrong with you, and you immediately jump to the conclusion that you have Alzheimer's disease.

The thought of getting Alzheimer's disease is enough to scare you into taking action in a preventative way if only you really knew what to do. In order to form a plan of action that would help to protect you from this dreaded disease you need to understand exactly what this disease is all about. Unfortunately, there is not too much medical knowledge around. Why is this so?

Doctors, by the very nature of their healing system, refuse to see diseases as the result of poor nutrition, or that they may be caused by the American diet. It lies within a protective belief system because if they were to accept that the human body is the result of what goes into it, then they would have to accept that changing the input would change the results. This would also validate what the health experts say: most diseases can be healed, controlled and/or prevented with good nutrition.

Those of us in the natural healing arts know that Alzheimer's is a disease that is the result of poor nutrition and bad circulation. Let us first look at the circulation aspect. The blood is the lifeline of the body. It feeds each and every cell within the entire system. When it comes to the brain, it can only present the nutrients that the brain requires because blood does not enter into the brain matter. There is a protective envelope called the blood-brain barrier, and its purpose is to prevent blood from passing into the brain. The blood-brain barrier accepts the nutrients that the brain needs and passes those through so that the brain can feed and nourish itself. There are chemicals in the environment, the marketplace, in our food, air, and water that may be able to transverse the blood/brain barrier.

Now if the blood is thick with cholesterol and triglycerides then the amount of nutrient-rich blood is severely restricted and the amount that passes by the barrier becomes even less. When this happens you can begin to imagine how little of the available nutrients are able to feed the brain, so it is no wonder that the brain is starving to death, dying a little bit each day. This may be the main reason that people begin to forget.

This brings us to the next area of concern, memory or your ability to recall information when you need it. The mind works because of neurotransmitters. Neurotransmitters are nutrients that act as "switches" in the brain. They allow the electrical nerve impulses to pass, and permit all of the functions of the body to take place in proper sequence.

You can begin to imagine what can take place when the brain does not have an adequate amount of neurotransmitters, or the nutrients available to make them. In electrical terms you would have a power failure or a device would not work properly and may even burn up. The brain is confronted with the same kind of situation. It does not make the right or complete connections and, therefore, there is a "short." The mind goes blank or it begins to plug into an old, disconnected memory (or circuit). We call this confusion, disorientation, lapse of memory, senility, and of course, Alzheimer's disease. But there is a way to fortify the brain with the proper amount of nutrients necessary to create neurotransmitters because neurotransmitters, like enzymes in the body, are the result of biochemical constructions.

Alzheimer's, senility, dementia, and general memory problems have different causes. I choose to believe that they are fundamentally the result of malnutrition. There are many theories out there as to what causes Alzheimer's. One of the theories is that aluminum is in the brain, and once aluminum gets into the body it cannot be chelated out, but science is not sure. If you think about it many of us grew up eating out of aluminum cookware and glassware, such as the old spun aluminum glasses of the 1950s.

Another theory is based on findings of a protein plaque that they have discovered in the brains of Alzheimer's patients. What is interesting about this is that so many prescriptions and over the counter drugs are bound to a protein in order for greater efficacy within the body because this guarantees the product gives a result.

One of the most important nutrients for the brain is oxygen; 25 percent of all the oxygen that you breathe goes to feed your brain. Oxygen is carried through hemoglobin to the blood-brain barrier. There the oxygen is passed into the brain environment, and oxygen helps to nourish the brain along with other nutrients.

If we take into consideration that the number one killer in the country today is cardiovascular disease, primarily clogged arteries, then it is easy to see that there is not enough oxygen-rich blood flowing to the blood-brain barrier. The arteries are so constricted that not enough blood is reaching the barrier to pass oxygen to the brain. Consequently, it is my belief that Alzheimer's, senility, and dementia are oxygen starvation problems.

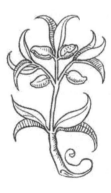

NUTRIENTS, AMINO ACIDS, HERBS AND OTHER SUBSTANCES TO SUPPORT GOOD MEMORY

Nutrients	Amino Acids	Herbs and Other Substances
Choline	L-Glutamine	Acetylcholine
Folic Acid	L-Glutachione	Glutamic Acid
Inositol	L-Methionine	Gotu Kola
Lecithin	L-Taurine	Madagascar Periwinkle
Magnesium	L-Tyrosine	PABA (Para Aminobenzioc Acid)
Manganese		Phosphatidyl Choline
Niacin/Niacinamide		
Pantothenic Acid		
Potassium		
Selenium		
Unsaturated Fatty Acids		
Vitamin B-1		
Vitamin B-6		
Vitamin E		
Zinc		

Choline. Known as a fat burner and works to dissolve fats in the bloodstream.

Folic Acid. Essential for mental and emotional health.

Inositol. Co-functions with choline as a fat burner.

Lecithin. Excellent fat metabolizer.

Magnesium. Plays an important role in neuromuscular contractions.

Manganese. Helps nourish the nerves and brain. Aids in the utilization of choline.

Niacin/Niacinamide. Improves circulation and reduces the cholesterol level in the blood. Niacin is important for improving memory.

Pantothenic acid. Important for healthy skin and nerves and vital in cellular metabolism.

Potassium. Unites with phosphorus to send oxygen to the brain. Also functions with calcium in the regulation of neuromuscular activity.

Selenium. A natural antioxidant that appears to preserve elasticity of tissue by delaying oxidation of polyunsaturated fatty acids.

Unsaturated Fatty Acids. Makes it easier for oxygen to be transported by the bloodstream. Helps perform a vital function in breaking up cholesterol deposited on arterial walls.

Vitamin B-1. Beneficial effect on mental attitude and a healthy nervous system. Linked with improving individual learning capability.

Vitamin B-6. Promotes the normal functioning of the nervous and musculoskeletal systems.

Vitamin E. Causes dilation of the blood vessels, permitting a fuller flow of blood.

Zinc. May be involved in binding a certain substance in a certain part of the brain so that it is there to perform its function. That part of brain contains a considerable amount of zinc.

L-Glutamine. Readily crosses the blood-brain barrier in the brain where it is quickly converted into glutamic acid. Serves primarily as a fuel for the brain, which also keeps excess amounts of ammonia from damaging the brain.

L-Methionine. Helps nourish brain cells and supports choline's role in promoting thinking ability.

L-Taurine. Both a neurotransmitter and mood elevator.

L-Tyrosine. Stimulates production of norepinephrine, the "alertness" brain chemical, and has a role in sharpening learning, memory, and awareness, elevating mood and motivation.

Acetylcholine. Most important of the body's neurotransmitters (brain chemicals that carry messages between neurons, facilitate learning, memory and intelligence). Key role is maximizing mental ability and prevents loss of memory in aging adults.

Glutamic Acid. Principal amino acid contributor to brain-energy supplies.

Gotu Kola. Specifically to improve memory and longevity. Excellent oxygen carrier.

Madagascar Periwinkle. Carries more oxygen to the brain than any other herb known.

PABA. Works to allow electricity to jump from nerve ending to receptor sites.

Phosphatidyl Choline. Acts as a fat metabolizer and is converted into acetylcholine, a neurotransmitter.

SYMBOLOGY OF MEMORY PROBLEMS

Most memory issues are caused by a lack of nourishment—specifically oxygen that symbolically represents spirit. Spirit lives in the heavens, and heaven is what we breathe.

Everything around us is heaven because it is air. Senility and those types of memory issues are indicative of where one has lost their faith. They have lost their ability to be in control of their life because over time they have succumbed to man-made concepts, values, standards and ideals. They are no longer feeding themselves enough of true spirit; they are no longer bringing adequate amounts of oxygen to the brain.

One of the reasons why exercise is so vitally important for the human being is because it oxygenates the body and brain. By oxygenating the body, by bringing spirit into the body, a person becomes inspired, and when a person is inspired there is nothing that they cannot do. Oxygenation also feeds the mind/brain/body. Once again we can see that being engulfed in spirit, and nurturing self with spirit, you become inspired and can think and see clearly. Another unique thing about oxygen is that cancer cannot live in an oxygenated body. Symbolically, that is beautiful because it tells us that when we have spirit in our life, and a true working faith, we know that we can handle whatever it is that comes our way, and we have no doubt.

Oxygen/spirit in the body has multiple purposes, and it demonstrates the truth of us being spiritual beings in a material body. Through being a spiritual being and operating from a position of personal power, a person goes forward in life dealing with whatever it is they are confronted with in a masterful way. There is a Universal Teaching that states: "You are never placed in a situation that you cannot master." You have to keep in mind that you are constantly co-creating your reality with the Creative Continuum/God. Your mind is an electromagnetic generator, and you are constantly sending out electromagnetic waves. What is important about that is the understanding that everything in the universe is composed of atoms. Atoms make molecules, and molecules make physical reality. Every atom has a positive or negative charge, just as magnetic poles repel or attract each other, our subconscious expectations send out electromagnetic waves. They either repel or draw things to us in order to fulfill our subconscious expectations. You attract and repel things based on expectations you have regardless of whether or not these things are beneficial. This is the importance of truly understanding self and understanding the concepts one works with as well as the patterns of behavior. Another Universal Teaching is, "know what you are looking at then none of the mysteries are hidden from you, everything is revealed." In reality everything is a symbolic representation of thoughts in action.

Symbology of the Nutrients

Choline and Inositol. Two B vitamins that should also be a part of every formula that is designed to nourish the brain. These two nutrients are considered lipotropic vitamins, and as such they participate in the destabilization of fats. It is interesting that fat is a fuel for the mitochondria, the energy producing "engines" within every cell, and helps the body to stay healthy in many other different ways. However, when there is excess fat, it becomes a form of defense, protecting the body and the ego of an individual. Fat is used by some as a form of defense, a way of being "unattractive," or in terms of power, "throwing their weight around."

When we look at choline symbolically, it represents inner-strength, and inositol represents integrity. Both of these energetic forces are essential for good memory because by having inner-strength you are not afraid to look within, you are not afraid to look back in order to see ahead, and you have the ability with integrity to draw on your past strengths and your past successes in order to bring them into the future. This is what the mind is constantly doing, looking back to the past to see how it dealt with a similar situation to the current one we are faced with. Thus, it sets in motion those energies that will help it in terms of fulfilling the subconscious expectations. Drawing on past behavioral responses the person will complete the cycle as before.

This is why reading a symbol is so vitally important. It gives the person the opportunity to change their personal history, which takes us to the cliché: "History repeats itself." Personal history is of the same nature. By reading symbols, you have the opportunity to change the outcome and, thus, create a new response to an old stimulus, and this new result will lead you to move forward in life.

Folic Acid. A part of a formula because symbolically it represents a fortifier, and as such it gives us the strength to fortify and strengthen the mind, and it helps to strengthen courage and determination. Folic acid fortifies against the forces that would prevent forward movement.

Magnesium and Pantothenic Acid. Both share a very similar symbolic representation and that is inspiration. Magnesium is the solid or manifesting aspect, and Pantothenic acid is the energetic part that helps the manifestation become real. Pantothenic Acid is essential in memory function from a symbolic point of view because it provides the individual with the energy of inspiration. It inspires one to move forward, to have the confidence and courage, and to know that they can handle anything and everything that they are confronted with.

Manganese. On a chemical level, helps the body in terms of utilizing choline. As we have stated, choline represents inner-strength and manganese represents the will of getting things done.

Again, with memory it is a matter of not only recalling how to do something, but also having the will to get it done. Whether or not a person can manifest the energy of intent will determine the strength of their will to move forward and get a project, event or situation accomplished.

Niacin/Niacinamide. Is included in a formula for its symbolic interpretation of openness and receptivity. In doing so it allows the mind, from a memory point of view, to be open and receptive to looking back to the past and gaining insights. The Universal Teachings state that we should draw on our past successes because when you can remember your past successes then you have the opportunity to bring those insights and understandings as well as that experience into the now, and by doing so you are further guaranteed the ability to succeed at whatever you are doing and wherever it is that you are at the moment.

Niacin, as a nutrient, aids memory in playing a vitally important role. It acts as a vasodilator opening up the arteries and allowing more blood to flow to the blood-brain barrier. This provides more oxygen, which nourishes and enhances your memory so that you can draw on your successful past.

Potassium. Symbolic of balance and harmony, specifically in regard to material considerations. When we look at potassium symbolically with the understanding of what it does and realize how it works with phosphorus (courage) to send nourishing oxygen (spirit) to the brain, and when the brain functions at optimal levels, generally speaking, the mind would have greater clarity and be able to see things clearer through that clarity which would allow for making better decisions, decisions that would help maintain balance and harmony between the material, spiritual, male and female that all dwell within the self. It is also important to see the role of balance and harmony when potassium works with calcium (strength). When you apply strength in a balanced way, whatever it is that you approach will end up having a balanced and harmonious result.

Selenium and Zinc. These are important from two different perspectives. Zinc, symbolically representing support and fundamental expression in life, gives a person their working faith. A working faith is a matter of reminding oneself and drawing on past successes. That tells the person that they can succeed in what they are currently involved in. Selenium protects the cells of the brain and helps the detoxification process, thus, it symbolically helps eliminate doubt. What is doubt other than toxic thoughts that undermine an individual's courage and confidence? One can begin to see how vitally important selenium is as well as all of the nutrients that we have discussed in terms of facilitating better memory.

Unsaturated Fatty Acids. Symbolically represent substance. When you look at substance you can see that there are many different interpretations and levels, but fundamentally, it is the essence of something. Unsaturated fatty acids carry oxygen (spirit) to the brain. The more spirit, the more faith, the more courage, the more confidence, the clearer the mind, the easier the recall to utilize the Universal Teaching, "look back in order to see ahead," as well as drawing on past strengths in order to create a successful future in any endeavor. By providing substance of character, substance of mind and substance of faith to the brain, memory is enhanced because, again, there is no fear of looking back or not wanting to look at anything because the individual is coming from a position of strength, always seeking to understand, always looking to see what cannot be seen and always looking to understand the energy behind what is being seen.

Vitamin B-1. Raises your mood and helps with learning. Symbolically, it is a facilitator and it allows the person to process transactions within the self that are going to position the self in a better place. It allows the facilitation of memories from the past, again based on another Universal Teaching which states: "Draw on past successes."

Vitamin B-6. Serves two roles in memory. First, it is used as a source for communication in the sense that it is beneficial for the nervous system. It helps in transporting the energies of thought as electricity from nerve ending to receptor site. Secondly, it works in terms of protection and regulation because it helps us in regulating our emotional responses to given stimuli. Of course, the more you are aware the more control you have over those kinds of patterned, behavioral responses. Some responses, if the emotions are not controlled, will lead to and manifest as disharmony on many levels.

Vitamin E. Symbolic of self-confidence. One of the ways vitamin E demonstrates itself is that it is an excellent antioxidant. Since we say that oxygen represents spirit, we need to clarify that singlet oxygen is oxygen that is not balanced. It is seeking an electron in the outer orbit in order to become complete. So, when we look at vitamin E as self-confidence we are really talking about balance and harmony with self, without fear and doubt. When you think about that you begin to see how such a position would allow for greater memory because there is nothing to block out, nothing to avoid and nothing to hide from because one has the courage and confidence to be able to confront what one has to confront.

Menopause

Menopause is a naturally occurring phenomenon, happening to both men and women. In men, the transition is called "the male climacteric."[34] Most men, however, begin to exhibit slowly decreasing sexual functions in their late forties or fifties, and one study has shown that the average age for terminating inter-sexual relations was sixty-eight, though variation was great. This decline is related to decrease in testosterone secretion.

In women, the occurrence seems to take place between forty to fifty years of age. It is believed that the main reason for the physical changes is based on the concept that the ovaries are "burned out."[35] The burnout occurs because the primordial follicles decrease with age, and as they decrease in number, the ability of the ovaries to produce estrogen also decreases.

Interestingly, not all women experience the same physical reactions as their bodies go through this particular transition. Some women experience virtually no affects at all. There are many different reasons for this variance. Lack of exercise, emotional stress, and physical stress all can exaggerate the changes taking place. One of the most obvious influences is the nutritional status of the body, especially the adrenal glands.

Menopause is not a disease; it is a natural change within the female body when the body metabolically changes from being a potentially child bearing female to being gender-less, so to speak, or more male. There is a Teaching in the Gospel According to Thomas, in one of the many documents of the Dead Sea Scrolls, where Jesus said to them:

> When you make the two one, and when you make the inner as the outer and the outer as the inner and the above as the below, and when you make the male and the female into a single one, so that the male will not be male and the female (not) be female, when you make eyes in the place of an eye, and a hand in the place of a hand, and a foot in the place of a foot, (and) an image in the place of an image, then shall you enter [the Kingdom].

During menopause, or the "change of life," both genders no longer need to replicate the species, or further it through procreation. Menopause says, from a different point of view, that the purpose of life is multiple.

The most important thing in life is to further yourself, and develop your self on all four levels: Spiritual, Emotional, Social and Material/Physical. Once we go past the childbearing ages, we are supposed to move forward, concentrate on self, and elevate self to the next level.

When a person thinks, from a different point of view, that life can last up to 120 years, then by the time you are forty or fifty and going through the menopausal transition, the person will have gone through half of their life. Now they have the rest of their life to work on the self, to understand what their concepts and patterns are, so that they can master them.

Menopause is a natural transition and it is symbolic of change. The degree of difficulty within the change might be an indication of where your concepts are heavy. In other words, if a woman is very much into being a woman then it may very well be that the menopause might be difficult and uncomfortable because so much of her identity is wrapped up in her gender. But remember, menopause is a natural evolution, not a disease or condition.

ESTROGEN PRODUCTION

Estrogen is primarily produced in the ovaries. The reduction of the primordial follicles or the removal of the ovaries can, therefore, account for the menopausal experience for women. However, there is another set of glands in the body that produces both estrogen and progesterone; these are known as the adrenals. The health and vitality of the adrenals may be one reason why some women have an easier time with this natural transition.

PHYSICAL EFFECTS OF MENOPAUSE

The physical manifestations of female menopause are brought about because of the loss of estrogen production. The loss of estrogen often causes marked physiological changes in the function of the body. These changes include hot flashes, irritability, fatigue, anxiety, and occasionally, various mental/emotional states.

NUTRITIONAL CONSIDERATIONS

The first and foremost consideration in any normal transition within the body would be to nourish it so that it can maintain homeostasis. Like everything else in the body, homeostasis must be maintained in order to ensure good health. Homeostasis (homeo = same; stasis = standing still) is defined as balance and harmony within the body. It is the condition created when each cell in the body functions in an environment that is within certain physiological limits. Homeostasis is achieved when the body (1) has the proper amounts of gases, nutrients, ions, and water; (2) maintains the optimal internal temperature; and (3) has an optimal volume for the health of the cells. When homeostasis is disturbed, health may be affected.

ADRENALS

The adrenal glands sit on top of each of the kidneys. The glands have two parts: the cortex and the medulla. One of their roles is to produce hormones: mineralcorticoids, glucocorticoids, and the gonadocorticoids (better known as the sex hormones). The steroid hormones include the adrenal cortical hormones, hormone forms of vitamin D, and the androgens and estrogens (the male and female sex hormones). These hormones are the precursors to sex hormones which are symbolic of expression.

ESTROGEN

A woman's change of life can be very discomforting. The hot flashes, night sweats, mood changes, and other more subtle differences can be very annoying. These changes are all brought about because of the decrease/lack of hormone production. Estrogen is the one specific hormone medical science focuses on when a woman goes through menopause. Estrogen is found in the ovaries and adrenals, so even after menopause, estrogen production can still take place.

It is important to note two facts: (1) that many women may have had operations in which the ovaries have been removed; (2) the adrenals are considered the stress centers of the body, and are usually the first glands adversely affected by stress which will cause the adrenals to produce a less than adequate amount of estrogen. These facts make it necessary to work on three different nutritional levels:

♦ *If ovaries are present, nourish and rebuild, and re-stimulate estrogen production.*

♦ *Nourish and fortify adrenal glands.*

♦ *If ovaries have been removed then we must bring in natural herbs that contain estrogenic properties.*

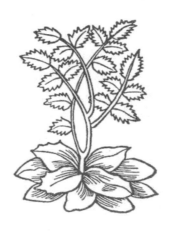

NUTRIENTS AND HERBS TO ASSIST IN RELIEVING NIGHT SWEATS AND HOT FLASHES

With these understandings in mind the following nutrients will be helpful.

Nutrients	Herbs
Calcium	Dong Quai
Iodine	Licorice Root
Pantothenic Acid	Passion Flower
Vitamin B-6	Unicorn Root
Vitamin C	Wild Yam Root
Vitamin E	

Calcium. In insufficient amounts, causes a decrease in estrogen production.

Iodine. Nourishes the thyroid.

Pantothenic Acid. Nourishes the adrenal glands.

Vitamin B-6. Excellent for women who are susceptible to finger/joint pain that often accompanies menopause.

Vitamin C. Found in large quantities within the adrenal glands. Also needed in sex glands as aging takes place.

Vitamin E. An antioxidant. Helps prevent oxidation of the hormones produced in the adrenal glands.

Dong Quai. Considered one of the best herbs for females because it does many different things within the reproduction system.

Unicorn Root. Cleanses and strengthens ovaries.

Licorice Root and Wild Yam Root. Have all been used to provide estrogen type properties to the body.

Passion Flower. Great for calming the nerves, much like a tranquilizer.

SYMBOLOGY OF MENOPAUSE

Menopause symbolically denotes the changing of a form of expression. In examining the process of what physically takes place there is a lot of insight to be gained. It also provides validation on a particular concept, that concept being: the ability to express oneself. It now has become a question in one's mind about being able to do just that, express one's self in a new and different manner since the expression of creating a child is no longer viable. The role of being female and male changes.

Symbolically, menopause is a time when the form of expression is to evolve and change for both genders. This change takes place at an age that it is, on one level, no longer necessary to bring children into the world. It seems that the Divine Intelligence of Life knows that there is a time for child bearing and raising and a time when the strain of doing that is unhealthy for the mature adult. It takes enormous amounts of energy and patience to raise a child, and is truly an endeavor for the young.

Menopause indicates that it is no longer necessary to propagate. At the same time children are a form of symbolic expression of self and unity, and the inability to do that makes one think that their ability to have an expression and communicate is over, yet that is not the case at all.

Menopause is an appropriate time to change. When one aspect of life is no longer necessary to maintain life or a particular level of life or lifestyle, then there is no longer a need for it. Through understanding the concepts that supported it and eliminating them, you become free from your influences. It is through this freedom that new levels of communication are discovered within the self that ultimately will manifest outwardly.

The ovaries, being symbolic of expression, demonstrate how all of it fits together. The ovaries are no longer producing eggs, the germs of expression, and, therefore, the body no longer needs to go through that particular form of cleansing, so the menses permanently disappears.

Another aspect of menopause, in the physical realm, is that the adrenal glands reduce their production of the precursors that form estrogen. One of the reasons that some women have a hard and uncomfortable transition may very well lie in the fact that the adrenals cannot manufacture enough, or properly formed amounts, of the hormones necessary in order to maintain a smooth transition. This could be the result of stress and/or malnutrition.

Since most people consume the standard American diet they have a tendency to be undernourished. Because they are malnourished, and do not have the nutrients necessary to manufacture adequate amounts of the precursors, the transition of change is difficult.

Looking at that symbolically it is easy to understand that when people go through life experiences and are unprepared for them, they have a difficult time. When they have not been nurtured in the true ways that they need to be nurtured, mentally, physically, spiritually, socially, or financially you can see the seeds of difficulty, dissention and disease. If people do not have the wherewithal in at least three of these five areas, then they are not totally prepared to deal with the challenges that life presents. That is not to say that they cannot master their situation, it only implies that it will be more difficult. By having at least three of the five needs fulfilled, an opportunity is created for an understanding of where personal work needs to be done.

The adrenal glands are the stress centers of the body, and because most people are stressed as well as nutrient deficient, the production of the hormones is decreased further, which makes the transition that much more uncomfortable.

The lack of hormones, which are symbolic of a lack of faith in self, does not necessarily mean that the individual is less capable of having an expression in any other arena. In fact, if anything it should help indicate that it is time for a new level, a higher level, a less material level of expression, thus, leaving room in the later years of life to pursue spiritual expression.

SYMBOLOGY OF THE NUTRIENTS

As discussed in the physical aspect of menopause, it is a biological transition. It is the term applied to the physical changes of going from one level of being to another. As in all changes in life, certain elements need to be present in order to make those transitions easy and comfortable. A great example would be in moving from one residence to another. A person can do it alone, with friends, or to make it really easy, they can hire a moving company.

Let us look at the symbology of the nutrients involved in making the menopause transition easy and comfortable.

Calcium. Symbolically allows drawing on strengths as a way of validating that the person does have the capability to change. Even though they may have lost one form of expression, a new one will present itself provided they have the desire and intent to manifest it.

Iodine. Symbolizes intent. As a new being emerges from menopause or andropause climacteric, this being must find new purpose. We use the term "being" because for some people, this change of life evokes many questions about how to move forward. The iodine provides the person with the intent to move forward. Once the mind is made up and strength and new forms of expression are visualized, these individuals are able to move forward and draw on their inner-strengths.

Pantothenic Acid. Symbolic of inspiration. Inspiration is essential for those who may feel their purpose or expression is no longer valid. Life requires inspiration in order to move forward to a new level of expression.

Vitamin B-6. Helps to regulate emotional and energetic expression, preventing loss of balance in either direction.

Vitamin C. Represents a sense of material and physical protection. In this regard it tells the woman that regardless of the fact that she is no longer at one level of expression, she is still viable and can move forward and express on other levels with a sense of wellness.

Vitamin E. Its antioxidant properties help prevent the hormones from becoming oxidized. That means it protects the hormones from becoming less effective in their functions. Vitamin E represents self-confidence, which relates back to the parallel issue in menopause: just as a woman is losing her ability of expression in one form, she can be confident of her ability of expression in other avenues. Vitamin E combined with pantothenic acid provides the woman with inspiration to move forward in her life.

Nerve and Muscle Function

Each time you talk with someone in the healing arts, you are bound to get different perceptions of the same truth, but there is one thing all healers agree upon, whether they are allopaths (commonly referred to as medical doctors), osteopaths, homeopaths, naturopaths, or faith/psychic healers, and that is that nerve transmission and proper muscle function is vital to good health.

NERVE FUNCTION

Without proper nerve transmissions, your body would die. The nerves act like telephone lines; they receive the messages from the brain and transmit, actually carry them, through nerve "lines" to their correct destinations. Each destination point then reacts in a very specific way, based upon the directive of the message sent from the brain.

The nerve endings are connected to organs, glands, and muscles. Each of these performs special functions that help you to live, for instance, the muscles contract and expand on a fairly regular basis, based on what they are told to do. The heart is another excellent example, its beating is stimulated by the electric current that flows through the nerve lines to the heart muscle; it contracts and then expands—one heartbeat.

MUSCLES AND MUSCLE FUNCTION

The muscles play an entirely different role than do the nerves. Muscles are a kind of tissue made up of fibers that are able to contract, causing and allowing movement of the parts and organs of the body.

There are two basic kinds of muscle tissue: striated and smooth. All skeletal muscles are striated, long, and voluntary. They respond quickly to stimulation but are paralyzed by any stopping of nerve supply. Smooth muscle, found in internal organs, is short and involuntary. It reacts slowly to stimulation but does not entirely lose its ability to contract if the nerves are damaged.

The heart muscle (myocardium) is sometimes called a third (cardiac) kind of muscle. However, it is basically a striated muscle that does not contract as quickly as the skeletal muscles, and is not completely paralyzed if it loses stimulation.

NUTRITIONAL NEEDS

Minerals play an important role in the transmission of impulses between the nerves and the cells that make up muscles. Minerals are part of all body tissues and fluids, and are important factors in keeping physiological processes going. They act in nerve responses and muscle contractions, regulate electrolyte balance, the making of hormones, and become parts of enzymes.

NUTRIENTS TO SUPPORT THE NERVOUS SYSTEM

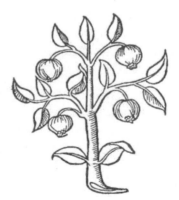

Nutrients
Calcium
Inositol
Magnesium
Niacin
Vitamin B-6

Calcium. A mineral necessary for strong, healthy bones and teeth. Other functions of the calcium ion include its influence in neuromuscular excitability and transmission of nerve impulses.

When calcium levels in the blood are low, symptoms of increased neuromuscular irritability, seizures, and cardiac cramps are possible.

Inositol. Necessary for hair growth, the metabolism of fats and cholesterol, and for the formation of lecithin.

Magnesium. Essential for the normal metabolism of potassium and calcium. Deficiency symptoms include muscle fasciculation (involuntary twitching), tremors, and muscle spasms.

Niacin. A B-complex nutrient that promotes growth and proper nervous system function. Deficiency symptoms include insomnia, tiredness, and nervous disorders.

Vitamin B-6. Necessary for the nerves, muscles, and digestion. A deficiency will cause nervousness and irritability.

SYMBOLOGY OF NERVOUS ISSUES

All nerve disorders are a symbolic form of a breakdown in communication. From a physiological perspective, the nervous system is a network for transporting electrical energy. Thoughts have their beginnings as either a conscious directive (like lifting your arm or picking up something), or an unconscious directive (like breathing). Each type of transaction is initiated by electrical impulses generated by the mind/brain. The brain is both an electromagnetic generator and a bio-computer: as it sends out magnetic waves, it also sends out electrical impulses through the nervous system to tell each muscle, gland, organ, and system what to do and when to do it.

Accomplishing life's tasks requires a lot of communication. You must be able to clearly express your wants, needs, and desires, and you also need the strength and courage to go after them. We use the terms "strength" and "courage" because when we go back to the biochemical and electrical flow of thought, we see that electrical impulses must jump from nerve ending to receptor site and that transference of electrical impulse requires the minerals calcium and magnesium. Phosphorus also plays a role, when confidence is required.

Each of us already pursues the fulfillment of our subconscious expectations. Remember, we are all seeking approval and based on that, we live our lives creating those situations that will validate who we think we are and how we are supposed to be. In communicating change or seeking to accomplish change, having complete muscular control over every variable helps you to consciously reach these goals, as opposed to just fulfilling your subconscious expectations.

If you or someone you know is afflicted by conditions that are synonymous with nervous disorders, including epilepsy, seizures, twitching, paralysis, cramping, or tremors, insight can be gained by examining the symbology of the body part involved.

Symbology of the Nutrients

When it comes to nervous disorders or issues that affect the nervous system, we are really talking about issues that affect the ability to communicate or to have control over events, situations, and emotions.

Nerves can be likened to telephone lines within the body. As a person thinks a thought it is converted from thought energy into electrical energy. That electrical impulse travels down the nerve (phone line) from the brain, it travels to the particular nerve ending, and then jumps to the receptor site on a gland, organ, or muscle. This movement completes the call, and that creates the desired transaction.

Calcium and Magnesium. These two minerals are essential in that transaction. Strength (calcium) and inspiration (magnesium) are required for everything to function properly in the body. (See also Cramps, Leg Aches, and Osteoporosis.)

Moving forward in life requires strength, even if you do not think about it during your daily routine, it is there working. Life also requires a degree of confidence in order to handle everything that is presented to you. From that perspective everything requires strength, and that is one of the reasons calcium is one of the most abundant minerals in the body; it acts as material support. Magnesium is also vital because you need inspiration to move forward in life.

Inositol and Niacin. Niacin symbolically represents openness and receptivity. Looking at the proper functioning of the nervous system from that point of view, as long as the mind is open to new thoughts and new ideas and you are receptive to moving forward with courage and confidence, you will be inspired. This allows for easier transmission of thoughts, which will help you to move forward.

Inositol is important to the nervous system for several reasons. First, inositol nourishes the myelin sheath that protects the entire nervous system. The nervous system, being the telephone lines within the body, communicates all needs, both necessary and desired on every single level.

Inositol symbolically represents integrity, and integrity is vital to the nervous system's efforts to transmit messages to every part of the body. Integrity is important in life, obviously, because it substantiates who you are and how you go about moving forward and accomplishing tasks.

Vitamin B-6. Improves nerve health. Deficiency symptoms include a tendency toward irritability and nervousness. Symbolically, B-6 represents protection as well as regulation, which would take care of those irritable feelings. This is especially true when you feel you are in control because in addition to being protected, you would also feel you have the strength to deal with any situation. Because B-6 also regulates emotions, so to speak, there should be no excitability, quick reactions, or loss of temper (an explosive reaction to a given stimuli).

Obesity

See Weight Loss and Water Retention.

Osteoporosis

Osteoporosis affects both women and men, although women more frequently suffer from the condition. Aside from age-related hormonal changes, one major cause of osteoporosis is a diet with high-protein content. Protein foods (meat, fish, foul, nuts, grains, etc.) leave an acid ash in the bloodstream, whereas fruits and vegetables leave an alkaline ash. Ash is the residue of metabolic processes. Eating a diet high not only in protein but in other acid-forming foods as well means that the calcium in the bloodstream will attempt to neutralize the acidity in order to maintain an alkaline state in the body.

The body's innate intelligence seeks to keep a slightly greater alkaline level because germs cannot live in an alkaline environment. This is a self-protective measure but to do so it uses up available bloodstream calcium ions, thus, forcing the body to pull from reserves from the bones or wherever else it can. This constant pulling of calcium from the bones contributes to the cause of osteoporosis.

NUTRIENTS, HERBS AND DIGESTIVE ENZYME TO SUPPORT BONE HEALTH

Nutrients	Digestive Enzyme	Herbs
Calcium	Betaine Hydrochloride	Alfalfa
Magnesium		Horsetail Grass
Phosphorus		
Vitamin A		
Vitamin C		
Vitamin D		
Zinc		

Calcium, Magnesium, Phosphorus, and Zinc. Essential for calcium assimilation.

Vitamin A. Vital to any growth and development (bone is constantly changing and being remodeled).

Vitamin C. Essential to production of collagen which is the substance that gives bone its flexibility.

Vitamin D and Betaine Hydrochloride. For calcium assimilation.

Zinc. Needed for the protein formation of bone.

Alfalfa. Contain easily-assimilated forms of calcium.

Horsetail Grass. For silica content.

SYMBOLOGY OF OSTEOPOROSIS

In considering the symbolic meaning of osteoporosis, calcium representing strength, and blood representing spirit, take center stage.

One of the more common man-made concepts is that eating meat will make our bodies stronger, yet the opposite is true. Meat, flesh foods, and other forms of protein actually debilitate the body, depleting its internal strength and rendering its bones more fragile through calcium depletion. This reaffirms that man-made ideas of strength are not valid because it is not true strength. It is similar to someone who uses bravado to hide insecurities.

It is noteworthy that some conditions and diseases affect particular parts of the body, while others attack certain functions, glands, or organs. In osteoporosis, the attack is on the body's fundamental support system—its bones. Symbolically then, osteoporosis occurs when a person feels a lack of strength to make changes or transitions. I pose it from that perspective because osteoporosis is something that manifests most often after menopause in women or andropause in men. Bones represent support, both physically and symbolically. Two of the key minerals in bones are calcium and magnesium, which represent strength and inspiration, respectively. These are two of the most important energies for living a fruitful, healthy life.

In both sexes, osteoporosis occurs because on a physical level, there is faulty restructuring or remodeling of the bones, due in part to a lack of hormones. Interestingly, it is also due in part to a lack of digestive juices, specifically betaine hydrochloride, and it is absolutely essential that betaine hydrochloride be present to get calcium ions into the bone matrix to rebuild bone. It is easy to understand how both men and women could have questions about their purpose after completing this major life transition. Questions about expression, abilities, and self-worth to name a few, and of course, none of this overtly manifests. Therein is the beauty of symbology.

Symbology is the living language of life. Symbols are the physical manifestations of both emotional and thought energies at work. Reading symbols helps you to see what cannot be seen—true thoughts and feelings in motion. Reading symbols also provides a glimpse of a possible future, one based on how a pattern of behavior would normally fulfill itself in the course of its cycle. Having clear vision in order to make proper decisions is one of life's vital goals. Clear vision comes about when you can see the energies at work, as reflected in the Universal Laws, upon which this work is based.

With osteoporosis, there is a depletion of strength. Contemporary culture's view of strength suggests that you need various attributes to be strong, including money, power, and certain dietary elements, specifically red meat and other flesh foods. The fallacy of that thinking is seen in the result of eating such a diet. High protein and acid-rich foods create an acid ash in the bloodstream though the process of digestion. This alerts the body to use calcium to neutralize the acidity in the bloodstream. This is done to help keep the body in a more alkaline state, which will not readily support germs, a catchall phrase for bacterias, fungi, and viruses. In this process of neutralizing the acidity, calcium is pulled from the bones, and because the American diet is somewhat mineral deficient, this creates the conditions that lead over time to osteoporosis.

Even though there is a push toward increased milk consumption, particularly among girls and women, milk does not truly satisfy the body's needs. Symbolically, the concept itself is false. The symbology of dairy products, milk specifically, implies the need for external support and sustenance (mother's milk) in order to be and grow strong. Drinking milk and eating meat is kind of a double whammy: milk symbolizes a mother's support, and meat symbolizes strength. The truth is both substances affect the body in different, but negative ways. Milk creates mucus, which can interfere with assimilation of nutrients, and meat creates an acidic environment, setting up conditions favorable for germs to take root and multiply.

Osteoporosis symbolizes great doubt both in one's strength to go forward and to be self-supporting in this new level of expression, and there is a greater tendency to relate to the past in terms of artificial sustenance and artificial strength.

SYMBOLOGY OF THE NUTRIENTS

The symbology of the nutrients is loud and clear. It implies that the individual is experiencing and working with a lack of faith in self. There is an underlying feeling of lacking strength, brought about because of feelings of a loss of expression.

Calcium. Nutritionally and symbolically, calcium (strength) is being depleted from the basic support system (skeleton). This is the result of the pursuit of a false sense of strength in the man-made teachings and presentations. The perfect example is drinking milk for calcium. As discussed previously, milk does not provide the body with the required amount of calcium.

When an individual has osteoporosis, he or she feels a lack in the wherewithal and strength to stand up and maintain the self as in the past. It is interesting that osteoporosis generally occurs when people are in their sixties and seventies. This is usually after menopause, when women, particularly, have lost their ability to express, or bring forth life in the symbolic form of a child. The expression from a female perspective of being able to conceive and create life is what gave women a subconscious sense of strength. When a woman feels she no longer has that capability, there can be a lack of strength in her expression.

Another consideration is that the U.S. Social Security Administration may soon lose its viability; it may not be financially able to provide the support that an individual needs in later years. The elderly cannot work and may be incapacitated, made to feel too old by a more "desirable" youthful society. These older citizens may come to feel they lack the strength and support that they need to be strong. Depending upon man-made sources of strength only depletes the body further, leaving the individual in a fragile state.

There are many components involved in rebuilding bone: calcium, magnesium, zinc, phosphorus, vitamin D, and betaine hydrochloride, also known as hydrochloric acid. Symbolically it is the strength, the inspiration, a working faith, and courage that support the person in each of life's endeavors; all of these elements combine both nutritionally and symbolically to create the whole support system.

Magnesium. Acts as a facilitator and represents inspiration. It assists in the assimilation of thoughts that lead to strength, and from a position of strength, all actions taken lead to a positive conclusion.

Inspiration and facilitation are essential for the development of strength (calcium) and courage (phosphorous).

Again, more calcium (strength) is retained when supplies of magnesium (inspiration) and vitamin D (insights/understandings) are adequate.[36] Profuse amounts of calcium are lost in the urine when magnesium is undersupplied, and the magnesium deposited in bones (symbolic of support) is given up reluctantly, even during a severe deficiency.[37] These facts indicate that magnesium, which is usually compromised,[38] is important in correcting bone abnormalities and is particularly low in diabetics.[39]

Phosphorus. Phosphorous is symbolic of courage. Too much phosphorus in the body blocks the absorption of calcium. When in their proper ratio to each other, calcium (symbolic of strength) and phosphorus (courage) work in tandem. We can readily see that when one has false courage or bravado they really are making up for feelings of not having strength. If one had true strength built on a solid foundation of a working faith, then there would be no need to boast, brag, or operate with a large ego. Such is surely the sign or symbol of a person who feels small within.

It takes courage in life to be able to break down and utilize to the fullest everything that comes your way. That is why phosphorous is so vital to good health; in matters of life, it is essential that courage and strength be in equal proportion.

Bone (support) contains 85 percent of the body's total phosphorous. This is why a well-nourished body is so important to success in life on all levels. Cells use the remaining phosphorous as a phosphate, demonstrating that courage and confidence come in many forms and energies. One never knows the level of courage another is demonstrating on a daily basis; what may look like weakness to one may be an exerted effort for another.

Vitamin A. The symbolic importance of vitamin A is the ability to see into the doubt that exists within the self. You could even say that vitamin A aids in self-examination by its role in improving (internal) vision. By helping you to see well, vitamin A gives you greater insight. Going into a situation totally prepared gives you courage and confidence. When those energies are at work for you, there is no doubt about your ability to master a situation.

Vitamin C. Increases absorption of iron, symbolic of faith and courage. Iron is contained in hemoglobin, which carries oxygen to the cells. It also removes carbon dioxide and carries it to the lungs. Oxygen is symbolic of spirit because air symbolically represents heaven and heaven is symbolic of the Creator's home or dwelling place. Tying together these insights, we can see that vitamin C (protection) is essential for faith, courage and strength to grow.

Symbolically, vitamin C protects us from those thoughts that undermine our inherent strength. When your courage and faith in self are compromised, doubt and fear set in, opening the door for frustration, anger, and resentment. Such developments can "eat you up," and consequently, can lead to cancer and many other different conditions and diseases.

Vitamin D. Symbolically, vitamin D's role in calcium absorption represents insight and, to a degree, understanding. This interpretation is based on vitamin D's integral part in the assimilation of calcium, which represents strength. Strength comes in two styles. The first is what we normally see in the world—bravado based on man-made concepts as to what strength represents. But there is also true strength, the type that is quiet yet runs extremely deep. People with true strength know that they can accomplish just about anything they set out to do.

Zinc. Symbolically, zinc represents those thoughts that contribute to supportive or fundamental expression and a working faith. Without a working faith and a positive means to express energy, there would be no growth on an individual's path. There would be difficulty in breaking down thoughts. Because of an inability to grow the self with full confidence and courage, the ability to express or reproduce is compromised, and in some cases, eliminated.

Pancreas Concerns

The pancreas is a gland designed to produce insulin and enzymes, some of which are used to digest proteins, fats, and carbohydrates. When problems develop in the pancreas, their results can be seen in the disruption of various functions throughout the body. If digestion is disrupted, constipation can result. If circulating blood sugar is not metabolized properly for fuel due to a lack of insulin or insulin sensitivity, it accumulates in the blood, and when the blood sugar levels remain high, diabetes can result. (See also Diabetes.) Keeping the pancreas healthy and strong should help to prevent these secondary problems in the body.

NUTRIENTS AND HERBS TO SUPPORT THE PANCREAS

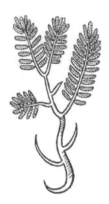

Nutrients	Herbs
Manganese	Cedar Berries
Selenium	Dandelion Root
Zinc	Gentian Root
	Goldenseal Root
	Licorice Root

Manganese. Stores of it are found chiefly in the human liver, kidney, pancreas, lungs, prostate gland, adrenals and brain.

Selenium. Supports the liver and pancreas.

Zinc. Plays a part in manufacturing of insulin in the pancreas.

Cedar Berries. Stimulate the pancreas.

Dandelion Root. Stimulates bile production, benefits the spleen and improves the health of the pancreas.

Gentian Root. Focus of activity is on those glands and organs involved in digestion, primarily the gallbladder and pancreas.

Goldenseal Root. Lowers blood sugar and stimulates the pancreas.

Licorice Root. Strengthens the pancreas and spleen.

SYMBOLOGY OF THE PANCREAS

The pancreas is interesting symbolically because of its role in manufacturing digestive enzymes and insulin, which help us to utilize the sweets of life. It symbolizes your ability to break down thoughts that are presented to you so that they can be effectively used.

Problems with the pancreas reflect difficulty in breaking down for digestion what is coming into your life. If you are facing a difficult situation and feeling overwhelmed, can it possibly be broken down and used for some better purpose, or is this event "indigestible"? Reframing the scenario, in reality, it is your belief system at work, and reality is only a reflection of what resides within, based on concepts. When the external is not flowing or working, it is a reflection of the conflict within.

SYMBOLOGY OF THE NUTRIENTS

The pancreas is a facilitator. It also assists in your being able to break down thoughts. In this way, you can utilize the strength and whatever kernels of growth are provided within those thoughts. The pancreas plays an important role in that process and the nutrients are the components that help it happen.

Manganese. Manganese represents will, specifically the determination to process a thought and use what it offers to help you move forward.

Selenium. Because of its role it in the detoxification process, is indicative of protection. Just as selenium supports the pancreas as it regulates what is good or bad for the body, so does it act to provide clarity about the nature of thoughts presented to you. The pancreas works in conjunction with the liver to break down and eliminate potentially harmful substances in the body. Symbolically, they also work together to eliminate and protect you from the toxic parts of thoughts.

Zinc. Symbolically, zinc represents support and a working faith. This is illustrated when the pancreas is creating insulin, providing the body its fundamental fuel source, glycogen (sugar). Zinc, via insulin, indicates that you have the ability to truly and effectively utilize the sweets that life provides.

As an indicator of a working faith, zinc is in harmony with the symbolic function of the pancreas, which is the ability to break down thoughts. The pancreas manufactures insulin to help the body utilize sugar, and it also creates digestive enzymes to help break down the food. This is mirrored in the mental processes required to confidently process thoughts to maximum benefit.

Parasites

Parasites enter the body through different channels. It could be from the water a person drinks or from being in a river or lake that is infected with parasites. Most parasites enter the body through the food we eat; meat is one of the major culprits of introducing parasites into the intestinal environment.

There are many different schools of thought in relation to parasites and the role that they play in creating disease. LaDean Griffin, noted healer and author, has stated that she feels parasites are a cause of diabetes. Her theory is that they invade the pancreas, thereby interfering with its functioning. In this way, the insulin-producing capabilities of the pancreas are reduced, and excessive sugar builds up in the bloodstream.

Another healer feels that parasites are the cause of tumors and cysts. Still others believe parasites in the intestinal tract rob the body of needed nutrition, thus, lowering its health and vitality, and this sets in motion the receptivity for disease.

Regardless of what role or roles you believe parasites play in illness, it is still prudent to eliminate them from the body, and the easiest way to do it is with herbs.

HERBS TO ASSIST THE BODY IN ELIMINATING PARASITES FROM THE INTESTINAL TRACT

Herbs	
Black Walnut	Pau D'Arco
Butternut Root Bark	Pumpkin Seeds
Garlic	Wormseed
Papaya Seeds	

Black Walnut. Used to expel various kinds of worms. Has high tannin content.

Butternut Root Bark. Most mild and efficacious laxative known. Used also as a treatment for liver disorders (as practiced extensively in homeopathy) and intestinal sickness. It increases the manufacture and secretion of bile and the activity of glands in the walls of the intestinal tract.

Garlic. Increases resistance to bacterial infection and has been proven to have this effect on multiple germs. Combats the following fungi: Candida albicans, microsporum, and epidermophyton.

Papaya Seeds. Used extensively in Mexico as a way of ridding the body of parasites and worms.

Pau D'Arco. Used in all situations that deal with bacteria. Fungi cannot grow around this tree.

Pumpkin Seeds. High in zinc and it is employed to kill parasites.

Wormseed. Also known as Jerusalem Artichoke. Known for its ability to kill parasites.

SYMBOLOGY OF PARASITES

Parasites are symbolic of a thought that one has accepted and lived with, even though the thought is actually detrimental. It is those thoughts that rob a person of power and strength.

The presence of parasites in the intestinal environment means that many of the nutrients required to help build the body and maintain health will be consumed by those parasites. Also parasites, like every living entity, produce metabolic wastes that also affect the health of the host's body. Since the body's immune system was not strong enough to prevent the parasite from taking hold, it is unlikely that the detoxification system will be strong enough to overcome the toxicity generated by the parasites to help the body maintain a healthy environment.

Parasites are symbolic of those thoughts that appear at first take to be okay or maybe even good for you. But when they are incorporated into your being and life, they slowly steal the strength you need to survive. However, having a parasitic infection just may be an indication that a person does not believe he or she is strong enough to combat the "forces," environment or situation. The environment and thoughts being presented undermine the health, ultimately causing debilitation to a degree that the person cannot move forward in dealing with the current situation, or any situation. The individual becomes weak and depleted.

The same thing symbolically could be said for those with Candida, chronic fatigue syndrome, or fibromyalgia, conditions that also leave the individual with very low energy levels and a lot of discomfort. Symbolically, we would have to look at a lack of inspiration as one of the foundations for Candida, chronic fatigue, and fibromyalgia. When inspiration is present in life and there is something to look forward to, there is no tiredness or lethargy; there is nothing but joy in abundance for doing what you want to do.

Parasites border on the same kind of a situation. Thoughts end up debilitating and they sap strength, energy, desire, and inspiration for moving forward to a new level of being as a powerful, positive individual.

Premenstrual Syndrome

Premenstrual Syndrome (PMS) has generated a lot of interest over the past few years as medicine and nutritional science have debated whether to acknowledge the existence of this condition.

In keeping with the philosophy of nutritional science that each disease or discomfort results from nutritional deficiencies, supplementation offers one of the more sensible approaches to countering the common symptoms of PMS. The most commonly reported symptoms include fluid retention, bloating, painful breasts, headaches, backaches, skin eruptions, mental depression, irritability and lethargy.

Interestingly, many of these symptoms are the same for Candida, and some women have a discharge prior to their menstrual cycle. Is it possible that as the body prepares to cleanse, it experiences a level of stress sufficient to lower the immune system, thus, allowing the Candida to temporarily flourish? Any change in the body's internal balance can create stress, and stress attacks the body by taxing the adrenal glands, which secrete hormone messengers that tell the other glands how to perform or what to manufacture.

All the body's glands and systems are interconnected and interdependent. That is why a proper nutritional balance is so vital to attaining and maintaining health. A strong nutritional state also greatly reduces or eliminates the opportunity for disease to take hold.

NUTRIENTS AND HERBS TO SUPPORT AGAINST COMMON SYMPTOMS ASSOCIATED WITH PMS

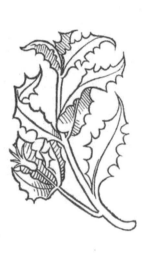

Nutrients	Herbs
Calcium	Blessed Thistle
Iron	Corn Silk
Magnesium	False Unicorn Root
Pantothenic Acid	Horsetail Grass
Phosphorus	Licorice Root
Potassium	Parsley
Vitamin B-1	Squawvine
Vitamin B-6	Suma
Vitamin C	Valerian Root
Zinc	Watermelon Seeds
	Wild Lettuce

Calcium. Acts as a calming agent and relieves backaches.

Iron. Depletion can cause a variety of symptoms, including fatigue, an inability to concentrate, paleness, and lack of muscle tone.

Magnesium. For the assimilation of calcium. Relaxes muscles and nerves.

Pantothenic Acid. Nourishes the adrenal glands. Helps to provide energy.

Vitamin B-1. Known as the "morale vitamin" for its beneficial effect on the nervous system and mental attitude.

Vitamin B-6. Helps maintain the balance of sodium and potassium, which regulates body fluids and promotes normal functioning of the nervous and musculoskeletal systems.

Vitamin C. Along with zinc and vitamins B-6 and B-3 (niacin), this nutrient is a vital co-factor in the production of additional GLA (GAMA Linolenic Acid).

Zinc. Another co-factor for GLA.

Blessed Thistle. For headaches and any kind of female problem.

Corn Silk. Used extensively for the reduction of fluids.

False Unicorn Root. Helps in reducing headaches and depression.

Horsetail Grass. One of the best sources of silica that is essential for calcium assimilation and utilization. Silica also transmutes into calcium.

Licorice Root. Estrogenic activity.

Parsley. Excellent for reducing fluid retention.

Squawvine. Good for the feelings of morning sickness or nausea. Also contains significant amounts of the amino acid tryptophan, known for its calming effects.

Suma. Invigorates the female hormonal balance without disturbing effects.

Valerian Root. Valerian root and its major constituents, called valepotriates, have marked sedative, anticonvulsive, hypotensive, tranquilizing, neurotropic, and anti-aggression properties.

Watermelon Seeds. Good for reducing fluids.

Wild Lettuce. Has a sedative effect on the central nervous system.

Symbology of Premenstrual Syndrome

PMS gives us lots of symbolic material, and it provides insight and understanding about what the sufferer is going through.

Looking first at the symptoms of PMS, muscular cramping is one of the most common. During a cramp, the muscle contracts and becomes locked in that position. In order for the muscle to relax and contract normally, calcium and magnesium must be present. (See also Cramps.) Symbolically, calcium and magnesium represent strength and inspiration, respectively. Consequently, PMS may symbolize that on some levels a woman has issues about being a woman; having an uncomfortable menstrual period could elicit all kinds of feelings related to the woman's concepts about female expression and womanhood.

In some instances of PMS, a woman may have a hormonal imbalance, which could cause a great deal of emotional sensitivity. More often than not, stress is going to tax the adrenal glands, and this will cause a change in the body's hormonal status.

In PMS, there are also issues with expression. Sensitivities, defenses, and hormonally linked emotional imbalances mean things can be taken wrongly. There can also be issues about cleanliness and possibly sex, again tied into the concepts of the expression of womanhood.

Another symptom is breast tenderness. Breasts often denote a female's concepts of or her feelings about being a woman. In general, breasts are tied into nurturing, motherhood, and femininity.

There are obviously concepts involved with the cleansing aspect from a female perspective such as sensitivity and defensiveness that could surround the menstrual cycle. As far as the menses go, having a period is natural, but the discomfort is not. The discomfort is tied into concepts one has about womanhood and the whole female expression.

SYMBOLOGY OF THE NUTRIENTS

It is interesting how something so natural can be so painful for so many women. A symbolic examination of the nutrients necessary to alleviate the pain and discomfort of premenstrual syndrome and the menstrual cycle sheds some insight.

Calcium and Magnesium, Phosphorus, and Potassium. These are the four minerals essential in eliminating cramping. The number 4 symbolizes advancement on the positive side and a blockage on the negative. (See also Cramps.)

PMS is related to the concept of strength—remember that the physical symptoms of cramping are caused by a lack of calcium and magnesium, which represent strength and inspiration. Almost everything in the body is muscle-driven. For movement to take place, muscles must act in harmony with each other. The realization of every task or journey undertaken by man is dependent on this harmonious movement. When a woman is inspired about her femininity and being a woman, she knows she has the strength to endure those things required for her gender's validation, and there is no need for cramps.

Studying the symbology of the minerals involved in muscular transactions will allow you to see all of the essential ingredients and energies for getting a handle on life, and these energies allow for the mastering of life itself.

With magnesium, we are looking at inspiration. Inspiration leads to flexibility of thinking; when you are inspired you seek more than one perspective. If you have and can manifest strength, courage, and inspiration in your every endeavor, you would be more open to seeing. You would be more flexible. There would be no muscle cramping on any level.

Phosphorous is symbolic of courage.   It takes courage in life to be able to break down and utilize to the fullest everything that comes your way. That is why phosphorous is so vital to good health; in matters of life, it is essential that courage and strength be in equal proportion.

Bone (support) contains 85 percent of the body's total phosphorous. This is why a well-nourished body is so important to success in life on all levels. Cells use the remaining phosphorous as a phosphate, demonstrating that courage and confidence come in many forms and energies. One never knows the level of courage another is demonstrating on a daily basis; what may look like weakness to one may be an exerted effort for another.

The presence of courage is always vital, with the amount needed depending on the current circumstance. Balance must be maintained, in the event of PMS, more courage is required.

Daily life requires an enormous amount of strength to cope with the energetic forces from the emotional, social, material, and physical levels. Should you be confronted by something that challenges your personal belief system, you would require courage to stand your ground and stay committed to your convictions. When these situations occur, you must also look closely at your convictions. Are they based on false, man-made concepts or on the insights and understandings that come from knowing Universal Truths? Do you have to defend your position and perceptions regarding how life is to be lived? This takes us to potassium.

Potassium symbolizes balance and harmony. It is essential for the physical functioning of the body, and reflects the need for balance between material and spiritual considerations. This illustrates the point that a fine balance must be maintained in all aspects. Life, like health, has to be maintained in proper balance, or it can become distorted. These distortions can lead a person to become so engrossed in the material plane as to become unbalanced. Were you to become potassium-depleted, you would begin to experience cramping and a tendency toward water retention. With water being symbolic of the material plane, we can see where the dependency or co-dependency on the material becomes dominant and overwhelming.

Iron. This mineral is an oxygen carrier, which is symbolic of spirit. It is also symbolic of emotional control. Faith in self is required to exercise emotional control.

Vitamin B-1. This B-complex vitamin is a facilitator of communication within the body. Of particular importance here is its role in bolstering morale and fostering a better mental attitude. Anything that can facilitate the journey through life is valuable because it relieves so much pressure on the person.

Vitamin B-6. With PMS, there is pressure and bloating, which are offset by vitamin B-6. While B-6 participates symbolically in both regulation and protection, in this case it is more of a regulator of fluids within the system. Water, which is symbolic of material life and considerations such as money or possessions, is retained as a matter of expression. People often use these objects to demonstrate that they are capable and powerful.

Zinc. Helps with various transactions within the body. Symbolically, it provides a working faith, a faith to know that one can get through the whole expression aspect of self on an emotional level. In this application there is not a conflict within about the role of being female, which ensures that a person can meet all the challenges and issues involved in expressing the self, particularly the aspects of gender.

Going through these cycles of life is easier than it might first appear because you already have all of the necessary ingredients within; it is just a matter of learning to see them, accept them, and build upon them. In the meantime, the woman must bring in external sources of knowledge to help her find what she is looking for within the self.

When you ingest something or do something externally, it is just a symbolic gesture of what is desired within the self. With regard to taking supplements, while the gesture is symbolic, the human body requires these things to function properly. At the same time, the Inner Self requires the symbolic significance that the nutrients provide.

Courage, a working faith, inspiration, the facility to move forward, protection, regulation—all of these energies and others must be present for the self to progress as easily and peacefully as possible.

Prostate Problems

Located directly under the urinary bladder and surrounding the superior portion of the urethra from its origin in the bladder, the prostate is the largest accessory gland of the male reproductive tract, and it is composed of muscular and glandular tissues. Similar in size and texture to a chestnut, it is a conglomerate of thirty to fifty small glands, from which sixteen to thirty-two excretory ducts open independently into the urethra.[40] These glandular units are surrounded by fibromuscular tissue that contracts during ejaculation. The gland is filled with nerve fibers, including sensory nerve endings that are scattered in the connective tissue.

The prostate slowly increases in size from birth to puberty, then grows at an increased pace, attaining a stable size during the third decade of life. It remains stable in size until about the age of forty-five, when further enlargement may occur. For reasons not yet completely understood, the prostate can frequently increase in size, at an older age, to a point that two out of three men reaching the age of seventy can suffer from some degree of urinary obstruction.

THE FUNCTION OF THE PROSTATE

The function of the prostate is to secrete a milky, slightly acidic fluid into the prostatic urethra, through its many prostatic ducts. The urethra is the terminal canal for the male reproductive and urinary systems, and serves as a passageway for the different fluids that interact to form semen.

Prostatic fluid contains enzymes that balance the acid levels of the interacting fluids and help in the movement function of sperm, the male transporter of life from the male to the female. Prostatic fluid also tempers acid levels in sperm stored in the ductis deferens. Sperm is acidic due to the metabolic end products, so the infusion of prostatic fluids into the ejaculatory duct serves to regulate the acidity of the sperm. Also, female vaginal secretions are acidic (with a pH of 3.5 to 4.0) and sperm do not become optimally motile until the pH of the surrounding fluids rises anywhere from 6 to 6.5. Prostatic fluids in the sperm neutralize the acidity after ejaculation, which would enhance the sperm's motility and fertility.

Many men over the age of fifty seem to suffer from an inflamed prostate gland. The inflammation is sometimes painful and almost always uncomfortable. By eliminating the physical causes, you may be able to increase the speed of healing. Another step would be to increase the use of those nutrients that are known to be beneficial to the prostate.

NUTRIENTS, AMINO ACIDS AND HERBS FOR PROSTATE SUPPORT

Nutrients	Amino Acids	Herbs
Magnesium	Alanine	Bee Pollen
Unsaturated Fatty Acids	Glutamic Acid	Gravel Root
Vitamin E	Glycine	Parsley
Zinc		Pumpkin Seeds

Magnesium. As a component of calcium homeostasis, magnesium works in the prostate to help with the utilization of calcium.

Vitamin E and Unsaturated Fatty Acids. Essential for glandular health; they work together in lessening of residual urine. Vitamin E protects unsaturated fatty acids from oxidation and plays a role in prostate support by protecting the fat-soluble vitamins: vitamin A, with its role in epithelial cells, and vitamin D, essential for maintaining prostate health.

Zinc. An essential mineral for normal prostate gland function. A component of semen; it is believed that at least 1 mg of zinc is excreted in one ejaculem. There are also major losses of zinc in the intestinal tract. Physiological functions of zinc include fertility, reproduction and sexual maturity.

Alanine, Glutamic Acid, and Glycine. Vital amino acids are important; their role in human nutrition is extensive and not fully known.

Bee Pollen. Contains various nutrients that strengthen and benefit the body.

Gravel Root and Parsley. Herbs used traditionally for their inflammation-reducing properties.

Pumpkin Seeds. High in zinc.

SYMBOLOGY OF PROSTATE ISSUES

Prostate problems stem from concepts related to reproduction, expression, impotence, an inability to perform, and the inability to live up to conscious expectations. Subconsciously, the man has feelings of inadequacy and doubts his ability to express himself.

All prostate problems, including cancer, result from the energies of anger, resentment, frustration, and guilt. These feelings have multiple causes; some come from feelings of inadequacy and others from an inability to perform.

The prostate is integral to fertilization because it produces a particular fluid that is injected into the vagina to create a sperm-friendly environment just prior to the sperm's release. Consequently, it is easy to see that faulty prostate function would also lead to faulty expression. Both would be built upon a man's doubt in his ability of masculine expression. He may also doubt or resent the specific concepts of manhood that are dominant in his family.

Remember, a male child is going to be either exactly like his father or the exact opposite. If the father was a prolific writer, then the child may be less inclined to pursue that career or mode of expression, and that certainly would be the case if the son felt inadequate or unable to compete against the father.

Prostate health depends on the overall subconscious concepts related to expression with which the man is working. Identifying them would help to illuminate what he needs to understand to resolve his prostate problems as they arise.

SYMBOLOGY OF THE NUTRIENTS

Symbolically, the prostate is tied into a man's expression of manhood and his ability to express the self. The nutrients involved in prostate health, especially those that reduce inflammation and support proper function, illustrate how the symbology of each nutrient helps to validate a man's self-expression.

Magnesium. Symbolic of inspiration. In this particular aspect it is there to help the body utilize the calcium, which can create sand, gravel or stones that will develop in the prostate gland. Calcium, being symbolic of strength, when not used properly, not incorporated into the self, creates problems—prostate stones, kidney stones. These are all issues where strength is not being utilized by the individual. Magnesium, by providing inspiration, allows you to utilize strength because when you become inspired it gives you another level of energy, another level of expression. It provides power in order to move forward, and by allowing the self to incorporate its strength into its movement, you can begin to see the relationship between magnesium and calcium in every muscular transaction and the utilization between strength and accomplishment, which is born out of inspiration.

Unsaturated Fatty Acids. Symbolic of character and substance. An individual requires these two qualities to be creative and expressive. It can be seen that for the totality of self to manifest positively all of the ingredients must be present in adequate amounts. Physical health is the result of being nutritionally sound, emotional or psychological health is based on the same principles.

When there are compromised levels of courage or confidence, or negativity about self is present in some small aspects of self, in time that doubt undermines self. When that happens, just like a nutritional deficiency, a problem will manifest in some way. Prostate problems are one such example.

The fact that so many men end up with prostate cancer indicates the anger, resentment, and frustration they feel about not being able to express themselves effectively. All of that can lead to guilt on some level, particularly when success in some form of expression is not present.

Understanding your own subconscious concepts and behavior patterns is vital to mastering any health condition.

Vitamin E. Symbolic of self-confidence. Self-confidence is required for you to be truly expressive and speak your mind, and is necessary for creativity and the bringing forth of life in a situation. Some situations and events in life require a greater degree of self-confidence than others.

Zinc. Vital to prostate health. It represents fundamental expression and having a working faith in self. When you have a working faith, you can handle anything with which you are confronted; you can be creative and expressive.

Almost 60 percent of men end up with prostate problems in life. We might ask if this happens because life beats them down or because, over time, they no longer feel they have the wherewithal to continue to perform at the levels they used to. Living life is a kind of battle; each of us constantly does battle and deals with the forces that come against the self, and these forces are generated both externally and internally. Part of the struggle is caused by each person's subconscious concepts and self-expectations.

A constant theme in this work has been how man seeks to fulfill subconscious self-expectations. Over time, this may result in a total loss of confidence in the ability for self-expression. This can also be true for those men who have acquired great wealth. Even though they may live in the midst of material opulence, it does not necessarily indicate that at an emotional and spiritual level there is true confidence, or a true working faith. All of their expression is tied into external validation and presentation. If they cannot express their manhood because the prostate is not functioning properly, it serves to remind us that the essence or who and what we are is internal, and that is what must be nourished.

By providing zinc, symbolic of a working faith, and vitamin E, which symbolizes self-confidence, we begin to see some of the energies at a symbolic level that may be lacking in prostate problems.

Stress, Tension, and Hyperactivity

It is often said that too much stress is a killer, both directly and indirectly. Too much stress is also known to cause heart attacks, high blood pressure, strokes, and depression. It contributes to lowered adrenal function and a depressed immune system. Stress creates physical tension. Tension is when the muscles contract and fail to relax. When there is tension in the muscles, this limits the amount of blood that can flow through the arteries, veins, and capillaries located in that area. When bloodflow is reduced due to tension, pain or cramping can occur in that area. Heart attacks are a specific example of what happens when blood is reduced to an area. It is also true that the consequences of elevated cholesterol levels are heart attacks.

Another good example of over stress and tension at work is the common headache. These are usually brought on by stress and once the muscles tense and bloodflow is reduced the headache begins. Blood carries oxygen and other nutrients to nerves and muscles, and when these become starved, they begin to experience pain.

Stress lowers the immune system by adversely affecting the adrenal glands, which subsequently can allow many conditions and diseases to flourish. The key reason for this is the adrenals are tied to the functioning of other glands by the adrenal-produced hormones.

The environment causes some forms of stress. This includes the air we breathe, water we drink, food we eat, and places we work. Because of all these different sources of stress, it is important to maintain an excellent diet and to fortify the body with those nutrients that will help the body deal with stress. A healthy and nutritionally sound body deals with the stresses of life from a position of strength. This means that although there is stress from many different areas in our lives, the body is not adversely affected by it.

Unfortunately, the American diet is so nutritionally deficient that it does not contain enough nutrients to keep the body fit and able. Stress depletes nutrients such as calcium, vitamin C, and the entire range of B-complex vitamins, and this depletion can cause feelings of nervousness, irritability, sleeplessness, muscle cramping, and other physical results. The best way to deal with these depletions is to provide the body with the nutrients necessary.

Hyperactivity is often the result of stimulating chemicals brought into the body via the diet. The body is over stimulated by these chemicals and when the mineral content of the body is too low hyperactivity manifests. The minerals act to maintain balance and harmony between the contractibility and relaxation of the muscles and nerves.

Nutrients, Amino Acids and Herbs to Nourish and Relax Nerves

Nutrients	Amino Acids	Herbs
B-complex Vitamins	L-Tyrosine	Hops
Calcium		Scullcap
Inositol		Valerian Root
Magnesium		
Niacinamide		

B-complex Vitamins. Water soluble vitamins that work together in the nervous system and are involved in energy production and fat and protein metabolism, all of which need to work properly for the nervous system to function.

Calcium and Magnesium. Work to nourish and relax nerves and muscles. Calcium is the dominant mineral-nutrient that is lost to stress. What is also interesting about stress is that when calcium is lost, it disrupts the relationship between sodium and potassium so that the individual immediately gains five to fifteen pounds of water.

Inositol. Acts in a calming way on the nervous system.

Vitamin B-6. Essential for healthy nerve endings.

L-Tyrosine. An amino acid known to elevate moods.

Hops, Skullcap, and Valerian Root. All used for ages to nourish, soothe and relax the nerves and muscles.

SYMBOLOGY OF STRESS, TENSION, AND HYPERACTIVITY

Stress is a multifaceted killer, and symbolically, it all comes down to the same thing: when we investigate the causes of stress, we can see that it is the result of how a person responds to what they see and hear.

If you question the validity of that statement, think of the last time you found yourself in an embarrassing situation. Your body went through a physiological and biochemical change. Your heart may have begun to race, and your stomach may have turned flip-flops. Only you can determine why you react in a particular way to such stimuli. We can see that stress is a result of concepts within the subconscious mind that cause people to act and react according to stimuli. Some of those stimuli trigger subconscious concepts and patterns of behavior that cause stress.

When the body experiences stress, the B-complex vitamins and calcium are depleted. We know calcium to be symbolic of strength. We can see that stress is the result of doubt at work, an uncertainty in our ability to handle a situation or to deal positively with a situation.

When we see or experience a stimulus, the mind immediately draws upon this Universal Teaching: "Look back in order to see ahead." The beauty here is that you have the opportunity to change the outcome of a situation if you are conscious and aware of how you have reacted in the past to similar stimuli. In all situations where there appear to be a new stimulus, remember that although it may appear different, it has a similar energy to previously known stimuli. Stimuli have one thing in common because they are all designed to do one thing, and that is they trigger concepts that you work with and your patterns of behavior. The stimulus is going to be the same energetically because it is in keeping with the individual's self-expectations. That, in turn, will trigger a behavioral pattern, which will fulfill the expectation.

The first step in dealing with stress is learning to identify the stimuli that create a responsive stress reaction, and you learn to do that by reading symbols. At this point, we are looking at the symbology of stress, and we can understand that it is built upon doubt and fear, as so many of our illnesses are, because it is elevated when we are out of balance and harmony.

The muscular tension caused by stress is symbolic of being rigid in relationship to what is going on at the moment. The rigidity of the muscles also indicates unwillingness or an inability to flow with the situation. When the muscles are tight they restrict movement.

Hyperactivity is symbolic of a loss of control. This, too, can also result from stress in the sense that it places an additional burden on a body deficient in minerals. The hyperactivity or lack of control is proportionate to the levels of nutrients in the body.

SYMBOLOGY OF THE NUTRIENTS

(See High Blood Pressure for stress.)
(See Nerve and Muscle for tension and hyperactivity.)

Thymus Concerns

The thymus gland is a key component of the immune system. It is here that thymocytes mature into two types of cells. One type of cell is called a T-cell. T-cells are phagocytes, white blood cells that are matured by the thymus gland. These cells are constantly patrolling, seeking out and destroying pathogens and cells that do not belong in the body. There are different types of T-cells that help keep the body safe from invasion and disease.

Your immune system is your first line of defense against many of today's diseases including cancer. Sickness begins at the cellular level, involving one or more cells at a time. The path towards disease starts here. When the thymocytes do not have a chance to mature into T-cells, there is no control over cell-mediated responses. To be on the safe side, especially with the threat of cancer, AIDS, and other diseases in the world, it may pay to ensure that this gland stays in top shape.

NUTRIENTS AND AMINO ACIDS TO SUPPORT THE THYMUS GLAND

Nutrients	Amino Acids
Beta-carotene (Vitamin A)	L-Arginine
Lecithin	L-Glycine
Zinc	

Beta-carotene (Vitamin A). Converted into a non-toxic form of vitamin A in the body; feeds and strengthens the thymus gland, which is instrumental in the body's response to infection.

Lecithin. Increases resistance to diseases by helping the thymus gland carry out its functions.

Zinc. Protects the immune system and supports the T-cells.

L-Arginine. A growth hormone that acts on the thymus gland to improve its ability to process T-effectors and B-cell lymphocytes.

L-Glycine. Necessary for the immune system, balanced growth of white blood cells, and health of the thymus gland, spleen, and bone marrow.

SYMBOLOGY OF THE THYMUS GLAND

You might say that the thymus gland, symbolically, is the essence of the immune system. Of course the immune system overall is complicated with many components and multiple processes taking place all the time. However, the all-important T-cells—the killer cells and the helper cells—are matured in the thymus gland.

From a biochemical perspective, the thymus is often called "the seat of power." You can see from a symbolic perspective that this is a faulty perception, even though the thymus is the power center of the immune system. The reason lies in the fact that it has nothing to do with real personal power, although it plays a major role in whether or not a person is continually sick. If you feel weak or lacking in personal power to deal with a given situation, then you may set yourself up for a sickness, such as a cold or flu. You may even stay sick, catching one condition right after the other. Are you one of these individuals who typically gets sick as often as the wind changes direction? This would indicate that you are dealing with doubt and uncertainty about the present and near future. You may be in an environment that is stressful and also one in which you may feel you are under constant attack and cannot defend yourself or speak out to stop the onslaught. There could be multiple reasons for you to think that you could not defend or express yourself. One reason could be age-related; a child is not able to withstand the judgments and criticisms received on a continual basis from a parent, though some people view rejection in the form of judgments and criticisms as a form of love. Nonetheless, it still has its physical effects on the individual. It is often the emotional forces in life that undermine an individual's health, and they are constantly seeking to defend themselves.

Immune or thymus-related conditions and diseases that might show themselves in other age groups would include allergies, acne, skin disorders, and autoimmune diseases. Such conditions could result because neither the thymus nor the immune system is up to par. The immune system and the thymus gland both may be malnourished due to poor dietary choices.

Looking at the symbology of the nutrients involved in nourishing both of these we can understand why that integrated system can become overloaded from external forces.

Symbology of the Nutrients

The thymus gland is considered the power seat of the immune system. (To see just how comprehensive its protective functions are and how many different nutrients it requires, refer back to Immune Health Concerns.)

Looking at the symbology of the nutrients, we can see that virtually every kind of energy is required to defend the self in life. The thymus gland plays a very important role because it is the site where T-cells are matured.

Beta-carotene (Vitamin A) and Zinc. Some of the most vital nutrients for the thymus gland are vitamin A and zinc. Examining vitamin A symbolically, we see first and foremost that it is a form of protection. Beyond that, it helps us to look within ourselves and to remove any doubt that exists. This is demonstrated by how vitamin A improves night vision; night is symbolic of preparation on the positive side and doubt on the negative side.

Of course, removing doubt implies that the person can see where it exists within the self. Life provides ample opportunity for introspection based on external events. An insight may occur due to some circumstance within an experience or transaction, and this, in turn, allows for an understanding to be realized from that insight. The insight may draw your attention to an aspect of what is going on, or you may have a thought about something, and the more you examine it, the more insight and understanding is achieved. These can lead to an awareness of the pattern and the concept that supports that particular pattern. Through the identification of the subconscious concept, its supporting patterns of behavior, and the surrounding doubt, a resolution can be found. As you understand all the elements, you will be able to control and eliminate them.

Vitamin A becomes a protective device because doubt is no longer functioning within the self. Doubt and fear are the two energies that open us up to illness and disease. When you think about the opposite of doubt and fear, which are confidence and courage, you can begin to see how life is a matter of an energetic attitude, or an energetic position, in dealing with the forces that one must confront.

Zinc acts in two ways. It is symbolic both of a very supportive role in health and awareness of a working faith. Once again, a nutrient validates that it takes faith in self to deal with life.

The people who are constantly getting sick because of a weakened immune system do so because they are under a heavy emotional attack or an attack of self doubt and uncertainty.

Bringing in the proper nutrients to build up the self, the thymus, and the entire immune system, makes a symbolic statement that you are becoming stronger and more confident, turning the doubt into confidence and the fear into courage.

Thyroid Problems

Often called the "master gland" or "power control center," the thyroid is vital because of its interactions with other glands. It is also involved in sexual development and maturity. Goiters often result from low iodine content within the thyroid, which fills with blood.

The thyroid secretes two hormones that influence the rate and processes of basic body metabolism and physical growth. There are two types of metabolism: catabolic and anabolic. In catabolic metabolism, the body is in the process of breaking down tissues, cells, and substances. These substances are simplified in their structure to speed up elimination, and release energy.

In anabolic metabolism, the exact opposite process is taking pace. New material is being created, and nutrients are drawn from the blood into the cells to repair and grow new cells. The chemicals in the blood are used in the process of converting chemicals into parts of living cells.

NUTRIENTS, AMINO ACIDS AND HERBS TO SUPPORT THE THYROID GLAND

Nutrients	Amino Acids	Herbs
Chromium	Tyrosine	Bladderwrack
Iodine		Irish Moss
Manganese		Kelp
Vitamin B-6		

Chromium. Can stimulate thyroid activity to initiate the mobilization of fat reserves for energy production.

Iodine. Essential for the manufacturing of thyroxin a thyroid hormone that helps influence and regulate metabolism.

Manganese. Essential for the formation of thyroxin, a constituent of the thyroid gland.

Vitamin B-6. Involved in nourishing the adrenal glands, reduces water content and inflammation. Excellent in metabolizing fats, proteins and carbohydrates.

Tyrosine. Plays an integral role in proper functioning of the adrenal, pituitary and thyroid gland.

Bladderwrack. Used effectively for thyroid problems.

Irish Moss. Provides iodine, and is a form of kelp.

Kelp. Contains iodine, in addition to other substances. The iodine nourishes the thyroid, parathyroid, pineal and pituitary, as it is a part of the building blocks of the thyroid hormone.

SYMBOLOGY OF A SLUGGISH THYROID

The functions of the thyroid gland show it to be a regulator of sorts. One could say that someone who is obese has lost the ability to regulate or control situations in his or her life. There may be an underlying feeling that the person is not up to the challenge at hand, and does not have the wherewithal or desire to regain control over the situation.

A sluggish thyroid warrants consideration on many levels, for instance, it is one aspect of obesity. Being obese or overweight has many different causes, all of which will have an emotional basis that will influence the functioning of the thyroid gland. If a person feels the need to protect himself from external forces, or people who are "attacking" him, then he is going to slow down his thyroid so that weight can be accumulated as a protective barrier. The person will feel secure from touch and hurt. Another causative factor for weight gain may be the need to have a sense of power, or to be able to throw one's weight around.

SYMBOLOGY OF THE NUTRIENTS AND VARIOUS HERBS

The thyroid helps to regulate the metabolism of the body. Symbolically, we can look at metabolism as the building up of stamina and endurance, plus the building up of protection and health on all levels. Metabolism also includes the breaking down and cleansing processes. This reflects the cleansing of negative, subconscious concepts that create weakness on some levels and allow other transactions to become lethargic in their function.

Vitamin B-6. With its symbolic representation of being a regulator as well as a protector, vitamin B-6 demonstrates how essential those energies are in helping an individual to maintain a feeling of well-being. When the thyroid is sluggish, it may be setting the body up to retain fluid and fats as a protective barrier because it seeks to protect the Inner Self from harm. It is building "power" to throw around.

The presence of B-6 in the mix works nutritionally and symbolically to help the body function properly.

Kelp and Iodine. Along the same lines is kelp, which provides iodine. On one level, iodine symbolically represents inspiration. When your metabolic functions are normal, they are able to do what has to be done in somewhat of an inspired mode, if not, lethargy and apathy are present.

Iodine also represents intent. It is important to mention that manganese also represents intent as well as the will to get the intent accomplished. Intent and the will to accomplish intent both require a metabolic energetic expense.

Iodine, like vitamin B-6, can also represent regulation. It regulates the approach to a situation or event, including people. It participates in regulating how the body responds to different stimuli.

Ulcers

There are multiple types and causes of ulcers within the body. Stomach ulcers are the most common and can occur within the stomach lining or in the duodenum, the first part of the small intestines. Ulcers can also affect the intestinal tract. When this happens, the colon is usually the first site where they manifest, generally as ulcerative colitis, but any segment of the intestinal tract can become ulcerated.

Ulcers can result from excess acid in our system. There is also a particular type of bacteria found by stomach ulcer sites which is believed to create the ulcers.

In either case, stress seems likely to play a part in the process. In fact, there is a particular type of internal ulcer called a stress ulcer, which is seen primarily in post-surgical or burn patients. When we look at stress we see that it affects many different functions within the body, and depletes nutrients.

Within the body, the adrenal glands are among those most directly impacted by stress. Stress diminishes their capacity to function, which can result in a less effective immune system. While in most instances, the immune system will hold things in check, when stress becomes too intense, bacteria and other latent or opportunistic conditions can become active. Ulcers, either from direct stress or lowered immune function, will flourish.

The herbalist Dr. John Christopher prescribed a remedy for internal ulcers: Mix one teaspoon of cayenne powder into a cup of hot water. Let it stand to room temperature and drink immediately before going to bed. By the next morning it seems that the ulcer will be gone. I have passed this suggestion along countless times and have heard that it works quite well. This treatment can last for years. Of course, if the original cause of the ulcer is not removed through understanding and control there is a great likelihood that an ulcer will reappear.

Two other approaches, not as "tasty" as the first, are to drink one ounce of aloe vera juice as often as possible, or to drink freshly made cabbage juice as often as possible. Keep in mind the potential for intestinal gases.

There are two other types of ulcers that a person can develop, but these are on the outside of the body: the diabetic ulcer, which usually is found around the ankle or on the feet, and bedsores, which usually develop in the skin over bony prominences in people who are bedridden or immobile for one reason or another. Both of these types can be handled in the same fashion. Pour granulated sugar or raw honey into the ulcer. Either of these substances literally feeds the cells from the top, and they create new, fresh skin. For bedsores, mix the sugar or honey with cornstarch, and make a paste. Hospital employees have told me that some hospitals employ this strategy along with mixing sugar and iodine and smearing it across new incisions in the operating room.

FOODS AND HERBS TO ASSIST THE BODY WITH ULCERS

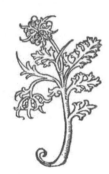

Foods and Herbs	
Cabbage Juice	Okra
Licorice Root	Slippery Elm Bark
Marshmallow Root	

Cabbage Juice. A natural antiseptic used to ease ulcer pain; heals ulcers.

Licorice Root. Relieves ulcer conditions, also used for flavor.

Marshmallow Root. Soothes mucous membranes. Internally, used to treat inflammation and mucosal afflictions of the genito-urinary tract.

Okra. A very old, traditional approach to healing ulcers. It may stem from the mucilage nature of the vegetable.

Slippery Elm Bark. Internally soothes irritated mucous membranes. Valuable for mucous inflammation of the stomach. Will help sustain ulcerated and cancerous stomachs.

SYMBOLOGY OF ULCERS

Ulcers are another condition brought about by stress, and are tied into the concepts of what you believe you can and cannot handle, what makes you upset, or what eats you up alive. Ulcers, regardless of where they are located in the body, are similar symbolically.

Certain concepts that you may deal with are incredibly distasteful, difficult to digest and assimilate. They metaphorically and literally will eat a hole in you. Symbolically, the causes of ulcers include being involved in ongoing situations that are impossible to stomach and digest. Because they are indigestible these situations symbolically sit in the stomach and eat at you. In an attempt to digest them, you may secrete too many digestive juices that, in turn, will eat away the stomach lining. You may find it hard to digest and assimilate a situation in order to process it, and when the situation is completely in opposition to your belief system, it may not be possible. In those cases, duodenal, or peptic,[41] ulcers can form.

The ulcers that form inside the cheek are an indication that there is too much uric acid in the bloodstream. Eating too much flesh food, dairy, most nuts, or grains causes the acidity.

When we look at American advertising, it implies that if a person eats meat then they are strong. Some advertisements even imply if you are eating hamburgers you have a happy family. The truth is that these things do not necessarily make a person strong or happy.

We persist in consuming particular kinds of diets in hopes that the emotional need will be satisfied, but it never is. Through over consumption of protein we create an acidic ash by-product in the bloodstream that affects the health of the body. Looking at that symbolically, we see that when you attempt something you cannot possibly accomplish because your subconscious concepts will not allow it, you could end up poisoning yourself with a bitter resentment. The bitterness manifests as acidity in the bloodstream, setting the body up for ill health. This happens because germs (negative thoughts) cannot live in an alkaline environment, but can in an acidic one. Alkalinity in the bloodstream is created through the consumption of fruits and vegetables.

In reality, fruits, vegetables, and all foodstuffs do hold some emotional value on some levels. Fruits and vegetables are nowhere near as powerful or as detrimental as the emotional concepts surrounding meat. As far as fowl and fish are concerned, there are entire cultural diets built around these two forms of flesh food. Once again we can see where emotional connections to family, cultures, and traditions can work against us in the sense that we seek approval and comfort on a daily basis. The truth is that true personal power is the only thing that will comfort an individual, and personal power is found within, not through the foods we consume. Personal power comes from the knowledge that you not only can handle, but that you can master any given situation in which you find yourself, without needing to resort to any artificial form of support.

Vision Problems

(See Cataracts; Glaucoma.)

Water Retention

Water retention, or edema, is a serious health problem. It directly contributes to obesity through the weight that is gained from water. Water retention can result from several things, but it generally stems from an imbalance in the potassium-sodium relationship. Stress can easily disturb this balance because it depletes nutrients, and calcium in this case, at an accelerated rate. If those nutrients are not replaced in meaningful amounts, problems can arise.

When calcium is depleted, the potassium-sodium ratio is disturbed, causing water to be retained. In fact, a person under stress will gain five to fifteen pounds almost immediately, and it will be all water. This extra water weight puts additional strain on the heart muscle and joints, and can influence emotional well-being.

NUTRIENTS, HERBS AND FOODS TO ASSIST IN REGAINING PROPER WATER BALANCE

Nutrients	Herbs	Food
Potassium (Amino Acid Chelate)	Buchu Leaf	Watermelon
Vitamin B-6	Corn Silk	
	Hydrangea	
	Parsley	
	Uva-Ursi	

Potassium and Vitamin B-6. Work together to maintain the fluid balance of the body.

Buchu Leaf, Corn Silk, Hydrangea, Parsley, Uva Ursi, and Watermelon. Excellent diuretics.

SYMBOLOGY OF WATER RETENTION

Symbolically, what is interesting about water retention and the impact of calcium depletion is that because of our tendency towards doubt and fear, we become more enmeshed in the material plane as a sense of security.

In truth, material things provide no security because material reality is fleeting; one day you can have all the money that you need, and the next day be unemployed and at the mercy of external forces. The Universal Teaching that applies here is, "that which you have in reserve can be gone." There is a parable in the *Bible*, known as the "golden talents," in which money is given to some servants, and each one uses it differently. The one servant who invested it and made money was given everyone else's money. This parable takes us to the Universal Teaching of "use what you have and more will be given."

Remember, you are never placed in a situation that you cannot overcome and master. Should you find yourself in tough straits, think back on that old adage about lemons and lemonade…and get squeezing! Making lemonade from life's lemons is the perfect metaphor because it underscores that negative thoughts and situations can be reframed simply by changing your perception about them. Take an incident that might appear negative on first blush and use it as an opportunity to learn about it and yourself. Why is the situation so distasteful? Has it happened before? What else can you change to avoid this in the future? Part of what you may come to realize is that our outward goals may be in direct conflict with our subconscious expectations of self.

Your subconscious expectations are built on who we think we are supposed to be in all situations, which may have no bearing on who we truly are or our ability to overcome and master.

SYMBOLOGY OF THE NUTRIENTS

Water retention symbolizes aspects of the material plane: holding onto it, acquiring it, or being more involved in the material plane. It also inflates—or bloats—the body, thus, making it larger. This can imply a need for protection. By making the body unappealing, the individual is spared certain physical interactions and emotional connections. This could be rooted in an uncomfortable experience from childhood.

As with weight gain, fluid retention could also indicate the need to express power by throwing one's weight around. A key physical, and also symbolic, difference here is that apart from fluid retention's contribution to the condition, weight gain is a matter of poor metabolism, whereas water retention represents an internal imbalance.

Potassium and Vitamin B-6. Water retention has its own nutritional requirements and symbolic interpretations. Both potassium and vitamin B-6 are fundamentals for balance and harmony in the material plane. Symbolically, both share the same energy, and that energy is regulation.

Vitamin B-6, which is a co-enzyme, and the mineral potassium, which is a co-factor, both work in helping the body to maintain proper balance. Symbolically, it indicates that you must have proper balance in dealing with life. You cannot be too materialistic nor should you be overly spiritualistic; taking either position or attitude is an indication of an imbalance.

Vitamin B-6 is involved in many transactions where the individual requires protection and regulation. It provides some protection from imbalances, but it is also involved in other aspects of thought. You might say that regulation leads to protection and that the consciousness of protecting self leads to having a balanced approach to life, one that reduces the possibility for exposure. An example of this would be playing outdoors during the winter. In this situation, it is best to dress in layers so that as you become overheated from play you can remove one layer of clothing. This will allow the body to maintain a fairly constant body temperature without the dangers of getting too cold or too hot.

Weight Loss

Weight loss is a major topic unto itself with many ways to approach it. There are psychological concerns as well as physiological, glandular effects at work in most everyone with weight issues.

Levels of stress affect weight as well. Stress depletes calcium, which disrupts the relationship between potassium and sodium, and five to fifteen pounds can be gained immediately through water retention.

Successful weight loss requires true desire and commitment to the goal. This leads to discipline, which leads to success. The most difficult aspect of weight loss is changing the diet, due primarily to the myriad of emotional attachments and associations we all have with foods. Some things are hard to give up, even when we know they are detrimental to our health.

SUPPLEMENTATION AS PART OF A WEIGHT-LOSS PROGRAM

In terms of incorporating natural supplements into weight-loss regimens, traditionally three basic approaches have been used: (1) diuretic-type herbs to reduce water content; (2) lipotropic vitamins, better known as "fat burners," to reduce fat and cholesterol levels in the blood as well as fat/cholesterol "deposits" against the walls of the arteries; and (3) natural appetite suppressants to curb the craving for food.

These approaches are effective, and each works well in its own right. They are great complements to a healthy diet and exercise program, which will all work together to help you get control of your weight and to maintain control.

NUTRIENTS, AMINO ACIDS, AND HERBS TO SUPPORT WEIGHT-LOSS PROGRAMS

The following will support your body in burning fat, increasing basal metabolism, and flushing excess fluids from the body.

Nutrients	Amino Acids	Herbs and Plants
Choline	L-Methionine	Kelp
Inositol		
Iodine		
Lecithin		
Potassium		
Vitamin B-6		

Choline, Inositol, and Lecithin. These factors are used to reduce the fatty deposits within the body by dissolving them. Lecithin acts as a carrier of fat molecules and pulls them out of the body.

Iodine. Essential for the manufacturing of thyroxin a thyroid hormone that helps influence and regulate metabolism.

Potassium. Acts as a diuretic by balancing fluids.

Vitamin B-6. Acts as a diuretic.

L-Methionine. An amino acid that aids the body in producing choline.

Kelp. Contains iodine, which nourishes the thyroid gland and helps to regulate metabolism.

SYMBOLOGY OF WEIGHT

Symbolically, we can look at weight from different perspectives. From one point of view, people will put on weight so as to be unattractive, unavailable or untouchable. In this case, there could be issues with abuse early on in the family, or a fear of commitment, relationships, or intimacy. By being obese and unappealing a person does not have to deal with those physical and intimate aspects of life. The weight is also a matter of protection; the individual gains weight to buffer them from the constant onslaught of negativity from those around them, whether it is family, friends, co-workers, or any other source. The weight provides a cushioning buffer zone.

Another perspective is the need to demonstrate authority. You know people who love to "throw their weight around" in given situations. In their mind their weight symbolizes power and authority.

If you have tried to lose weight and have been unsuccessful in your effort to return to a particular weight, think back to what you were doing at the point in time when you were at your target weight. Decide whether you are willing to give up any of your current power in order to return to that previous place and level of power.

SYMBOLOGY OF THE NUTRIENTS

The symbology of nutrients involved in weight loss reflects the characteristics that the over-weight person feels he or she is lacking. Remember that excess weight represents either a need for authority and power, albeit artificial power, or a desire to protect and isolate oneself, due to feelings of insecurity and fear.

The nutrients choline, inositol, iodine, potassium, and vitamin B-6 are the primary keys of proper weight maintenance. What do they represent symbolically?

Choline and Inositol. Let us start with the metabolic process, which in this case, reflects the breaking down or building up thoughts. With metabolism on the physical level, choline and inositol are the first to consider. Choline symbolically represents inner-strength, whereas inositol represents integrity.

Both of these characteristics are essential. It takes a lot of inner-strength to go within the self to begin to confront, understand, and resolve these issues. This is true because so many of us have been programmed to believe we are stupid, messy, inconsiderate, selfish, etc. For a refresher course in how that happens, just follow a mother around the grocery store and listen to how she addresses her children. The communication that is taking place instills concepts and reinforces others. Once that metabolic and psychological process occurs, the need to carry excess weight as a means of protection or artificial power is gone. The true, inner-strength can be seen.

Inner-strength is required to deal with whatever confronts you on a daily basis. Regardless of the situation, inner-strength will allow you to handle it.

Integrity is an interesting word because it means different things to different people. In this application, it represents solidity. The person is solidly fixed, unwavering and committed to a particular stance. Remaining committed to a particular path of change, such as weight loss, is very difficult. For so many people, the integrity of that commitment does waver because of the complex issues raised in the course of dealing with the underlying causes of excess weight. The hardest part of the commitment to weight loss is staying with a healthy diet, because our emotional attachments to food are so strong.

Iodine. This nutrient nourishes the thyroid. Iodine symbolizes inspiration, regulation, and intent. Being symbolic of intent, iodine emphasizes the need to be committed and to see the process through. Iodine stimulates and nurtures the production of thyroid hormones. While there is a need for stimulation to move forward in a weight-loss program, there is also the need to regulate food intake, another symbology of iodine.

Much like with the thyroid, where it takes a metabolic transaction to stimulate metabolism, it may take an emotional, spiritual, or physical/material transaction in order to manifest our intentions. Life is a matter of intent, but while we have intentions about everything, that does not necessarily mean we can manifest them. That is what life is about, manifesting your intent and bringing to fruition those things that you want in life, the things that will make you happy. The truth of that is what will really make you happy is to know yourself.

Inspiration is also crucial and provides the impetus for the energy to do battle with the forces confronting you, from both within and without.

Forces conveying messages such as, "you can't do it," "you don't have the right," "you don't have the authority," "you don't have the ability," or "you are unworthy" may even have been a factor in why you gained weight in the first place.

Potassium, and Vitamin B-6. These nutrients are both involved in regulation and protection with regard to weight issues, just as they are with water retention. (To read more about the need for regulation, see Water Retention.)

With weight, the need for regulation turns more toward regulating wants and desires, which are different than needs. We need to eat to fortify ourselves, and each of us needs to express the self. Yet, we can choose to express ourselves and still eat the foods that will support weight loss if we are willing to examine our attachments to foods and commit to changing our diet. There is a need for B-6 and potassium to act as regulators in this manner, especially with regard to material acquisitions, and weight is certainly that sort of an acquisition.

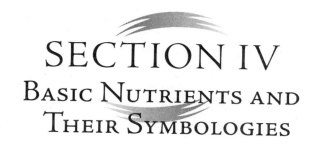

SECTION IV
BASIC NUTRIENTS AND THEIR SYMBOLOGIES

Biotin. This B-vitamin is necessary for manufacturing fats, metabolizing carbohydrates, and breaking down proteins into urea, which is expelled from the body as waste. It also converts the amino acids in protein into sugar, which provides energy for the body.

Biotin symbolizes liberation through cleansing in two ways. First is its role in energy production from proteins. Energy affords stamina and endurance to move forward. Symbolically, it represents being liberated from self-confining concepts, and allows growth and forward movement. Second is biotin's role in breaking down protein into urea. Here, we are liberating usable information (protein molecules) and eliminating useless and toxic concepts (urea).

Proteins are the building blocks of organic life; they are essential in making new cells, and are symbolic of thoughts. Needless to say, not all of life's building blocks—greed, desires, needs, for example—are healthy.

Urea, a liquid waste, is symbolic of our need to eliminate from our material selves those thoughts and actions that would create problems in our physical or financial life. Gout, a painful disease caused by buildup of uric acid crystals in the blood, is an excellent example of what happens when urea is not properly removed. It is symbolic of the unwillingness to change and eliminate those ideas not in keeping with growth and development. Gout can lead to arthritis (inflexible thinking) and to destruction of the joints. The inability to liberate your self from past ideas and concepts on how to act and react to every stimulus is eventually reflected as inflexibility and an inability to change and grow.

Calcium. This mineral is involved in the blood coagulation process, nerve and muscle stimulation, parathyroid hormone function, and in the metabolism of vitamin D. Calcium needs magnesium, phosphorus, and vitamins A, C, D and possibly E to function properly.

Calcium's major function is to work with phosphorus to build and maintain strong bones and teeth, and is essential for maintaining proper pH of the blood. Calcium eases insomnia and helps to regulate the heartbeat; a task researchers conclude is accomplished by calcium actually suppressing production and release of another nutrient, vitamin D-3.[42] Calcium is essential for the relaxation of nerve tissue, whereas magnesium is particularly involved with the normal function of the brain, spinal cord and all nerves.[43]

Symbolically, calcium is strength. It is responsible for the integrity of the bones (support) and teeth (ability to tear things apart for digestibility and assimilation). Healthy blood symbolizes strength in spiritual actions. From another perspective, everything we do is a spiritual action since our thoughts direct our conscious actions. The thoughts germinate into manifestation from deep within, seeking to fulfill self-expectations maintained deep within.

Sugar, symbolic of false promise (See also Chromium.), appears to increase urinary calcium excretion.[44] Some people allow material possessions to illustrate who they think they are, presenting them as reflections of accomplishments and material strength. An individual who builds on that basis is devastated when the money or material lifestyle is lost. One of the most dramatic illustrations of this concept can be seen in the Great Depression in the United States, when those who suffered financial ruin took their own lives. Of course, those with a strong working faith (symbolized by vitamin B-12) complemented with true strength can overcome such events.

Calcium's strength is further demonstrated in the coagulation, or clotting, process; strength prevents us from losing faith/spirit (blood). It is interesting to note here the symbolism of the other nutrients required for calcium (strength) to function properly: magnesium is inspiration, phosphorous is confidence, vitamin A is preparation or insight, vitamin C is protection or defenses, and vitamin D is insight and understanding. Scientists also think vitamin E, symbolizing self-confidence, must be present for proper assimilation and utilization of calcium.

The role of strength in regulating the emotions (heartbeat) is easily seen. If you feel you lack the strength to deal with life's issues, you are more likely to have excessive emotional reactions.

Insomnia, an event borne of fear, is also quelled by strength. When true strength exists, there is no fear, and preparation (sleep) can proceed, allowing the individual insights into energies at work.

Choline. Abundant in most animal tissues, it combines with fatty acids and phosphoric acid within the liver to form lecithin. Choline is also a part of the neurotransmitter, acetylcholine, a substance that relays electrical impulses throughout the nervous system. Choline is released at some neuromuscular and neuroglandular junctions, and at synapses between certain brain and spinal cord cells. In most parts of the body, acetylcholine leads to excitation.

Choline is associated primarily with the utilization of fats and cholesterol in the body, preventing fats from accumulating in the liver, and facilitating the movement of fats into the cells. It is essential for the nerves' myelin sheaths, the principal component of nerve fibers, which help to regulate and improve liver and gallbladder function, and aid in the prevention of gallstones.

Along with inositol and methionine, choline is considered a lipotropic, or fat-burning, vitamin. It is converted in the liver to betaine, a digestive element. Dietary fluctuations can alter plasma choline concentrations and affect the rate of acetylcholine formation.

Symbolically, choline represents inner-strength, and its biochemical transactions reflect this concept. When the substance combines with phosphoric acid (a form of courage) it produces lecithin (protection) to nourish and protect the myelin sheath covering of the nerves (communication). This allows for clean, strong signals to be sent.

We are communicating all the time on multiple levels. Physically, your brain is directing your body on functional and operational matters. It regulates everything based on a moment-by-moment intake and analysis of current biochemical and nutritional contents. Simultaneously, the mind evaluates all of the input being transmitted via sight, sound, and vibration. Collectively, these aspects have profound effects on the subconscious, and the conscious mind cannot handle all of the input. The mind channels different stimuli to different categories within the subconscious. Some are dealt with immediately in a conscious way, while others stimulate patterned responses to be carried out later. The mind will create the situation needed to fulfill the expectation of the particular concept that has been triggered by some of the input. Some results may not be seen for days, weeks, or even months; it takes time for the mind to move a person towards fulfillment of a concept or expectation.

Choline prevents fats (stored energy) from accumulating in the liver, which performs cleansing tasks for the body among other important functions. Looking at this symbolically, it is when energy is not being used in the pursuit of mastery that there is a doubt or fear at work. Otherwise, the action would move toward the attainment of mastery. People can appear to be busy, but they do not move forward on a personal level; they are engaged in busy work, which acts as a distraction from real progress.

Some believe that choline deficiencies may be responsible for high blood pressure. This symbolizes a lack of control over internal emotional responses to circumstances that trigger feelings of doubt in one's ability to handle the situation or face responsibilities. Muscular tension increases, raising the blood pressure.

Choline is often missing in people suffering from diabetes. Diabetes is symbolic on one level of the need for approval and the sweets in life. Diabetics are also seeking love. When a person lacks inner-strength, he or she will seek it outside the self. In the case of Type II diabetics, these folks bring in too much high-sugar food, and food in general. They do it to feel better about themselves, yet lack the inner-strength to utilize the sustenance they are receiving. The excess is stored as fat, which can, in turn, result in too much sugar in the blood-stream because it goes unutilized.

Overweight people also suffer choline deficiency. The reason for this is the fact that choline is a fat burner. It seems apparent that there is not enough choline in the system to keep up with the needs. Being overweight has several symbolic meanings, including the need for protection or to project authority.

Another choline-deficiency sign is nephritis, a kidney disorder. The symbology here is the inability to cleanse thoroughly. Cleansing of past concepts and toxic thoughts is necessary for good health.

Heart disease is another result of diminished levels of choline and other nutrients. A heart condition is the ultimate symbol for a lack of emotional control resulting from an absence of faith in self or inner-strength. At the other end of the spectrum is a heart attack, which can represent the ultimate in inward, emotional control to the point of breaking.

Inner-strength yields courage and confidence on some levels. As we age, we often give up using our inner-strength to accomplish things in life. Instead we depend on our external wealth and power, and as the ability to accomplish and accumulate in that arena diminishes, there is also an effect on the subconscious aspect of self. Some of these effects could manifest as forgetfulness.

Chromium. A trace-mineral essential for good health, chromium maintains normal levels of blood sugar (glucose), which acts as fuel for the body. Chromium has been shown to help dieters gain control over their appetites, especially cravings for carbohydrates. It also appears to help retain muscle tissue while shedding unwanted fat, and it even seems to suppress the notorious rapid weight gain after dieting. Chromium stimulates insulin action and among other things, causes a "full" message to be sent from the stomach to an appetite-regulating center in the hypothalamic region of the brain.

Symbolically, chromium reflects an ability to maintain emotional control because it can both raise and lower blood-sugar levels. When the emotions that elicit rage or anger get out of hand, the body burns more energy in response. It can become self-consuming, like cancer. When the dominant emotions lead downward to apathy and indifference, energy levels likewise shut down.

Chromium via the glucose tolerance factor has a strong insulin enhancing activity in the blood, therefore, effecting blood sugar. Blood is symbolic of spirit because it carries oxygen (spirit) to all the cells, while sugar is symbolic of promised richness in life. Because our western societies consume so much refined, white sugar (150 pounds-plus, per year, on average), which is void of nutritive value, the promise is false, empty on both physical and spiritual levels. This truth is borne out by the high incidence of diabetes worldwide.

Chromium helps one gain control over appetite (desire to consume/have) by being able to facilitate the messages being delivered with the use of insulin. Insulin is symbolic of courage and confidence, and with courage and confidence at work, the need for material possession to validate success in life is not as great. Success, after all, is measured by many standards and values.

Messages constructed with chromium help the hypothalamus (symbolic of regulation/balance/control) to regulate the degree of dependency that we express at any given time on the material plane. To see this concept at work, examine how the body retains water and fat; both are symbolic of our need for the material for sustenance.

Cravings for certain foods result from one of two mechanisms: either the need for a specific nutrient or for an emotional fix. Every food that is a part of our diet has a subconscious emotional equivalent. This is one reason it is so hard for people to change their diet, but most that do successfully change their diet also change their attitude.

Copper. This mineral helps the body to assimilate and use iron and plays a role in the making of hemoglobin, the blood cell's oxygen-carrying pigment. Copper is also involved in collagen synthesis. Its role in enzymes is vital to many functions, especially skeletal health where a deficiency would lead to demineralization of the bones.

It appears that copper symbolically represents inner-emotional support because it helps the individual to assimilate and use emotional control (iron). Inner-emotional support is needed in the regulation of emotional "fire," or anger, and in order for fire to exist there must be oxygen. With an emotional fire, the spirit (oxygen) feels and thinks it has no control over the situation, and the resulting rage within creates emotional (oxidative) damage to the self (cells). A loss of emotional control is based on fear and doubt in a given situation.

Through examining the skeletal system, we can see the symbology of strength and support at work; when inner-emotional support is lacking due to doubt or fear, however, it weakens the entire structure. The skeleton begins a demineralization of sorts, making the person feel as if he or she were dealing with the world from a position of weakness versus a position of strength.

A position of strength exists every time you go into a situation fully fortified and prepared as well as knowing that you have working faith and emotional control at hand.

Copper (inner-emotional support) also plays a role in myelin formation (protection), antioxidant protection, thermal regulation (heat is symbolic of fire/emotions), immune function (protection), and cardiac function (emotional physical center), to name a few.

All forms of copper enzymes in the body fundamentally do the same thing. They all consume oxygen and related compounds, such as super oxide radicals. This again demonstrates that inner-emotional support is necessary to keep the emotions under control, regulated, and balanced. If emotions remain bottled up, it can lead to cancer. Symbolically, cancer results from anger, frustration, guilt, or resentment; these energies "eat you alive."

Essential Fatty Acids. Linoleic, linolenic, and arachidonic acids are unsaturated, essential fatty acids (EFAs), which are essential for growth. New cells cannot be made without essential fatty acids.[45] Only linoleic acid must be obtained through the diet. The body can use linoleic acid to synthesize the other two.

Unsaturated EFAs are important for respiration of vital organs and make it easier for oxygen to be transported by the bloodstream to all cells, tissues, and organs. They help maintain resilience and lubrication of all cells, and combine with protein and cholesterol to form living membranes that hold cells together.

Essential fatty acids regulate the rate of blood coagulation and perform the vital task of breaking up cholesterol deposits on arterial walls. Fatty acids are essential for normal glandular activity, especially for healthy mucous membranes and nerves. They also function in the body by cooperating with vitamin D in making calcium available to the tissues, assist in the assimilation of phosphorus, and stimulate the conversion of beta-carotene into vitamin A.

Regarding the symology of EFAs, substance is the first word that comes to mind. Substance also refers to character, and of course, both are essential in an individual who seeks to grow into an enlightened being. Substance can be man-made—the manner in which our society judges a person based on status, wealth or formal education. It can also be true, spiritual substance—the knowledge that you have the strength and courage to handle and master whatever comes your way. New endeavors (cells) cannot be undertaken and accomplished without substance. Character helps one through all the phases of growing into someone of awareness.

Each of the body's organs, glands, and systems has a symbolic meaning. All of these physical aspects participate in the construction of your personal reality, both physically and symbolically. Spiritual substance provides the life force to invigorate, nourish, and cleanse the self. Essential fatty acids make it easier for oxygen (spirit) to be transported by the bloodstream (also symbolic of spirit) to all the cells. They combine with protein (building blocks of life) and cholesterol (stored energy) to form living membranes (protectors) that hold the body cells together.

Essential fatty acids (character) also regulate the rate of blood coagulation, a physical transaction that generally happens to prevent excessive loss of blood (spirit). It takes character to maintain self in the face of adversity. To be a "stand-up" person requires substance as a human being. Substance and character (EFAs) also function in life (the body) by cooperating with insights (vitamin D) in making strength (calcium) available; in assisting with the incorporation of courage (phosphorus); and in stimulating the conversion of preparation (carotene) into insights (vitamin A).

The fatty acids are involved in normal functioning of the reproductive system, the symbolic manifestation of self-expression. Some couples have a hard time conceiving, even when there is no physiological problem. The inability to conceive is due to the energies surrounding commitment to the relationship, fear of responsibility, and fear of being an authority figure (leader), to name a few.

Symptoms of EFA deficiency include reduced growth rate, abnormally scaly skin (revealing that defenses have hardened and the individual has lost sensitivity), and increased loss of water (material losses). Other deficiency-linked changes and their symbolic meanings include: a change in skin permeability (defenses, image), male and female infertility (failure to express), and increased susceptibility to infections (outside influences). It is easy to see how a lack of substance and character could lead to all those situations.

When vitamin E (self confidence) is under supplied, not only are iron (emotional control) absorption and hemoglobin formation impaired, but also the essential fatty acids forming part of the cell structure are so altered by oxidation that cells break down.[46]

Folic Acid. Folic acid is necessary for growth, cell division, and red blood cell formation. It helps with reproduction and is necessary for the health of the liver and glands. Folic acid is another vitamin that has a direct nourishing and fortifying effect on the "front line" of the body's defense system. Symbolically speaking, folic acid is a fortifier. It helps to fortify and strengthen every aspect of being.

The body requires every nutrient on a daily basis. The daily folate requirement is hinged to the daily metabolic and cell turnover rates. The requirement is increased by anything that increases metabolic rate (such as infection) and anything that increases cell turnover (such as malignant tumors). Gastrointestinal disorders are one sign of folate deficiency. It is symbolic of the inability to digest incoming thoughts. Some thoughts presented to us help us grow, when we have the courage to act upon them. Obviously, some thoughts work in the opposite direction.

Hair loss to the point of baldness is also a sign of insufficient folic acid. Hair generally returns following administration of the vitamin.[47]

Anemia, which is symbolic of a lack of faith or strength, is also a deficiency sign.

In fact, folic acid deficiency is linked to a particular type of large-cell anemia common among pregnant women. Here, we see another symbolic representation of a person feeling doubtful in her abilities. In this case, the doubt centers on the ability to produce a child, which in itself is an expression of manhood. "The expression of manhood" is a phrase that applies to both males and females. It has its origins in the book of Genesis where God says that he created man, male and female.

Another sign of diminished folic acid is retarded growth, which is symbolic on several levels. The first is doubt in one's ability to grow up and deal with issues. Along the same lines, it also indicates a fear of growing or moving forward into new situations. Doubt or fear creates feelings of being unfortified to deal with the upcoming energies in one's life.

Inositol. Closely associated with choline and biotin, inositol is effective in promoting the body's production of lecithin. Fats are moved from the liver to the cells with the aid of lecithin; therefore, inositol aids in the metabolism of fats and helps reduce blood cholesterol. It also prevents the fatty hardening of arteries and protects the liver, kidneys, and heart. Inositol is helpful in brain/cell nutrition, and is needed for the growth and survival of cells in bone marrow, eye membranes, and intestines. This nutrient is vital for hair growth and can prevent thinning hair and baldness.

The kidney appears to be the principal organ concerned with the turnover of inositol. It breaks the substance down into glucose, and ultimately carbon dioxide and water, plus other chemical compounds that the body may use. The most active form of inositol functions primarily at the membrane level.

Inositol represents integrity, which is closely associated with choline (inner-strength) and biotin (liberation, in a cleansing way). When you think about integrity's role in life, you can see how essential it is to have true inner-strength. It also takes a degree of integrity to examine the self honestly. As written in John 8:32, knowing the self is a necessary step in cleansing past concepts from the unconscious: "Know thyself, and the truth will set you free."

Integrity is a multileveled word. In some aspects, it signifies wholeness and completeness, while in others it means strength, commitment, and adherence. One can appreciate the role of integrity in biological transactions such as lecithin production. Lecithin (protection) nourishes and protects the nerves' myelin-sheath covering (communication). This allows clean, strong signals to be sent, which helps to ensure there are no miscommunications, regardless of subject matter.

Along the same lines as lecithin production is inositol's role in fat metabolism. Energy is produced from stored material (fat), and the amount of energy available to a body/person depends on many factors, one of which is inspiration. Inspiration combined with inner-strength and integrity makes for an energetic person.

The brain is the spiritual center from the perspective that mind is the connection between self and the Creator. The health of the spirit is dependent upon integrity. The brain stem and nervous system are covered with a myelin sheath, and this sheath is protected by inositol.

Inositol also plays a role in membrane strength, a line of defense. When the human defense system is healthy, it is possible to discern which thoughts are helpful and which are not, and negative thoughts (germs) can be devastating to the unprotected.

In the role of energy use, we can see adherence or commitment to a task at work. When you are committed to an endeavor, you always have the energy to do it. That energy may be high or low, and the scale is in direct proportion to the presence of the other nutrients in their symbolic forms, such as inspiration (pantothenic acid), intent (iodine), strength (calcium), courage (phosphorous), confidence (vitamin E), and insights (vitamins A & D).

Another aspect of inositol (integrity) at work is in the growth and survival of cells in bone marrow. Bone marrow is the true inner-strength of man, the body, and the symbolic man. Cells created within bone marrow become your bloodstream and immune system. The bloodstream carries spirit in the form of oxygen. Through strong immune function, your "temple" is protected from invasion. It is through spirit manifesting within as a working faith that protects us when we are aware. We achieve awareness through the reading of symbols, our personal guidance system. On the other hand, when we are in doubt is when germs have the opportunity to take hold within. This is because doubt and fear work at undermining strength and internal integrity. It is clear that self-knowledge is essential in the reality you are creating. The more aware you are of the concepts and patterns at work the greater the control over the creation that you generate. With awareness you are directing your will to manifest your intent.

Integrity also plays a role in perception. The eye is covered by a protective membrane which symbolizes that in all the ways you see things, you must seek integrity and truth. Appearances can be deceiving, but with protected and sound vision, clarity is possible.

Another area in which integrity is essential to well-being is in the symbology of the intestinal tract. The membrane that covers its internal lining is designed to protect us from invasion and to ensure uptake of only those thoughts\nutrients that would be beneficial for us.

Iodine. This is the primary micronutrient that nourishes the thyroid gland, and is one of the building blocks of thyroid hormone. Many bodily functions depend on this gland and its hormones. The thyroid regulates a person's mentality and speech, and aids in the condition of the hair, nails, skin, and teeth. Thyroxine is a hormone produced in the thyroid that controls many processes in the body. When thyroxine production is normal, carotene conversion to vitamin A, protein synthesis, and carbohydrate absorption from the intestines all work more effectively.

Iodine regulates the body's production of energy, promotes growth and development, and stimulates the rate of metabolism. The metabolism is a strong factor in the body's ability to burn fat.

Symbolically speaking, because of its essential role in thyroid health, iodine represents inspiration, intent, stimulation, and regulation. The thyroid's symbology is regulation/motivation. The thyroid manufactures and secretes two hormones that tell the body at what speed to operate. The thyroid hormones themselves are symbolic as messengers of action.

The thyroid is affected symbolically by attitudes stemming from image and expression. It is situated in the neck in front of and on each side of the trachea, and is close to the larynx. Therefore, it plays a part in your balance between material and spiritual considerations. Interestingly, people with sluggish thyroids generally are overweight. From a symbolic interpretation, this would indicate the person is imbalanced in their dealings with life, based on doubt and/or fear. The weight could be symbolic of authority, defenses, protection, and a desire to keep people at an emotional distance.

On the other hand are those with a hyperactive thyroid. These folks cannot gain weight, and, therefore, have a hard time maintaining a balance that will give them the strength to deal with life. This imbalance of strength also comes from doubt and/or fear. In both instances, the root concept would need to be understood to determine which force was at work in creating the imbalances.

Iodine regulates the body's production of energy. When inspiration is at work in your life, you have all the energy you need to stimulate action. With balance, the action is regulated so that an even keel is maintained on the path to success.

Iodine promotes growth and development, and also stimulates the rate of metabolism. Here we see that a consistent metabolic rate as demonstrated in perseverance, leads to accomplishment in a material sense.

Iodine is inspiration, symbolically speaking, because without inspiration there would be no motivation for growth and development. Without inspiration generating enthusiasm, you would have no energy or desire to do and to accomplish.

Iron. Essential for the enzymes involved in energy release, immune function, transport of oxygen to cells, and the removal of carbon dioxide.

Numerous aspects of the immune system's response are affected when the body's iron supply is low. Deficiencies impair the formation of immunological tissues and organs, reduce the synthesis of immunologically active proteins such as antibodies, and alter the formation of general protein synthesis. Iron deficiencies result in impaired cellular activity and cell-mediated killing such as granulocyte phagocytosis and NK (natural killer)[48] cytotoxicity.

Iron-deficiency anemia is common. Hemoglobin, many enzymes, and a substance known as myoglobin, which carries oxygen in muscle cells, cannot be produced without iron. Even a mild deficiency so limits enzyme and myoglobin production that chronic fatigue, headaches, and shortness of breath can occur long before anemia develops.[49]

Symbolically, iron represents emotional control. From this perspective we can see how emotions would affect energy. If the emotions get out of control because of a lack of faith (anemia), all kinds of repercussions can occur. Whereas emotions that are controlled beyond a balanced perspective can create feelings of anger. This is one causative factor in the development of cancer. The physical manifestation of this is in the fact that men who retain too much iron are usually susceptible to getting colon cancer. When emotions are low and imbalanced, then the individual is exposed to outside forces (negative suggestions, thoughts, put-downs) that could lead to illness. This is demonstrated by the role iron plays in supporting the immune system.

Low iron means a diminished amount of oxygen is available to the cells. This translates to lack of faith and lack of inspiration, another way of saying energy. It takes oxygen to make fire (also symbolic of emotions.). Fire, or combustion, is essential for all living transactions. Spirit is involved in everything we do, and emotions give us the "juice" to utilize the spirit within.

Magnesium. Involved in many essential metabolic processes, magnesium activates enzymes necessary for the metabolism of carbohydrates and amino acids, and helps promote absorption and metabolism of other minerals such as calcium, phosphorus, sodium, and potassium. Magnesium plays an important role in neuromuscular contractions and helps regulate the body's acid-alkaline balance. This mineral helps the body utilize vitamins C, B-complex, and E. It aids in bone growth and is necessary for proper functioning of the nerves and muscles, including the heart. Magnesium is crucial in the conversion of blood sugar into energy.

Symbolically, magnesium acts as a facilitator and represents inspiration. It assists in the assimilation of thoughts that lead to strength, and from a position of strength, all actions taken lead to a positive conclusion. When you act out of fear, doubt, or a lack of self-confidence, the seeds for failure are sown. One Universal Teaching that deals with strength, taken from Matthew 25:29, is appropriate to mention here: "For unto every one that hath shall be given, and he shall have abundance: but from him that hath not shall be taken away even that which he hath." In more modern parlance this means to use what you have, so that more will be given, otherwise, what you have and do not use will be taken from you. The lesson is clear: if you have a particular faculty or a way of thinking and you chose not to utilize it, you will no longer have access to it. And at that point, it can and will begin to work against you.

Inspiration and facilitation are essential for the development of strength (calcium), courage (phosphorous), regulation (sodium) and balance (potassium). Furthermore, magnesium is necessary to activate enzymes containing vitamin B-6 (regulation and protection). Blood magnesium is particularly low in diabetics.[50]

Of particular interest is the way in which magnesium (inspiration) decreases the need for vitamin B-6 [51] (protection), and can also help skin problems (defenses/protection/image). Rats exhibit marked hair loss when magnesium is inadequate.[52] This is significant because hair symbolizes strength and personal power, developed over time through past accomplishments.

There is another type of power—man-made—that unlike personal power is based on illusion, as are all man's teachings. The illusion is that material or physical strength will get you through anything and acts as a statement of your power/success. Just ask any wealthy person or "strongman" if this concept holds true for them in dealing with their problems. Only true personal power prevails in all situations.

Again, more calcium (strength) is retained when supplies of magnesium (inspiration) and vitamin D (insights/understandings) are adequate.[53] Profuse amounts of calcium are lost in the urine when magnesium is undersupplied, and the magnesium deposited in bones (symbolic of support) is given up reluctantly, even during a severe deficiency.[54] These facts indicate that magnesium, which is usually compromised,[55] is important in correcting bone abnormalities and is particularly low in diabetics.[56]

Manganese. Essential for the formation of thyroxin (symbolic of a specific form of activation), which is a hormone produced by the thyroid gland. Manganese helps certain white blood cells carry out phagocytosis, the process whereby the cells ingest and destroy toxins. Manganese also helps maintain sex hormone production, and nourishes the nerves and the brain.

Additionally, manganese aids in the utilization of choline; activates enzymes necessary for utilization of biotin, thiamine, and ascorbic acid; acts as a catalyst in the synthesis of fatty acids and cholesterol; and plays a part in protein, carbohydrate, and fat production. It is also necessary for normal skeletal development, the production of milk, and the formation of urea, a part of the urine.

Symbolically, manganese represents will, just as iodine represents intent. These are the two fundamental aspects of self necessary to master the material plane. If you are clear about your intent and you can see something becoming reality, then your will makes it happen. We already operate under the influence of will and intent on a subconscious level; this is how we create our reality. By gaining control over will and intent, you will manifest your vision at a given point in time. Like anything else, though, that vision can evolve and change over time.

We can see will at work in the role white blood cells (defenders/protectors) play in exercising the body's will to survive. We use our awareness on both conscious and subconscious levels to protect us from harm. We do some harm to ourselves on a conscious level, while other forms of harm are due to the invasion of negative suggestions that become thoughts. Manganese, as will, supports the immune system in its efforts to protect the body.

Manganese helps maintain production of sex hormones (self-expression). Without the driving force of will behind all our efforts, we would not be able to express ourselves. In its nourishing of the nerves (communication) and brain (spiritual center), we find all forms of communication and thought are enhanced and given power to manifest through the energies of both will and intent.

Another great example of will at work is seen in studies with radioactive manganese which show that while enzymes involved with muscular contraction contain this nutrient,[57] too much manganese (manganese poisoning) leads to shaking paralysis.[58]

Although this may appear a contradiction of will, sometimes even though determined to do something you can be frozen in place by your own doubt and fear. You might verbally pursue a goal, yet fail to move forward, resulting in frustration.

It is interesting that a deficiency in iron (emotional control) leads to increased manganese absorption. It demonstrates that sometimes people use the emotional force of will as bravado in place of a true working faith coupled with emotional control. This is seen in people who have material resources yet do not move forward from a personal- power perspective.

Mild dermatitis (image/defenses); slowed growth of hair (strength), nails (defenses), and beard (image); occasional nausea and vomiting (the inability to accept and digest thoughts that have been presented); decreased phospholipids and triglycerides (energy); and moderate weight loss (inability to protect self, feelings of powerlessness) can all be directly attributed to a lack of will power, courage, and confidence.

Niacin. A B-complex nutrient, niacin promotes growth and nervous system function. It also helps to maintain health of the skin and digestive system and is critical to the metabolism of fats, carbohydrates, and proteins. Niacin has been used to alter the blood's fat content to help prevent coronary artery disease. It is also necessary for the synthesis of sex hormones.

One way niacin works in the body is to dilate the blood vessels, allowing blood freer access to the extremities. As a vasodilator, niacin also allows more blood to flow to the blood-brain barrier where oxygen is fed to the brain; consequently, niacin is important for improving memory.

Symbolically, niacin represents openness and receptivity, due in part to the role it plays in growth. You cannot grow and ascend, if your mind is closed. Niacin, through the expansion of the arterial system, allows more blood and more oxygen to the brain. Oxygen represents spirit or faith in self, and with faith in self, you are more apt to be open to new ideas.

Niacin's role in nerve function symbolically allows for greater internal communication, essential for individual growth. Communication with the Inner Self is necessary to draw on guidance for handling future situations.

Niacin is integral to metabolism, both the breaking down and the building up of energies that come into a person's life. If niacin is lacking, there is a correlate block to moving forward. The metabolism slows, and there is a tendency to gain weight—in itself symbolic of a defensive, doubtful position in life.

The cardiovascular system is also affected by niacin. Symbolic of the life of the body, the cardiovascular system is responsible for the delivery of the blood throughout it. The blood is symbolic of spirit because it carries oxygen to every single cell. The heart, the center of the cardiovascular system, symbolizes emotions.

Blood, the body's lifeline, represents spirit within the material realm and carries all nutrients to each cell within the body. It feeds and cleans the body, carrying away potentially destructive toxins. Likewise, toxic thoughts left within the mind to operate freely as patterns of behavior will ultimately destroy a person's health and life and must be eliminated from the system if there is to be true growth.

Because niacin dilates the blood vessels, its symbology of "opening up" is clear. For example, niacin allows blood freer access to the hands and feet. Hands are symbolic of the ability to handle situations, while feet are symbolic of direction. When the extremities are not constricted and are fed the required amounts of blood for optimal function, it symbolically gives the individual more courage and strength, because of the symbology of blood.

When the digestive system is functioning well, it is easier to break down new thoughts and ideas. The ability to consume and digest them, and to immediately utilize the knowledge they contain is the result of being open. While being open and receptive can lead to greater understanding, you must exercise discretion about what you allow to enter. Accept nothing on blind faith. Rather, question everything that comes your way, be it vitamins or thoughts.

A lack of niacin can lead to gastrointestinal disorders, which can symbolize an inability to digest new thoughts and ideas for growth.

Dermatitis is another sign of deficiency. The condition can lead to dry skin and symbolizes a person who is hard to touch or reach.

Nervous disorders symbolically represent a difficulty in communicating on all levels within the self as well as with others, while muscular aches represent a lack of courage or confidence in the ability to participate in an event or in life.

Loss of appetite, also the result of a niacin deficiency, represents a lack of desire. Desire stems from a mind stimulated by receptiveness to new ideas.

Insomnia is symbolic of an inability to prepare for tomorrow, fear of the unknown, or fear of death, while fatigue indicates a lack of desire or enthusiasm.

Halitosis, or bad breath, is also indicative of niacin deficiency. Bad breath comes from sick gums, decaying teeth, or poor internal health. Either way, it reflects an unwillingness to bring new ideas into the body or system. Old ideas on how to eat, think, act, and react are patterns of behavior that are stagnating the body. Toxins are building, and bad breath indicates an imbalance and disharmony within, on multiple levels.

Pantothenic Acid. Occurs in all living cells. It stimulates adrenal hormones important for healthy skin and nerves; plays a vital role in cellular metabolism; participates in the release of energy from carbohydrates, fats, and proteins; and plays a role in the utilization of other vitamins, especially riboflavin (vitamin B-2). It is an essential constituent of co-enzyme A, which forms active acetate and acts as an activating agent in metabolism. Pantothenic acid is essential for the synthesis of cholesterol, steroids (fat-soluble organic compounds), and fatty acids. It is important in maintaining a healthy digestive tract and reduces the toxic effects of many antibiotics.

Pantothenic acid nourishes the adrenal glands, the stress centers of the body. When the body is under stress, the adrenals produce hormones to help it maintain balance and harmony despite the taxing effects of the stress. The adrenal glands' two distinct parts, the cortex (outside) and the medulla (inside), produce hormones to deal with long-term stress and short-term stress, respectively. The adrenal medulla is actually part of the nervous system, modified to secrete the "emergency" hormones adrenaline and noradrenaline.

The adrenals are quite sensitive to pantothenic acid deficiency: the glands shrivel and fill with blood and dead cells, cortisone and other hormones can no longer be produced, and the many protective changes characteristic of countering stress do not occur.[59] Even a slight lack of pantothenic acid causes a marked decrease in the quantity of hormones released.[60] The adrenals also support immune system health, and when they are overtaxed, the immune system subsequently becomes less effective.

Symbolically, pantothenic acid represents inspiration. It nourishes the adrenal glands, which are symbolic of courage and confidence. The adrenals produce hormones (messengers) that tell the body to perform many essential functions. These include biochemical functions such as the converting of cholesterol into sex hormones. This family of hormones is symbolic of expression as well as image. Some messengers tell the body to take quick actions based upon quick decisions of an immediate threat. This is reflected in the "flight or fight" concept.

When you face a vast force or feel overwhelmed, you may go into either a subtle or overt state of doubt and fear. The reaction that creates this fear is based upon how your feel about yourself and your ability to deal with the situation at hand. The part of the body that reacts to the fear impulse is the adrenals, which send out messages in the form of hormones to the appropriate body parts so they know how to react.

Courage and confidence are vital to every activity in life, and these attitudes stem from internal inspiration. From a nutritional perspective, pantothenic acid is the nutrient that participates in energy production. Energy, symbolic of enthusiasm in this case, represents inspiration. That inspiration, built on courage and confidence, is important and supportive of every transaction in which you will engage. This will lead to growth on many levels including the physical, because pantothenic acid plays a role in physical growth.

The most important aspects of growth are the mental expansion and achievements made in life. Without inspiration to seek and discover new insights, understandings, and self-expression, there cannot be true emotional, spiritual, social, or material/financial growth.

People deficient in pantothenic acid show a simultaneous decrease in secretions such as hydrochloric acid, a digestive enzyme essential for breaking down food (thoughts). Indigestion results from this deficiency.

If you lack inspiration, you do not have the desire to examine and question what is being presented to you, which can, in turn, lead to deficiencies and other symptoms with their own symbolic meanings.

For example, the loss of the vitamin B-1 (unity) and pantothenic acid (inspiration) can result in decreased circulation (a condition conducive to clotting) and degeneration of the heart muscles (inability to maintain emotional control in situations).

Low levels of pantothenic acid can also cause fats to burn at only half their normal rate.[61] Stored fat cannot be changed to energy without vitamin B-6[62] (protection and balance); rats deficient in this vitamin utilize both protein and fat so ineffectively that they become grossly obese.[63]

Cancer cells, the symbolic results of anger, frustration, resentment, or guilt, have a much lower content of vitamin B-2 (symbolic of balance and harmony) and pantothenic acid (inspiration) than do normal tissues, and taking these vitamins protects the body without stimulating the growth of malignancies.[64] Symbolically, when a person is inspired, and in balance and harmony within, there is no room for any of the root causes of cancer.

Phosphorus. Phosphorus performs more functions than any other mineral in the body. In its phosphate form, it helps the muscles work; helps the body break down and convert fats, carbohydrates, and proteins into body structures; and is involved with keeping the nerves and blood healthy.

Phospholipids, such as lecithin, break up and also transport fats and fatty acids. They also prevent the accumulation of too much acid or alkali in the blood, facilitate cellular osmosis (passage of substances through cell membranes), and promote secretion of glandular hormones.

Phosphorous is symbolic of courage. Too much phosphorus in the body blocks the absorption of calcium. When in their proper ratio to each other, calcium (symbolic of strength) and phosphorus (courage) work in tandem. We can readily see that when one has false courage or bravado they really are making up for feelings of not having strength. If one had true strength built on a solid foundation of a working faith, then there would be no need to boast, brag, or operate with a large ego. Such is surely the sign or symbol of a person who feels small within.

It takes courage in life to be able to break down and utilize to the fullest everything that comes your way. That is why phosphorous is so vital to good health; in matters of life, it is essential that courage and strength be in equal proportion.

Bone (support) contains 85 percent of the body's total phosphorous. This is why a well-nourished body is so important to success in life on all levels. Cells use the remaining phosphorous as a phosphate, demonstrating that courage and confidence come in many forms and energies. One never knows the level of courage another is demonstrating on a daily basis; what may look like weakness to one may be an exerted effort to another.

The presence of courage is always vital, with the amount needed depending on the current circumstance. Balance must be maintained, in the event more courage is required. This is analogous to maintaining proper acid-alkaline ratios in the blood. Acidity could be looked at symbolically as thoughts that will consume you, eating away at your strength, courage, and confidence while simultaneously stimulating anger, resentment, frustration, and maybe guilt. All of these thoughts and emotional energies are symbolic of cancer. Alkalinity is the exact opposite. Here your thoughts are weakened and undermined, and you have a hard time absorbing strength and courage from external sources. People who get kidney stones usually have alkaline urine that also contains bacteria and large amounts of ammonia.[65] Calcium crystals, which cannot dissolve in alkaline urine, are, therefore readily deposited as kidney stones.[66] The kidney is symbolic of elimination and regulation. In this case, the stones represent strength that was not accepted or used, but could not be eliminated because there was a need for it in the body.

Potassium. Potassium and sodium help regulate water balance within the body by regulating the distribution of fluids through the cell walls. This mineral pair also works together to help normalize the heartbeat and nourish the muscles. Potassium is necessary for normal growth, to stimulate nerve endings for muscle contractions, and to preserve proper alkalinity of the body fluids. Potassium also aids in healthy skin and assists in the conversion of glucose to glycogen. It functions in cell metabolism, enzyme reactions, and in the synthesis of muscle protein from amino acids. Potassium stimulates the kidneys to eliminate toxic wastes, and unites with phosphorus to send oxygen to the brain.

Potassium represents proper balance and harmony in material considerations. Excess materialism leads to a tendency to retain fluids. Balance and harmony in the spiritual sense are the keys to flexible thinking. When there is balance within, you can bend in any area or direction without the fear of falling over or losing balance.

Interestingly, persons with diabetes frequently are deficient in potassium,[67] which is needed to utilize sugar.[68] In this application, it is apparent from the symbology of diabetes (inability to utilize sustenance and make use of available resources) that diabetics are lacking potassium and the ability to attain balance and harmony.

Potassium (balance and harmony) and magnesium (inspiration) are vital in helping to prevent heart (emotional center) attacks,[69] while a lack of the substances allows clots to form in the heart and brain (spiritual center) alike.[70] A potassium deficiency causes contractions of the intestinal muscles to slow markedly or these muscles may become partially or completely paralyzed.[71] When we are out of balance, it is difficult to correctly process incoming material; the body's building process, therefore, becomes imbalanced, with weakness on many levels.

Since potassium stimulates the kidneys to eliminate poisonous body wastes, it demonstrates that balance and harmony in one's thinking is essential for eliminating obsolete, detrimental thoughts. Potassium (balance and harmony) unites with phosphorus (courage) to send oxygen (spirit) to the brain (spiritual center).

Selenium. While selenium's overall role is not well understood, its most important known role is as a component of glutathione peroxidase, an antioxidant enzyme. Symbolically, selenium represents both protection and cleansing. The protection mode is demonstrated in numerous transactions within the body, most notably in its part in constructing glutathione, a free-radical scavenger.

Free radicals damage DNA (the blueprint for the cells) by stealing electrons from molecules of the amino acids they attack. When you latch onto an idea that is not beneficial, it robs you of your energy (electrons). It also creates a false sense of faith that, likewise, will not support us in true endeavors. This is why free radicals, also known as singlet oxygen, are so detrimental. Interestingly, the body generates singlet oxygen as well. In some cases, the immune system uses them for its own transactions. In this case we can see the spirit (oxygen) acting on behalf of our body in a different way.

Also noteworthy is the fact that toxins in our environment are the cause of free- radical generation. The air (symbolic of spiritual thought) is polluted, the water (symbolic of our material life) is polluted as well as depleted, and the foods we consume are loaded with chemical additives. These man-made poisons, like other man-made thoughts, concepts, and ideas about how to think and live are, likewise, polluted. Their producers have only one aim: ensuring profitability for the companies that grow, package, and sell the food we eat.

Look at the thoughts that you consume on a daily basis. It is easy to see that society's priorities are imbalanced when its most important concern is profit.

As a protector of cells from free radical damage and as a cleansing agent, selenium is found in the highest concentrations in the liver and kidneys. Very little is found in the brain and lungs. This tells us that symbolically, selenium is more involved in material dealings than in spiritual thinking.

One sign of selenium deficiency is hemolytic anemia (lack of faith). Similarly, if we do not cleanse man-made teachings from our consciousness, we are doomed to remain weak or to become so by following man's ways and depending on the material and not the spiritual for sustenance. Even though man talks about being spiritual, his actions may say otherwise.

The inability for self-protection leads to the destruction of red blood cells (lack of spirit (oxygen) carriers), and immune dysfunction. In truth, it is hard to defend yourself against attack from the outside, when you are unprotected in your thinking about material life.

Selenium is a potent anti-carcinogenic agent. Because the causes of cancer are rooted in anger, resentment, frustration, and/or guilt, it is easy to see how inadequate cleansing and protection of certain emotional concepts would cause these energies to be present. The protection aspect of selenium is also verified in those emotional conditions that create change.

As in the police car and telephone examples, emotions cause internal biochemical changes, which can set the stage for the development of mutant cells.

With selenium supplementation, there is a strong trend toward improved clinical outcome of cardiovascular health.[72] Cardiovascular health deals with emotional responses to given stimuli. Once a stimulus is experienced via sight, sound, or feel, it triggers a subconscious responsive action. Often, these actions are designed to fulfill self-expectations; the mind begins to set up events and circumstances to create the needed response. The end result might be a heart attack or another equally detrimental emotional response.

Vitamin A. This antioxidant vitamin performs so many crucial functions necessary for good health that deficiency of the nutrient is a major public health problem.[73] Essential for all vision, particularly night vision, vitamin A is also important for the outer cellular layer of tissues, including skin, bones, and organs. It is also essential for the mucous membranes, thin sheets of tissue cells that cover or line various parts of the body including the mouth, digestive tube, breathing passages, and the genital and urinary tracts. Vitamin A is essential for healthy skin, teeth, and gums. It promotes growth and vitality and is necessary during pregnancy and lactation.

Vitamin A and beta-carotene do not carry the risk of toxicity posed by ingesting high amounts of fish liver oil.[74] Vitamin A and beta-carotene have proved to protect against cancer in humans.[75] Higher intakes of carotene[76] and vitamin A[77] are associated with a lower risk of cancer, and beta-carotene has been found to have specific anti-tumor activity in animal studies.[78] Synthetic forms of vitamin A have been used to correct pre-cancerous conditions[79] and to treat cancer.[80] It has also been successful in the treatment of acne,[81] night blindness associated with primary biliary cirrhosis,[82] gastric ulcers,[83] and photo-dermatitis.[84]

The symbolic importance of vitamin A for night vision is the ability to see into the doubt that exists within the self. You could even say that vitamin A aids in self-examination by its role in improving (internal) vision.

Nighttime has different symbolic interpretations. The first is doubt, which emerges from the difficulty in seeing clearly through night's darkness. Lack of clarity is synonymous with doubt in all situations. A second interpretation of the night is that it is a pause in the cycle, a time of rest for the physical body to repair and the Spiritual Self to prepare for the upcoming day. This Universal Teaching, "life is a movement and a rest," is also illustrated by the seventh day of creation, as depicted in the *Bible*. Another is that nighttime is a period of preparation, a window during which the mind stills and organizes itself for the tasks of the new day. If we recall the Universal Teaching that "every action generates a reaction" and that patterns of behavior are triggered by the events of the day just ending, then it is important for the mind to take the time to analyze these events and begin to formulate an appropriate response. This form of preparation is built upon the understanding that certain patterns of behavior have been triggered by events and stimuli experienced during the day. The mind analyzes these events and begins to formulate a plan for responding. In addition to responding, it is also projecting ahead and emitting energies that will help to bring about events that will fulfill expectations based on subconscious concepts.[85]

With proper vision, you can avoid the doubt and frustration that accompanies preparing for a situation. Vitamin A helps you to see well, giving you greater insight. Going into a situation totally prepared gives you courage and confidence. When those energies are at work for you, there is no doubt about your ability to master a situation. This has a positive effect upon the image. People who suffer with skin blemishes such as acne are experiencing self-doubt as they are going through a particular cycle or phase in life. Without the doubt and fear, the reflection of inner-confidence will show in improved complexion.

Because it supports the mucous membranes and feeds the thymus gland, another aspect of vitamin A's symbology is that it is instrumental in protecting you from invasion by outside forces. The thymus is an immune center from which T-cells rush out to do battle with foreign invaders. On a physical level, this can be allergens, germs, bacterias, viruses, fungi, or environmental toxins. These forces can also be thoughts, attitudes, or energies from others that you willingly brought into your consciousness and realm of reality to meet subconscious needs.

Vitamin A promotes growth and vitality. You cannot have true personal growth or even vitality without self-confidence on all levels. When you feel good about yourself, your immune system gets a boost and stays strong, too. Both aspects help you feel more protected from outside forces, allowing you to move forward with courage.

Additionally, vitamin A is necessary during pregnancy and lactation. Not all females or males can produce children; pregnancy is the result of many factors in a couple's life, including positive feelings about self-expression, the ability to provide for a child, and the capacity to nourish another being. Each of these elements stem from one's subconscious feelings of being in control. Feelings of personal power and being protected from outside forces are also present.

Teen pregnancy is an exception to these conditions. Some teen mothers have healthy babies, despite their own immaturity, negative self-concept, or the possible stigma of bearing a child out of wedlock and at such a young age. Teenage mothers may also harbor feelings of rejection for the child because the baby's father may have abandoned her, or she may feel the child has wrecked her life.

The fact that they were able to conceive validates that their courage and confidence for self-expression within our society, which has its own ideas about taboos such as teen pregnancy, baby abandonment, or infanticide—all situations with their own symbolic significance. (For more on this topic, see Section I: From the Inside Out.)

Vitamin A serves so many functions that the symptoms of deficiency are many and varied. Defective teeth and gums symbolize an inability to properly break down incoming energies into digestible fragments. Foods represent thoughts, and certain foods have emotional attachments for each individual. A propensity for eating specific foods could further damage the teeth or gums. Sweets, for example, are the comfort food of choice for someone who is conditioned to receive a sweet goody for doing a good job; in order to feel better at any point in life, such a person might turn to sweets to recapture this emotional high. As sweets destroy the teeth and set up gum infections, the self-image can only worsen. This scenario is similar to that of acne, which is also affected by vitamin A.

Dry hair and skin are also tied to image. Hair symbolizes strength, while dry skin represents both image and the ability to protect self, reflecting a lack of confidence.

Allergies may affect an overly sensitive person whose lack of self-confidence makes it difficult to accept new ideas. One by-product of allergies is sinus trouble, which is symbolic of blocked spiritual intake (air/heaven) and a lack of faith in self. Loss of smell represents an inability to protect the self from negative thoughts. Smell is a tool to protect the body from consuming a foodstuff or continuing to inhale a substance that could cause discomfort, disease, or even death.

Retarded growth is another telling symbol of vitamin A depletion wherein self-doubt and its companion, fear, have literally hindered or stifled growth. Because vitamin A represents the ability to see clearly, it greatly reduces or even eliminates doubt and fear, allowing growth and development on many levels.

Susceptibility to infections is another deficiency sign. Being in a state of doubt or fear lowers our resistance to intrusive energies generated either by a concept triggered within or from external elements, such as when others seek to impose their concepts upon us.

B-complex Vitamins. These nutrients help the nervous system function and are also essential for healthy skin, muscle tone, hair, and eyes. Additionally, they are required for proper functioning of the liver and gastrointestinal tract, and for metabolism of carbohydrates, fats, and proteins. They are also known for their critical role in basic, cellular energy production.

When the body is deficient in specific B-complex nutrients, the symptoms include a poor appetite; rough, dry skin; fatigue; dull hair; constipation; acne; or insomnia.

Overall, the B-complex nutrients represent confidence and courage on multiple levels. These two attributes contribute to many other emotions. If we think of vitamins as representing the positive aspects of particular emotions, their negative aspects are readily apparent as deficiencies associated with specific B-complex vitamins.

Vitamin B-1. Necessary for a healthy mouth, skin, eyes, and hair, vitamin B-1 is also needed for carbohydrate metabolism. Vitamin B-1 is essential for nerve tissues, muscles, digestion, and for normal heart function.

Symbolically, vitamin B-1 acts as a facilitator. It facilitates communication on two levels by ensuring the health of the mouth. The mouth is the portal through which you provide material sustenance for the well-being of your body, and is also a primary structure for communication, a vehicle used for self-expression.

Vitamin B-1 facilitates a good image through the maintaining of healthy skin. Skin performs several functions for the body. First and foremost, it is something that all people can see, the "face" you present to the world, quite literally. It is also the body's largest organ of elimination.

B-1 regulates body temperature, preventing heat loss or overheating. In this respect, B-1 as a facilitator helps to maintain control over emotions. The emotions can create anger under certain conditions, but B-1 allows venting of anger through expelling or eliminating moisture (laden with impurities from the system) through healthy pores.

B-1 protects your internal health and your eyes (how you see the world); it also maintains healthy hair (strength). You can readily see its role as a facilitator of a strong, healthy image. It also enhances communication along the nerve lines (transmission lines for the body). Thoughts, even subconscious ones, are converted to electrical energy that is transmitted over the nerve network, facilitating transactions, such as muscular relaxation or contraction/constriction.

It also facilitates digestion (the breaking down of thoughts) and the ability to control emotions. This is particularly reflected in its role in maintaining the heart, which symbolizes emotions.

If the body is deficient in vitamin B-1, you may begin to suffer from depression or fatigue (usually the result of a lack of inspiration or nothing to facilitate a good feeling/desire), constipation (the inability to let go of the past, holding onto old ideas), shortness of breath (doubt of one's ability to do a certain project/commitment), numb hands and feet (unsure of direction [feet] or inability to handle the situation [hands]), or a loss of appetite (no desire to partake of material life; withdrawal).

Children can also suffer impaired growth due to vitamin B-1 deficiency.

Vitamin B-2. This nutrient, also called riboflavin, functions as part of a group of enzymes in the breakdown and utilization of carbohydrates, fats, and proteins. It is important for cell respiration, and it aids in the formation of red blood cells and antibodies. It also supports good vision. Riboflavin is necessary for the production of an enzyme involved in the lens physiology's protective mechanisms.

Symbolically, vitamin B-2 represents courage. It works with vitamin B-1 in supporting eye, skin, and hair health. Symbolically, these elements involve the need for confidence and courage. If either one is lacking, it would impact not only the way you see yourself and others, but also the way they would see you.

B-2 assists the body in utilizing the food it consumes. Foods represent thoughts. Some offerings are beneficial, while others offend the taste buds. Just as they help protect our physical bodies from ingesting toxic substances, the taste buds are also one of the first lines of defense in protecting the body from invasion by toxic thoughts. It is interesting then that so much of our food is loaded with sugar or salt. If it appeals to the taste buds, some people might consume willingly or be tricked into consuming poison. This is one reason why healthcare costs in the United States are among the highest in the world.

If we are presented with thoughts that are not in keeping with our normal way of thinking (our subconscious belief system), and we lack the courage to look more closely at these thoughts, we could miss their potential benefits. We will not be able to digest it or even break it down in order to assimilate it and gain sustenance from it. That is not to suggest all thoughts are of value; some thoughts are detrimental to well-being.

Foods also have a personal, emotional value to each person, with each food item carrying its own special, emotional connection. Eating certain things makes a person feel good, and that is one reason it is difficult for some individuals to change their diet; it would mean giving up those emotional feelings of well-being.

Vitamin B-2 aids in the formation of red blood cells, which carry oxygen to every part of the body. This is essential for all the cells and, particularly, for the brain. The brain symbolizes the material body's spiritual center, and it is through the mind that the power of spirit operates.

Oxygen is symbolic of spirit, which dwells in the air/heaven. Just as oxygen feeds fire, the more spirit the body has, the more energy it has available to it. Those who suffer B-2 deficiency often experience dizziness as a result of lack of oxygen to the brain, symbolic of a lack of spirit or self-confidence to handle tasks at hand.

Vitamin B-2 demonstrates how vital courage is to health because of its role in the production of antioxidants that act on the level of the cellular membrane, which keep cells intact and healthy.

This nutrient also inhibits cataract formation in the eyes. Cataracts can distort vision to the point of blindness. Symbolically, this reflects fear of seeing the future because of doubts about where it might lead. To move forward in life one must be able to make clear choices, free of distortion. Vitamin B-2 (courage) must be present for growth and forward movement.

Eye problems, in general, are another sign of the need for B-2 (courage). We view life through a filter of subconscious concepts that shade everything; therefore, everything is distorted. People see what they want to see, and they may lack the ability to clearly discern what they actually do see.

One B-2 deficiency sign is mouth inflammation, which could impact one's ability to take sustenance or communicate effectively with others. A sore tongue also represents difficulty in self-expression. When courage is lacking or doubt is present in a person, then others may not be able to hear that individual clearly on any level.

Poor digestion reflects an inability to break down all the thoughts and energies coming at or into the person, and the dry, hard skin of dermatitis symbolizes defenses and a need for protection.

Vitamin B-6. This nutrient is extremely vital owing to its role in antibody and red blood cell production. The presence of vitamin B-6 also increases the number of T-cells and white blood cells that support immune response by ingesting foreign matter that has invaded the body. It is required for proper absorption of vitamin B-12, production of hydrochloric acid, and magnesium assimilation. It acts as a co-enzyme in the utilization of carbohydrates, fats, and proteins. It releases glycogen from the liver and muscles for energy. Interestingly, 50 percent of the body's total B-6 is concentrated in muscle tissue.

B-6 aids in the conversion of the essential amino acid tryptophane to niacin and is necessary for the synthesis and proper action of DNA and RNA. The balance of sodium and potassium, which regulates body fluids and promotes the normal functioning of the nervous and musculoskeletal systems, is maintained by B-6. It is necessary for healthy skin, nerves, muscles, and aids in digestion. In pregnant women, vitamin B-6 helps to alleviate morning sickness, but without the toxicity associated with drugs.[86]

Symbolically, vitamin B-6 represents regulation as well as protection. Both are demonstrated by how the vitamin helps maintain adequate numbers of white blood cells, the body's main defense against invaders that could cause harm or disease.

Thoughts are much the same. They are forces that are invading the personal belief system. Some ideas require regulation by emotional response, and others, a protective mode so as not to destroy a current position or stand on issues/concepts. These regulating, protective thoughts are necessary to keep the body in a state of good health because thoughts actually change its biochemistry in response to external stimuli or emotional responses to a given event.

Drivers often experience this response when involved in a near accident. The normal, fearful response includes a racing heart and a sick, sinking feeling in the pit of the stomach. Both of these physical events are triggered by hormones manufactured and released in response to the visual and auditory cues, which are tied to a subconscious concept.

As a co-enzyme, B-6 is involved in the digestive processes; as such, it symbolically acts as a regulator, assisting you in breaking down thoughts that are presented. Through examining the thoughts, you can determine what is useful and what is not. By regulating the emotional responses, damage can be prevented to the self as well as to the body.

Another example of B-6 as a regulator is seen in how it releases glycogen from the liver. Glycogen is a form of sugar that the body uses for fuel. This is akin to regulating one's emotions, energy output, and enthusiasm.

Because it aids in the conversion of tryptophane to niacin (opening up), we can see that being in control of emotions through the regulation of energies makes it easier to open up to new ideas.

Vitamin B-6 is also necessary for the synthesis and proper action of DNA and RNA. Once again, regulation and protection are at work keeping our integrity whole. RNA and DNA are the blueprints of our cells telling them how to recreate themselves as well as how to perform their particular functions. When we are deficient in nutrients, we are symbolically deficient in the ability to protect ourselves, to perform correctly, and regulate our growth.

Muscle weakness is a sign of B-6 deficiency. Muscles are symbolic of the strength that is available to you to apply control and handle any given situation. Without strength, you may believe yourself helpless in dealing with the forces or energies of life. The truth of this perception is seen in the physical fact that a deficiency of vitamin B-6 (protection) leads to impaired immune response, but what you may not have considered is the importance of regulated thinking in regard to gaining strength. Symbolically, this is the inability to defend the self from the thoughts, judgments, and opinions of others. A deficiency will also cause nervousness, based on fear and doubt in one's ability to deal with a situation.

Learning disorders are another sign and are symbolic of an unwillingness to stretch the mind to embrace new ideas or participate in new endeavors. They stem from a fear that by accepting new levels of awareness, you may become vulnerable through also having to take on more responsibility for which you feel unprepared.

Dermatitis or acne can also occur. Skin is the first external protector of the internal environment, and embodies the image that is projected. Hair loss is another possibility, also tied symbolically to strength or image.

Disorders of the mouth are symbolic of the vulnerability felt without the protection of B-6. The resulting doubt and fear lead to poor communication or the inability to "chew" on new thoughts.

Depression can result from a lack of self-confidence. Protection issues, victimization, and feelings of helplessness against the world are connected symbolically with B-6 deficiency.

Anemia symbolically reflects a lack of spirit and can also be caused by low levels of B-6. Again, we can see that when you feel unprotected, you are at the mercy of life and are not prepared to meet challenging situations from a position of strength.

Arthritis is another condition resulting from doubt and fear, and is symbolic of inflexible thinking. An individual feels unable to go beyond certain parameters in handling or dealing with situations, so he or she remains locked into old ways of thinking, thus, creating inflexibility. The particular joints or bones afflicted by arthritis give an indication as to where the sufferer's issues lie. Knee joints, for example, reveal doubt in your ability to "straighten up" and deal with the pressure of a situation, usually something involving material support or financial direction. The wrists also deal with mobility in terms of how you handle situations. If your wrists are inflexible, you may have limited choices on movement of the hands. When that occurs it also limits your flexibility in handling everyday situations.

Severe insomnia is yet another symptom of a B-6 deficiency. Symbolically, it is the inability to prepare for upcoming events. Insomnia is usually a doubt or fear-based issue. It has been induced in a group of volunteers through diet made deficient in vitamin B-6.[87]

Men deficient in vitamin B-6 may become impotent because of feelings of vulnerability, which hamper self-expression. The penis is symbolic of the expression of manhood. During extreme stress, the sex urge and sperm production diminish. Both of these symptoms, brought on by physical or emotional stress, demonstrate how a lack of faith in self diminishes the creative aspects as well.

Vitamin B-12. This nutrient helps form normal red blood cells and a healthy nervous system, for which it supports production of myelin, the sheathlike covering that protects the nerves. B-12 plays a role in making folate available to cells and helps the body to more effectively metabolize fats, carbohydrates, and proteins. It also accelerates the production of bile salts, thereby decreasing blood cholesterol levels.[88] Symbolically, B-12 acts as working faith. Without faith and fortification (folate), new life (red blood cells) and expression (cells; a reflection of self) would not take root and produce viable results.

It takes an internal working faith, which stems from past successes, to truly accomplish the difficult things in life. As taken from Matthew 25:14-29, the Universal Teaching based on the parable of the golden talents to use what you have been given in order to receive more or not to use it and risk losing it all is a great example of having and working with faith.

Interestingly, B-12 reserves take decades to be depleted; the substance is readily conserved and recycled by the body. Similarly, working faith is also a constant, and when it is used daily to deal with life's situations, it grows stronger. By contrast, when doubt becomes part of a person's daily habit, then anemia (lack of spirit) can result. In other words, the person would be lacking in faith. This would manifest as low B-12 reserves in the body.

Vitamin B-12 protects the nervous system. This symbolically translates into a working faith, which protects us from the emotional reactions that come from being overly sensitive. An individual may experience extreme emotional reactions if there is doubt in his or her expression. The over-reaction, in itself, can lead to major problems.

That is one of the reasons for turning the other cheek; nothing constructive can come of feeding an angry person's energy by responding to a verbal attack. Once you do respond, and negative, counter-productive energy is released, there is no calling it back until it has fulfilled the expectation of both parties. You cannot possibly know the other person's expectations, and you may even be unsure about your own, unless you have mastered your concepts. You can control the exchange to a great degree by simply not engaging in it.

When vitamin B-12 is working in the arena of metabolism—the building up or breaking down of stuff—you can see how an internal, working faith is integral to the process. Without it, how difficult would it be to fully utilize all that is available to you? Doubt limits perception regarding what is available, and an external, blind faith will not provide the true sustenance needed to accomplish life's difficult tasks or growth.

It is noteworthy that B-12 helps in the production of bile salts, which are necessary to emulsify fats for better utilization by the body. Symbolically, with a working faith, the fats of life (stored energy) are easily used to accomplish one's goals.

Faith inspires. The fact that B-12 decreases cholesterol in the blood tells us that the natural inclination of spirit and inspiration is to not be hindered in any of their forms of expression, either within or without. When there is too much cholesterol in the blood, the amount of oxygen (spirit) available to the cells diminishes.

Vitamin C. Also known as ascorbic acid, this antioxidant vitamin's uses are numerous. It increases the absorption of iron and is essential for healthy teeth, gums, bones, and collagen production. Vitamin C supports immune function, strengthens blood vessels, and helps to nullify the toxic effects of heavy metals, such as lead, which are often found in drinking water.[89] Large concentrations of vitamin C are found in the adrenal glands where it is essential for adrenaline formation. Intense stress rapidly depletes vitamin C levels in the adrenals.

Vitamin C is symbolic of two major aspects of the material plane. On one level, it represents material/physical protection, much like another free-radical scavenger, vitamin A. Vitamin C protects the body within the material plane from those forces and elements that are natural to the material existence. Collagen production and immune system support are the primary examples of this type of protection.

On another level, vitamin C represents our obvious, yet rarely considered, dependency on the material plane. The reality is we could not live very long without essential physical elements such as air, water, or food. As spiritual beings encased in a material vehicle (body), we need material/physical sustenance to survive, as represented by water (material life). We also need spiritual sustenance, as represented symbolically by air (spiritual life). Both are necessary for human survival.

Vitamin C increases absorption of iron, symbolic of faith and courage. Iron is contained in hemoglobin, which carries oxygen to the cells. It also removes carbon dioxide and carries it to the lungs. Oxygen is symbolic of spirit because air symbolically represents heaven. Heaven is symbolic of the Creator's home or dwelling place. Tying together these insights, we can see that vitamin C (protection) is essential for faith and courage/strength to grow.

Free-radical damage occurs because of electron transfer, a process during which an oxygen atom readily gives up its outer electron or seeks to bond with another; the second electron taken randomly to balance the two protons in its nucleus. This disrupts electrical flow and energy for both the oxygen atom and for the original structure or location of the stolen electron. Electron transfer occurs because virtually everything in nature—from the smallest atom to the human body—seeks harmony and balance.

The body's billions of cells are constantly exposed to these renegade radicals, which are created by normal body chemistry and other external stimuli, such as air pollution and cigarette smoke. The physical damage to the body attributed to free radicals is believed to be wide ranging and a major deterrent to good health. The body goes to great lengths to absorb essential elements necessary to keep a sufficient level of protection against the cell damage caused by oxygen free radicals. Cells damaged by free radicals have a tendency to deteriorate and age more rapidly than healthy cells and can also lead to disease. Vitamin C helps the body neutralize these elements.

Symbolically, vitamin C protects us from those thoughts that undermine our inherent strength. When your courage and faith in self are compromised, doubt and fear set in, opening the door for frustration, anger, and resentment. Such developments can "eat you up," and consequently, can lead to cancer and many other different conditions and diseases.

A friend brought up the point that very few animals require vitamin C in their diet. In fact, most animals make vitamin C in their liver, but humans lack an enzyme needed for the conversion of glucose into vitamin C. Symbolically, this is very interesting. It appears most animals do not have to be concerned about the sweetness (glucose) of their lives; the need to convert what is being presented to them into a beneficial substance, therefore, is of no importance.

Humans, on the other hand, think about our lives and all that this comprises. It seems that we must be able to assess what is being presented and to be able to use it in a healthful/helpful way. When we cannot, or when we are not presented with those thoughts that can be converted, we end up in a weakened state, possibly manifesting as a disease. In this case, when vitamin C is lacking, the disease, scurvy, may develop.

One common symptom of vitamin C deficiency is muscular weakness. Without that protected feeling, you may feel you do not have the strength to deal with whatever you are facing at the time. Another symptom is anemia; this represents a lack of strength, faith, and courage. Appetite loss, another symptom, reflects a lack of desire to partake of the offerings of the material plane. Slow-healing wounds are yet another symptom, and reflect a person who is dealing with emotional hurts that are also slow to heal, and also is slow to forgive and move on. Fractures, a vitamin C issue, symbolically denote a feeling of weakness and vulnerability in the area symbolized by the broken bone. The symptom of bleeding gums deals with image and communication, and indirectly reflects an inability to break down incoming data.

People with a low resistance to infections are also vitamin C compromised. Infections are symbolic of external thoughts that are in conflict with your internal belief system. They also represent the result of encountering opposing expectations. Susceptibility to bruises or skin hemorrhages is another sign and reflects an individual's sensitivity to external forces, things other people say and do, while swollen joints represent a fear-based inability for flexible thinking.

Vitamin C accelerates the rate of cortisone production, appears to improve its utilization and delay its breakdown, and alleviates many of the limitations resulting from a pantothenic acid (inspiration) deficiency.[90,91,92,93] Apparently, because large amounts of vitamin C are used to detoxify harmful substances formed in the body during stress, greater than normal quantities are lost in the urine during these times.[94]

Epidemiological evidence overwhelmingly shows that high dietary vitamin C helps provide protection from multiple-site cancers.[95,96,97,98] Vitamin C is widely accepted for its ability to prevent the formation of stomach carcinogens.[99,100] The stomach is the place where the digestibility of thoughts begins. If the subject/topic is uncomfortable and hard to stomach, it will first be rejected here.

Therapeutic doses of vitamin C have been successfully used to treat early vertebral disk lesions.[101] The vertebrae are aspects of the spinal column, which is symbolic of support. One can see that protection from attack is essential in supporting the self. Vitamin C has been used to decrease capillary fragility in diabetics.[102] This is another example of protection coming to the aid of the body against the misconceptions associated with diabetes. Diabetics, themselves, may harbor some of these misconceptions—that they do not have the strength or the right to enjoy the sweetness of life, for example.

Diabetes symbolically represents several energies at work, one being the need for a little sugar in life, i.e., love. Additionally, it reflects failure to utilize resources completely, stemming from a need to gather and hold on to the material. This may be reflected as being overweight or having a lot of money but not using it for self-benefit.

A major function of vitamin C is its nonspecific role as a detoxifying agent;[103] for nearly thirty years it has been known to prevent the toxicity, allergic reactions, and anaphylactic shock caused by drugs.[104] It also appears to react with any foreign substance reaching the blood,[105] and if generously supplied, it nullifies the toxicity of fluorine,[106] saccharine and other artificial sweeteners,[107] lead,[108] benzene,[109] carbon tetrachloride,[110] and excessive vitamins A and D[111] as well as drugs.

In a single year no less than forty-five research projects reported that vitamin C rendered harmless a wide variety of bacterial toxins and inhibited the growth of whatever bacteria it failed to destroy,[112] its action was nonspecific in that it was deadly to all types of viruses[113] and bacteria,[114] and that while small amounts could bring some immunity,[115] huge doses were much more effective. All of this validates vitamin C's symbology as a protector.

Vitamin D. This fat-soluble vitamin is known as the "sunshine vitamin" because the action of the sun's ultraviolet rays converts a form of cholesterol present in the skin into vitamin D. This nutrient must be present for the assimilation and utilization of calcium. In fact, vitamin D is so effective in helping the body assimilate calcium that it has been used by itself to dissolve joint and spinal calcium deposits.

Vitamin D aids in the absorption of calcium from the intestinal tract and in the breakdown and assimilation of phosphorus, which is required for bone formation. It helps synthesize those enzymes in the mucous membranes that are involved in the active transport of available calcium. Of particular importance for the normal growth of children, vitamin D also helps the body maintain a stable nervous system, normal heart action, and normal blood clotting. All of these functions are related to the body's supply and use of calcium and phosphorus. Vitamin D is best utilized when used in conjunction with vitamin A.

From a symbolic perspective, vitamin D's role in calcium absorption represents insight and, to a degree, understanding. This interpretation is based on vitamin D's integral part in the assimilation of calcium, which represents strength. Strength comes in two styles. The first is what we normally see in the world—bravado based on man-made concepts as to what strength represents. But there is also true strength, the type that is quiet yet runs extremely deep. People with true strength know that they can accomplish just about anything they set out to do. They know this because they have proven it to themselves time and time again, even when man-made situations appeared beyond their control and abilities. With insights and understandings, strength is easily achieved. Without them, it would be virtually impossible to achieve true strength.

Look at how vitamin D is manufactured in the body. It requires sunlight, which is symbolic of insight and seeing clearly. Nothing is hidden in the light, especially if you have the eyes to see.

Vitamin E. Because it plays a role in a wider variety of body functions than almost any other nutrient,[116] vitamin E has been described as a "guardian angel"[117] which protects the essential fatty acids, carotene, vitamin A, the B-complex vitamins (indirectly), and the pituitary, adrenal, and sex hormones from being destroyed by oxygen.[118] In fact, vitamin E markedly reduces the need for oxygen;[119] allows fewer cells to be harmed when blood vessels have been cut, mangled, or burned;[120] and increases the number and speed of formation of new blood vessels into a damaged area.[121] Vitamin E strengthens the capillary walls and, thus, decreases clotting.[122] It also strengthens the heart muscles,[123] and its action is said to be similar to that of digitalis.[124]

Symbolically, vitamin E equates to self-confidence and a reduced need for external support in matters of faith; it builds working faith, the solid, in-dwelling faith of self-reliance that stems from personal experience. Man will never be able to overcome himself without first going within and communing with the spirit.

One of vitamin E's important roles is that of a free-radical scavenger, or antioxidant. Free radicals in the body are at work destroying aspects of the DNA, your blueprint for who you are. In your mind, random, negative thoughts can also act to destroy who you are. A lack of confidence can set up both the mind and body for invasion, confusion, fear, lack of control, and degeneration.

The body is a wondrous reality of symbolic significance. It tells us moment by moment where we are. Symbology is the way in which to understand the communication from your Greater Mind, a.k.a. the subconscious. Without vitamin E (self confidence) blood cells (carriers of faith [oxygen/spirit]) break down,[125] or severe liver (cleansing) and kidney (also a cleansing organ, as is skin) damage can occur.[126] Low vitamin E levels also impair iron absorption and hemoglobin formation. Essential fatty acids forming part of the cell structure also become so altered by oxidation that the cells break down.[127]

Fat is life. Life is born out of cellular division. The dividing of cells is based on many different factors including essential fatty acids. The problem is that we have been taught that all fat is bad, when in reality, the best approach is to avoid hydrogenated oils and fried foods, and use polyunsaturated fats and oils.

Symbolically, the ability to draw in and utilize strength is compromised by our inability to absorb iron. Because the body cannot carry oxygen/spirit to every aspect of self, the ability to learn from external experiences is also compromised.

Other consequences of vitamin E deficiency in humans include nearsightedness (the inability to focus or to see one's future path clearly) and crossed eyes (not seeing things "straight on," as they truly are). Both have been corrected by large amounts of vitamin E.[128]

Finally, in all varieties of laboratory and farm animals, inadequate vitamin E results in degeneration of the testicles (expression of manhood);[129] in human males, the motility and fertility of sperm (self-expression/power) are in proportion to the amount of vitamin E present in semen.[130]

Vitamin K. Necessary for the formation of prothrombin, a chemical required for blood clotting, vitamin K is vital for normal liver functioning and is an important factor in vitality and longevity. It is involved in phosphorylation, a process in which phosphate combines with glucose and passes through the cell membranes, where it is converted into glycogen to provide energy reserves for the body.

Vitamin K symbolizes commitment. For example, a combination of vitamin K (commitment) and calcium (strength) is necessary to prevent blood loss. When blood (spirit, the foundation of confidence) is lost or anemia sets in, it symbolizes an individual experiencing a lack of faith (spirit/oxygen). Along the same lines, we can see that it takes a commitment (vitamin K), confidence (phosphorous/phosphate) and energy (glycogen) to produce the stamina to accomplish certain feats.

The liver, symbolic of cleansing as well as regulation, requires a commitment to function properly. Without commitment there cannot be a true cleansing, nor can there be regulation of those elements in life that would cause imbalances, because imbalances can lead to emotional turmoil and overreaction

Zinc. This mineral has many different functions within the body, ranging from taste and smell to supporting metabolism and reproduction. It is a constituent of at least twenty-five enzymes involved in tissue respiration, digestion, and metabolism, including the one needed to break down alcohol. (Low serum concentrations of zinc are associated with alcoholic cirrhosis.) Zinc also aids in the digestion of phosphorus, protein, and carbohydrates.

Necessary for burn and wound healing, zinc plays a key role in normal tissue development including cell division, protein synthesis, and collagen formation.[131] Zinc is essential in the synthesis of nucleic acid for both DNA and RNA, the blueprints of the body.

Zinc is involved in the synthesis and action of insulin, binding to insulin and enhancing its activity; insulin promotes fuel storage because the brain requires glucose, and accelerates the membrane transport of sugars, which increases four times in normal hearts and six to seven times in diabetics.[132]

Zinc plays an important role in nourishing the thymus gland as well as liberating vitamin A from the liver. A component of male reproductive fluid, zinc is also involved with prostate gland functions.

Symbolically, zinc represents those thoughts that contribute to supportive or fundamental expression and a working faith. This is seen in its role as a component in digestion, metabolism, rebuilding, tissue development, respiration, cell division, and insulin production. Without a working faith and a positive means to express energy, there would be no growth on an individual's path. There would be difficulty in breaking down thoughts. Because of an inability to grow the self with full confidence and courage, the ability to express or reproduce is compromised, and in some cases, eliminated.

Working faith and self-expression, likewise, are essential to the healing of emotional wounds (as well as burns and tissue wounds). Fire is symbolic of the emotions, which when out of control are all consuming. That is why anger is a causative factor in the development of cancer. When a person has a working faith and a comfortable form of expression they are able to turn adversity into opportunity.

Phosphorous, symbolic of courage and confidence, needs zinc (expression and working faith) to function properly. Insights and understandings (vitamin A) can support the awareness of defenses (thymus gland), once vitamin A is liberated from the process of cleansing and conversion (liver).

Interestingly, zinc (expression and a working faith) works to protect the self from invasion of negative substances (thoughts) via a heightened sense of smell or taste. Smell, a function of the nose, is symbolic of spiritual intake. Your nose should have the ability to prevent you from inhaling or incorporating a false (man-made) aroma, symbolic of a certain thought, into your life. Industry has fooled the nose just as man-made teachings have fooled people into thinking that the appearance and smell are more important than the substance or essence of it.

The taste buds accomplish essentially the same task. Man-made industry has tainted virtually everything humans consume with a false sweetness that does not satisfy and ultimately creates more problems, such as diabetes, characterized by an excess amount of sugar in the blood. Zinc, as a participant of insulin, adds faith and expression to the mix, and insulin symbolizes moderation coupled with courage and confidence.

A zinc deficiency could cause diarrhea (the need to immediately eliminate a thought or the inability to draw strength and power from what is being presented), lethargy (a lack of inspiration or motivation), dermatitis (expression or appearance issues), mental disorders (the inability to cope), skin lesions (another example of a lack of expression and faith causing image issues), anorexia (inability to acquire substance), loss of taste (inability to protect self or to discern), growth retardation (small stature, feelings of weakness), and sexual immaturity (the inability to express). If attitudes about the self do not change, this type of person would become sterile.

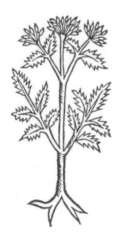

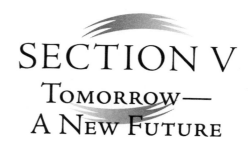

SECTION V
TOMORROW—
A NEW FUTURE

1. THE RETURN TO HEALTH

Wherever you are today is the result of where you have been, on multiple levels. You have probably heard this sentiment expressed as "you are what you eat" or "you are what you think." Both statements are true. That is why it is important—if not essential—to truly understand the root causes of both your physical and mental condition. This understanding will speed recovery and assist in bringing the body back to a point of balance and harmony, which is reflected within as excellent mental and physical health, and outwardly as happiness and well-being.

Nutrition, materially and spiritually, is of the highest concern. From a spiritual perspective, the questions you ask yourself will generate answers to questions that shed light on issues related to your illness. Once understood, these same issues will lead to changes in your life. Including proper nutrition as part of your program of change will also facilitate the healing process on both a physical and spiritual level.

From a dietary perspective, I wholly recommend a vegetarian diet because it is the one diet loaded with living foods. Living foods are those foodstuffs that do not require cooking for consumption. Cooking partially destroys food's synergistic healing properties, and cooked food also requires additional amounts of energy for your body to process and digest. Living foods, on the other hand, still have their own enzymes intact and will work to digest themselves, meaning the body does not have to work as hard to get the nutritional benefits.

Two particularly important vegetarian foods to include in the diet are sprouts and tofu, a soybean curd. Sprouts are rich in micronutrients, while tofu is a great source of protein, which allows you to cut down on meat, fish, and fowl consumption. Tofu metabolizes into amino acids that are necessary for the health of the immune system as well as the rest of the body.

2. CHOICES

Many different approaches to healing are available in the world today. Each person can pursue his or her choice of healing paths. Of course, there are no guarantees that (1) they will find the help and relief they seek, or (2) that their family and friends will accept their course of action.

Every society and culture instills within its members mental norms or mores as to what is acceptable, i.e., what is expected, what will work, and what is useless. Here, too, there are no guarantees that any of these societal, cultural perceptions are correct. There is, however, one truth that will always prevail, regardless of the system. It is this: the body heals itself.

The body is derived in a four-layer process. First, there is spirit, followed by mind, brain, and body. The spirit is that inner part of man in which dwells the Divine Aspect of the Creator. The mind is the aspect of self that receives data from both our material senses and Spiritual Self, guiding us accordingly. The brain converts the spiritual input, or thought energy, into physical action. The brain is the bio-computer that runs the body, and the body is a mirror-imaged, physical manifestation of our thoughts, reflecting the Divine, Inner/Spiritual Self (subconscious mind beneath our ego subconscious) and the materially driven Outer/Ego Self (conscious mind). When the beliefs and values of our Inner and Outer Selves are in conflict, all ailments or diseases are born.

As discussed previously, the brain is a bio-computer and an electrical energy converter that keeps all bodily functions on an even keel. The mind operates this bio-computer much like a driver guides his car. Were you a pedestrian crossing the street and encountering a speeding car, your mind would tell your brain to pump out the adrenalin and get those feet and legs moving fast. The brain obliges, and you move to safety. Thus, all physical actions and reactions begin within the mind and are communicated to the brain, which makes necessary adjustments to the body, some of them creating disharmony. Only when you uncover the thoughts in your mind that motivate the brain to create conditions conducive to ill health will you realize the opportunity for true self-healing.

This brings us back to the purpose of this Work: learning to see thoughts in action. Phyllis and I know from our personal experiences and from those reported to us by other people that this system will not fail to bring about excellent health as well as peace, balance, and harmony within. It can all be accomplished by understanding the self.

There comes a time for many people when they begin to question. They search for what they feel is the truth about life and living. Eventually, they discover that good health is synonymous with life, and later still for some comes the understanding that anything not in accord with the Divine Principles of Living will create dis-ease.

Looking around today, we see degenerative conditions such as cardiovascular disease, cancer, and AIDS killing record numbers of people. Why? There are many reasons, but the essence of the problem is this: man does not live in harmony with the Divine Principles (Universal Teachings) that were given to him in the *Bible* and other great works of faith.

The *Bible* tells us that the Creator has no beginning or end (a divine clue to help man understand himself and the world). What in our world could possibly fit the description of having no beginning and no ending? Only one thing meets that definition…energy. Energy can neither be created nor destroyed; it can only be changed from one form to another. Energy, then, is a manifestation of the Creator.

We know that man, like everything else, is a vessel for energy. Measuring or charting that energy as it flows through the body via a number of electrically based diagnostic tests is one way to reference a human's state of health. Our brain waves can be read by viewing the graph created by the electroencephalogram (ECG). Heart rhythm currents, likewise, can be read from an electrocardiogram (EKG).

Because man was created in the image of the Creator's energy, he also has the ability to create. Indeed, man's creative aspect is readily visible to us, especially when we look at the marvels of technology. It is unfortunate that in achieving these milestones, man failed to employ the wisdom of the Creator to prevent the pollution also evident in our environment today.

The Creator-energy is the foundation of man, his source of power, his essence, and his Creator Self. This essence is the foundation of health or sickness. If the energy flow within a man is harmonious, then longevity can be anticipated because there would be no energy depletions, diseases, blockages, or disharmonies. On the other hand, internal disharmonies and energy blockages can cause a disruption within the body and lead to disease and even death. Since the body is the physical manifestation of thought-energy, only thought-energy can restore it to balance and harmony.

Remember, the mind uses the brain/bio-computer to manipulate the body, and through our thoughts we also compel body actions, such as walking, running, swimming, and talking. We think about something that we want to do, consciously or unconsciously, and then we do it with the help of our body. The process that makes this possible is thought. Thought is energy, which is converted by the brain into electrical messages and transmitted throughout the body.

Consider this analogy. A person dials a telephone number (thinks a thought), it goes to a switchboard (brain), and is forwarded by the transmission lines (nerves) to the person being called (area of the body). The "call" has been placed. The call is the mutually harmonious result of two different directives at work. These types of calls, or thoughts, have the same ability to disrupt the body's normal homeostasis mechanisms, allowing us to become ill. Here is how: Our bodies are covered with millions of bacteria at all times. It is only when we are involved in something that creates a conflict between our directives (desires of the Ego Self and Creator minds) that we create an opening in our regulating mechanisms. In this way, we let a germ enter. A germ (or thought) can come from anyone, even a friend or relative. They could present a thought that would create disunity, discomfort, disharmony and disease within the self.

After seeking out the internal, disharmonious thoughts that you accept as truth, what can you do to protect yourself and restore your body to excellent health? Since the body is energy manifesting in physical form, it is necessary to use complementary energy to help it regain balance and harmony. What is complementary energy? There are two types that we need to incorporate. One is positive affirmations based on understandings to change misconceptions, and the other is living food! Living foods in addition to their other advantages, also have a higher energy level than cooked, frozen, or canned foods. Living things contain life within them. By following natural dietary laws, we stand a better chance of restoring our bodies, and of quickening the spirit. Degenerative diseases are a result of our diets, our inner-thoughts, and the environment in which we live. These elements are, themselves, a symbolic representation of our own thoughts, accepted and projected outward. Remember, "know thyself, and the truth will set you free."

3. CHANGES

Now the real work begins. In reading this information you, hopefully, have arrived at many insights and understandings. This is the beginning of a new life for you. Changing habits and thought patterns that create problems will not be easy, yet it is possible. Remember the Universal Teaching that you are "never placed in a situation that you cannot master."

This means you now have in your mind and in your hand the tools that will allow you to make changes guaranteed to improve the quality and quantity of your life, particularly in terms of realizing vibrant health. You now stand on the brink of exercising control over the forces that contributed to negative health problems. You could become a Metaphysician.[133]

Through conscious control, you will evolve into the next aspect of your True Self. In turn, you will inspire and help others to seek understandings and incorporate them into their daily life. As human beings, we teach by example, not words. This is why it is taught in Matthew, chapter 12:33, that "the tree is known by his fruit."

Throughout this work the terms, concepts, patterns, and belief systems[134] have been mentioned. Recall that concepts are the ideas you maintain about yourself which, along with subconscious expectations, lead to behavioral patterns that eventually become ingrained and dominate your actions. A concept is a personal belief about self that you are trying to prove through self-fulfilling of expectations. Once the expectation is fulfilled, you have proven the self-concept as true and valid.

A pattern of behavior is how you normally respond in a given situation to certain stimuli. For instance, every time you stick your finger near a fire, you pull it back as soon as you feel the heat. This is a programmed response to a given stimuli, or history repeating itself. For that to remain true, your personal history must follow a prescribed plan of action, or pattern of behavior.

In your quest for self-mastery, you must know and understand your belief system, including its concepts and patterns of behavior. I assure you it is not as difficult as it may sound.

You will have guidance from the Creator in gaining control over your Outer Self, given in the form of a living language called symbols. These symbols give you the opportunity to see clearly and to understand fully these words, from the Gospel According to Thomas: "Know what is in thy sight, and what is hidden from thee will be revealed to thee. For there is nothing hidden which will not be manifest."

Once you learn to read symbols and see your patterns clearly, you can go out and do the work that you are here to accomplish. You will be able to do this with control, and eventually, with mastery.

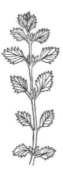

Epilog

You must be clear about where you are coming from in all matters, whether it is the outer Ego Self or the deeper, inner Spiritual Self that is seeking to manifest. If you would like additional information/support about all of the manifestations and aspects of those two selves, Ego and Spiritual, write the publisher to learn about other services available by the author to help your understandings grow deeper.

If you are ready to continue on the path to Self and seek to become a Metaphysician, meet with a group of like-minded people or would like to listen to my podcasts contact me at: symbolreader@msn.com.

Until then, be well.

Michael

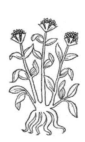

Notes

1. H.B. Allen, P.R. Gross, A.M. Klingman, J.J. Leyden, O.H. Mills, R.I. Rudolph, "Oral Vitamin A in Acne Vulgaris," International Journal of Dermatology 20(4) (1981): 278.

2. M. About-Khair, S. Fathi, M. Wahid, "Zinc in Human Health and Disease," Ric. Cl. Lab. 18 (1988): 0-16.

3. Shils, Young: 1299.

4. B. Leibovitz, B.V. Siegel, "Ascorbic Acid, Neutrophil Function, and the Immune Response," International Journal for Vitamin and Nutrition Research 48(2) (1978): 159.

5. R. Anderson, "Effects of Ascorbate on Normal and Abnormal Leucocyte Functions," International Journal for Vitamin and Nutrition Research 23 (1983): 23.

6. E.H. Ruddock, M.D., G.P. Wood, M.D., Vitalogy (1919).

7. T. Kummet, F.L. Meyskens, T.E. Moon, "Vitamin A: Evidence for Its Preventive Role in Human Cancer," Nutrition and Cancer 5(2) (1984): 96.

8. M. Lepper, S. Liu, C. Maliza, W.J. Raynor, A.H. Rossof, R. Shekelle, "Dietary Vitamin A and Risk of Cancer in the Western Electric Study," Lancet (1981).

9. E. Bjelke, J.J. Gart, G. Kvale, "Dietary Habits and Lung Cancer Risk," International Journal of Cancer 31 (1983): 397.

10. M.M. Matthews-Roth, "Antitumor Activity of Beta-carotene, Canthxanthin, and Phytoene," Oncology 39 (1982): 33.

11. J. Gouveia, F. Gros, T. Hercend, G. Lemaigre, G. Mathe, G. Santelli, et al, "Degree of Bronchial Metaplasia in Heavy Smokers and Its Regression After Treatment with a Retinoid," Lancet i (1982): 710.

12. D.S. Goodman, "Vitamin A and Retinoids in Health and Disease," New England Journal of Medicine 310(16) (1984): 1023.

13. P. Katz, R.S. Panush, G. Powell, et al, International Journal for Vitamin and Nutrition Research 53 (1982): 61-67.

14. G.T. Deusch, S.D. Waksal, C.S. Wilson, Nutrition, Host Defenses, and the Lymphoid System in Advances in Host Defense Mechanisms 2 (New York: Raven Press, 1983).

15. P. Fraker, Surv. Immunol. Res. 2 (1983): 155-164.

16. H.W. Felter, The Eclectic Materia, Pharmacology and Therapeutics Eclectic Medical Publications (1983, first published in 1922).

17. Discover (February 1984).

18. Journal of the American Dietetic Association (March 1985).

19. New England Journal of Medicine (January 5, 1978).

20. Science News (October 13, 1984).

21. Science (January 14, 1977).

22. Braverman, Pfeiffer, Healing Nutrients Within (1987).

23. W.R. Beisel, "Nonspecific Host Factors—A Review," Malnutrition and the Immune Response (New York: Raven Press, 1977).

24. C.G. Neumann, "Nonspecific Host Factors and Infection in Malnutrition," Malnutrition and the Immune Response (New York: Raven Press, 1977).

25. B. Leibovitz, B.V. Siegel, "Ascorbic Acid, Neutrophil Function, and the Immune Response," International Journal for Vitamin and Nutrition Research, 48(2) (1978): 159.

26. R. Anderson, "Effects of Ascorbate on Normal and Abnormal Leucocyte Functions," International Journal for Vitamin and Nutrition Research 23 (1983): 23.

27. W.R. Beisel, "Single Nutrients and Immunity," American Journal of Clinical Nutrition 35(2nd Supplement) (1982): 417.

28. M. About-Khair, S. Fathi, M. Wahid, "Zinc in Human Health and Disease," Ric. Cl. Lab. 18 (1988): 0-16.

29. R.A. Anderson, et al, "Chromium Supplementation of Human Subjects: Effects on Glucose, Insulin and Lipid Variables," Metabolism 32(9) (1983): 894.

30. Anal. of Ophthalmology (July 1979).

31. McGraw-Hill, Nutrition Almanac (1979).

32. The Journal of Holistic Medicine (Fall/Winter 1981).

33. Optometric Monthly (August 1983).

34. Arthur C. Guyton, M.D., Textbook of Medical Physiology 6th Edition (Philadelphia: W.B. Saunders Company): 1002.

35. ibid: 1016.

36. M.S. Seelig, The American Journal of Clinical Nutrition 14 (1964): 342.

37. I. J. MacIntyre, Chronic Diseases 16 (1963): 201.

38. M.S. Seelig, The American Journal of Clinical Nutrition 14 (1964): 342.

39. H.E. Martin, et al, The Journal of Clinical Investigation 26 (1947): 216.

40. W.M. Bloom, M.D., Don Fawcett, M.D., A Textbook of Histology (Philadelphia: W.B. Saunders Company, 1975): 848.

41. A peptic ulcer occurs when the lining of these organs is corroded by the acidic digestive juices which are secreted by the stomach cells. A peptic ulcer of the stomach is called a gastric ulcer, an ulcer of the duodenum is a duodenal ulcer, and a peptic ulcer of the esophagus is an esophageal ulcer.

42. D. DiPette, P. Grelich, A. Nickols, et al, "Dietary Calcium Supplementation May Lower Blood Pressure by Alterations in {1, 25} Vitamin D3," Clinical Research 36 (1988): A425.

43. E.H. Back, et al, Archives of Disease in Childhood 37 (1962): 106.

44. A. Bishop, N.J. Blacklock, J.E. Morris, J.A. Thom, "The Influence of Refined Carbohydrate on Urinary Calcium Excretion," British Journal of Urology 50 (1978): 459.

45. P.P. Swanson, Fed. Proc. 10 (1951): 660.

46. H.N. Marvin, et al, Proceedings of the Society for Experimental Biology Medicine 105 (1960): 473.

47. R. Gubner, Arch. Derm. Syph 64 (1951): 688.

48. Natural killer (NK) cells are small lymphocytes that originate in the bone marrow and develop fully in the absence of the thymus that can react against and destroy another cell without prior sensitization to it. NK cells are part of our first line of defense against cancer cells and virus-infected cells.

49. E. Beutler, The American Journal of the Medical Sciences 234 (1957): 517.

50. H.E. Martin, et al, The Journal of Clinical Investigation 26 (1947): 216.

51. S.M. Gershoff, et al, The Journal of Nutrition 73 (1961): 308.

52. L.A. Maynard, et al, The Journal of Nutrition 64 (1958): 85.

53. M.S. Seelig, The American Journal of Clinical Nutrition 14 (1964): 342.

54. I. MacIntyre, Journal of Chronic Diseases 16 (1963): 201.

55. M.S. Seelig, The American Journal of Clinical Nutrition 14 (1964): 342.

56. H.E. Martin, et al, The Journal of Clinical Investigation 26 (1947): 216.

57. G.C. Cotzias, et al, The Journal of Clinical Investigation 37 (1958): 1269.

58. "National Research Council: Manganese," National Academy of Sciences (Washington, 1973).

59. F.S. Daft, et al, Public Health Reports 55 (1940): 1333.

60. H.F. West, Lancet ii (1985): 877.

61. V.H. Cheldelin, et al, Journal of the American Chemical Society 43 (1951): 5004.

62. C.W. Carter, et al, Biochemistry Journal 49 (1951): 227.

63. Y. Kotake, The Journal of Vitaminology 1 (1955): 73.

64. E. Mascitelli-Coriandoli, Nut. Abst. Rev. 30 (1960): 451.

65. D.S. Kushner, The American Journal of Clinical Nutrition 4 (1956): 561.

66. R.S. Goodhart, M.G. Wohl, Modern Nutrition in Health and Disease (Philadelphia: Lea & Febiger, 1955).

67. Nutrition Review 10 (1952): 163.

68. J.W. Holler, The Journal of the American Medical Association 131 (1946): 1186.

69. G. Rouser, The American Journal of Clinical Nutrition 6 (1958): 681.

70. P.M. McAllen, British Heart Journal 17 (1955): 5.

71. Nutrition Review 14 (1956): 295.

72. E. Jussila, M. Kaariainen, S. Kemila, H. Korpela, J. Kumpulainen, et al, "Effect of Selenium Supplementation After Acute Myocardial Infarction," Research Communications in Chemical Pathology and Pharmacology 65: 249-252.

73. Adrianne Bendich, Lillian Langseth, "Safety of Vitamin A," The American Journal of Clinical Nutrition 49 (1989): 358-371.

74. Adrianne Bendich, "The Safety of Beta-carotene," Nutrition and Cancer 11 (1988): 207-214.

75. T. Kummet, F.L. Meyskens, T.E. Moon, "Vitamin A: Evidence for Its Preventative Role in Human Cancer," Nutrition and Cancer 5(2) (1984): 96.

76. M. Lepper, S. Liu, C. Maliza, W.J. Raynor, A.H. Rossof, R. Shekelle, "Dietary Vitamin A and Risk of Cancer in the Western Electric Study," Lancet (1981).

77. E. Bjelke, J.J. Gart, G. Kvale, "Dietary Habits and Lung Cancer Risk," International of Journal Cancer 31 (1983): 397.

78. M.M. Matthews-Roth, "Antitumor Activity of Beta-carotene, Canthxanthin, and Phytoene," Oncology 39 (1982): 33.

79. J. Gouveia, F. Gros, T. Hercend, G. Lemaigre, G. Mathe, G. Santelli, et al, "Degree of Bronchial Metaplasia in Heavy Smokers and Its Regression After Treatment with a Retinoid," Lancet i (1982): 710.

80. D.S. Goodman, "Vitamin A and Retinoids in Health and Disease," New England Journal of Medicine 310(16) (1984): 1023.

81. H.B. Allen, P.R. Gross, A.M. Klingman, J.J. Leyden, O.H. Mills, R.I. Rudolph, "Oral Vitamin A in Acne Vulgaris," International Journal of Dermatology, 20(4) (1981): 278.

82. A.C. Bird, C.M. Kemp, L. Lyness, S. Sherlock, R.P. Walt, "Vitamin A Treatment for Night Blindness in Primary Bilary Cirrhosis," British Medical Journal 288 (1984): 1030.

83. S. Benedek, G. Deak, T. Javor, P. Kenez, G. Mozsik, L. Nagy, I. Patty, F. Tarnok, "Controlled Trial of Vitamin A Therapy in Gastric Ulcer," Lancet ii (1982): 876.

84. S. Klaus, M.M. Mathews-Roth, J.J. Norlund, M.A. Pathak, "New Therapy for Polymorphous Light Eruption," Archives of Dermatology 108 (1973): 710.

85. A person's life, when lived without understanding, is operating on "automatic." This means that they are responding to events, situations and people from a "patternistic" form of behavior. Patterns are a repetitious series of learned responses. These in turn influence how you will react based on how you have handled a similar situation in your past. If it is the first time you have encountered this particular type of situation, then you will scan your memory banks to see how your mother or father dealt with a similar situation. The choice that you make will depend upon which parent you seek to emulate or reject. Your reaction will be in keeping with that plan that you are automatically trying to create. Therefore, you will end up with "predetermined" results. All that you go through in a given day triggers patterns and programmed responses within you. What you are seeking to do, at a subconscious level, is to fulfill your patterns. These patterns come complete with expectations about yourself that you try to fulfill. Patterns are built upon concepts. Concepts are the foundation of ideas about who you think you are supposed to be, and this is based on an ego point of view.

86. G. Baum, E.L. Boxer, J.H. Davidson, N. Lawrence, J.B.R. Lewis, D.J.R. Morgan, T.E.S. Stowell, "Meclozine and Pyridoxine in Pregnancy Sickness," Practitioner 190 (1963): 251.

87. R.E. Hodges, et al, The American Journal of Clinical Nutrition 11 (1962): 181, 187.

88. Nutrition Review 20 (1962): 213.

89. C. Hill, "Interactions of Vitamin C with Lead and Mercury," Annals of the New York Academy of Sciences (1980): 262, 355.

90. B.H. Ershoff, Nutrition Review 13 (1955): 33.

91. Nutrition Review 15 (1957): 185.

92. A. White, Annals of the New York Academy of Sciences (1958): 72, 79.

93. Nutrition Review 10 (1952): 217.

94. L.P. Dugal, et al, Endocrinology 44 (1945): 420.

95. A.J. Tuyns, "Protective Effect of Citrus Fruit on Esophageal Cancer," Nutrition and Cancer 5(3-4) (1983): 195.

96. S. Wassertheil-Smoller, et al, "Dietary Vitamin C and Uterine Cervical Dysplasia," American Journal of Epidemiology 114(5) (1981): 714.

97. S. Graham, J. Marshall, C. Mettlin, D. Shedd, M. Swanson, "Diet in the Epidemiology of Oral Cancer," Nutrition and Cancer 3(3): 145.

98. L.N. Kolonel, et al, "Rise of Diet in Cancer Incidence in Hawaii," Cancer Research Supplement 43 (1983): 23, 97.

99. S.R. Tannenbaum, "Reaction of Nitrite with Vitamins C and E," Annals of the New York Academy of Sciences 355 (1980): 267.

100.M. Eagen, S.S. Mirvish, L. Wallgave, et al, "Ascorbate-Nitrate Reaction: Possible Means of Blocking the Formation of Carcinogenic N-Nitroso Compounds," Science 177 (1972): 65.

101.J. Greenwood, "Optimum Vitamin C Intake As a Factor in the Preservation of Disc Integrity," Medical Ann. District of Columbia 33(6) (1964): 274.

102.W.J.H. Butterfield, B.D. Cox, "Vitamin C Supplements and Diabetic Cutaneous Capillary Fragility," British Medical Journal (July 26, 1975): 976.

103.Nutrition Review 15 (1957): 185.

104.M.B. Sulzberger, et al, Proceedings of the Society for Experimental Biology and Medicine 32 (1935): 716.

105.Nutrition Review 4 (1946): 259.

106.R.D. Gabovich, et al, Fed. Proc. 23 (1964): T450.

107.M.M. Thompson, et al, The American Journal of Clinical Nutrition 7 (1959): 80.

108.H. N. Holmes, et al, Journal of Laboratory and Clinical Medicine 24 (1939): 1119.

109.B. Ekman, Acta Pharmacology Toxicol. 3 (1947): 261.

110.E.L. Hove, Proceedings of the Society for Experimental Biology and Medicine 77 (1951): 502.

111.E.B. Veddis, et al, The Journal of Nutrition 16 (1938): 57.

112.I.J. Kligler, et al, Journal of Path. Bact. 46 (1938): 619.

113.F.R. Klenner, Tri-State Medical Journal (July, 1954).

114.I.J. Kligler, et al, Journal of Path. Bact. 46 (1938): 619.

115.K.E. Burkhaug, Acta Tubercul. Scand. 13 (1939): 45.

116.H.A. Mattill, Nutrition Review 10 (1952): 225.

117.D.H. Roderuck, et al, Annals of the New York Academy of Sciences 52 (1949): 156.

118.H.A. Mattill, Nutrition Review 10 (1952): 225.

119.H.A. Mattill, Nutrition Review 10 (1952): 225.

120.D.H. Roderuck, et al, Annals of the New York Academy of Sciences 52 (1949): 156.

121.P. Mecray Jr., The American Journal of Clinical Nutrition 3 (1955): 461.

122.S.R. Ames, et al, Inter. Rev. Vit. Res. 22 (1951): 401.

123.B.A. Schottelius, et al, American Journal of Physiology (1958): 193, 219.

124.W.M. Govier, et al, Journal of Pharmacology and Experimental Therapeutics 88 (1946): 373.

125. H.M. Nitowsky, et al, Bulletin of the Johns Hopkins Hospital 98 (1956): 361.

126. H.A. Mattill, Nutrition Review 10 (1952): 225.

127. H.N. Marvin, et al, Proceedings of the Society for Experimental Biology and Medicine (1960): 105, 473.

128. C. Desusclade, et al, Presse Medicale 67 (1959): 855.

129. P.L. Harris, et al, International Congress on Vitamin E (1955).

130. G. Sillo-Seidl, Nut. Abst. Rev. 33 (1963): 812.

131. M. About-Khair, S. Fathi, M. Wahid, "Zinc in Human Health and Disease," Ric. Cl. Lab. 18 (1988): 0-16.

132. M.J. Henderson, H.E. Morgan, C.R. Park, et al, Recent Progress in Hormone Research 17 (1961): 493-538.

133. A Metaphysician is someone trained in the Art of Metaphysical Naturopathy. This is following the path of nature in all physical matters and understanding the forces at work on an energetic level, beyond the physical.

134. The belief system under which every person operates is the result of programs that are based on man-made teachings. These teachings are not in keeping with Spiritual Truth or Universal Law, but rather are the ideals, standards, and guides for living that help man control and dominate others. The problem—aside from the fact that these teachings are inherently destructive—is everyone has accepted them as true.

The role of the sexes is an excellent example of a misconception in practice. According to society standards, the male provides for his family while the female takes care of the home and the children. Some religious sects even practice the belief that the female is lesser in the eyes of the Creator and, therefore, she has no voice of her own. She is told to listen to her husband and follow his instructions. The truth is that males and females were created equally. In the first book of Genesis, it is written: "So God created man in his own image, in the image of God created he him; male and female created he them."

INDEX

Page numbers in bold indicate the primary discussion of a topic.